Medicine and
the reign of technology

Medicine and the reign of technology

STANLEY JOEL REISER

Assistant Professor and Director,
Program in the History of Medicine,
Harvard Medical School, and
Clinical Associate in Medicine,
Massachusetts General Hospital

CAMBRIDGE UNIVERSITY PRESS

Cambridge
London   New York   Melbourne

Published by the Syndics of the Cambridge University Press
The Pitt Building, Trumpington Street, Cambridge CB2 1RP
Bentley House, 200 Euston Road, London NW1 2DB
32 East 57th Street, New York, NY 10022, USA
296 Beaconsfield Parade, Middle Park, Melbourne 3206, Australia

© Cambridge University Press 1978

First published 1978
Reprinted 1979

Printed in the United States of America
Typeset, printed, and bound by Vail-Ballou Press,
Inc., Binghamton, New York

Library of Congress Cataloging in Publication Data
Reiser, Stanley Joel.
Medicine and the reign of technology.
Bibliography: p.
Includes index.
1. Medicine – History.
2. Medical innovations – History.
3. Medical instruments and apparatus – History.
4. Diagnosis – History.
5. Medical innovations – Social aspects.
I. Title. [DNLM: 1. Technology, Medica.
2. Diagnosis – Instrumentation. W26 R375m]
R145.R44   610'.9'03   77-87389
ISBN 0 521 21907 8

To Katharyn

Contents

Illustrations

Preface

The process of determining a patient's ailment from his symptoms is crucial in medical care. For the physician and the patient, this process or diagnosis is not only the starting point of their relationship as therapist to subject, as human being to human being, but it also determines the course of any future medical intervention.

This book describes some of the technological advances made in the art and practice of medicine during the past four centuries, and shows how those advances altered the methods of diagnosing illness; and how new methods, in turn, have altered the relation between physician and patient and have influenced the systems of providing medical care and treatment. The book concludes that modern medicine has now evolved to a point where diagnostic judgments based on "subjective" evidence – the patient's sensations and the physician's own observations of the patient – are being supplanted by judgments based on "objective" evidence, provided by laboratory procedures and by mechanical and electronic devices. The book attempts to trace the historical development of how this happened, and, along with the resulting gains, points out the potential losses to the sick patient, to the physician as clinician, and to society.

The development of some of the major technological advances of diagnosis is described – the microscope, the stethoscope, the thermometer, the increasing knowledge of bacteriology and biological chemistry, X-ray devices, electrocardiographs, and the most recent automated devices such as the computer. The reliability of the evidence thus produced is discussed, as well as the hazards involved in its unquestioning acceptance.

The physician discovers illness in people by means of a variety of diagnostic methods, each of which focuses his attention on a different aspect of the disease from which his patient suffers. The kind of diagnostic method chosen is shown to affect the physician's perception of the nature of an illness, because it necessarily selects some aspects of illness and excludes others.

The growing supremacy of technology in medicine is discussed, and how it has led to the rise of the specialist and to the centering of medical care in hospitals; and thus to the decline of the general practitioner and an increasing alienation between doctor and patient.

A large number and variety of factors influence medical care and the use of technology, some of them being philosophy and religion, economic and political systems, social and cultural values. This book does not seek to discuss the totality of the factors that are a part of the growth of medicine and technology. It focuses, mainly, on the thoughts and actions of doctors and patients as they have responded to the availability of new diagnostic technology, and on the process by which a technical advance is accepted or rejected. Further, I have not attempted to discuss all the diagnostic methods that are a part of medical history. I examine a selected number of techniques, chosen for their importance in the evolution of diagnosis, and for their illumination of the themes of this book. My analysis is confined principally to developments in Great Britain and the United States, and, from the early twentieth century on, chiefly to those events that shaped American medical care.

Modern physicians, more than men and women in other professions dealing with people, must now use technology intimately, continually, and expertly. The physician has become a prototype of technological man. By studying his behavior over the past four centuries, as technology has been incorporated into the most significant of his professional duties, I hope to point out some of the dangers, as well as the benefits, inherent in the general relation between man and machine.

In exploring this aspect of medicine, I have used a large number of primary sources, and hence owe particular thanks to those who have helped me locate the necessary material. At the Francis A. Countway Library, whose magnificent collection of medical works almost invariably yielded the information I sought, I am particularly indebted to Harold Bloomquist, who was the librarian from 1969–75, Richard J. Wolfe, curator of rare books, his assistants, and Elaine Ciarkowski, circulation librarian. The rest of the staff at the Countway, too numerous to name individually, were always obliging and gracious to me. The Archives of the Massachusetts

General Hospital were generously open to me through the efforts of Mr. James Vaccarino and Mr. Martin Bander.

I gratefully acknowledge those institutions which furnished the financial support necessary to write this book: the National Institute of General Medical Sciences through a grant to me while a graduate student, the Josiah Macy, Jr. Foundation through their support of the Program in the History of Medicine at the Harvard Medical School, the Joseph P. Kennedy, Jr. Foundation through their aid to the Kennedy Interfaculty Program in Medical Ethics at Harvard University, and the Milton Fund of Harvard University for the award of a helpful small grant.

To Mrs. Sarah Mills, Mrs. Susan Brooks, Ms. Deborah Shelkan, and Ms. Barbara Goroll, the secretarial assistants whose help has been indispensable during various stages of the book, go my profound thanks.

A number of people have kindly given advice and criticism to me during my work on this book. But I wish to acknowledge my special gratitude to Professor I. Bernard Cohen and his wife, Frances Davis Cohen, Mrs. Lyle Gifford Boyd, Dr. John D. Stoeckle, Dr. Audrey Davis, Professor Everett I. Mendelsohn, Professor Barbara Gutmann Rosenkrantz, Professor Bernard Barber, Mr. Eric Valentine, Ms. Alison M. Bond, and my wife, Katharyn Dancer Reiser.

STANLEY JOEL REISER

Boston, Massachusetts
December, 1977

*Medicine and
the reign of technology*

1 *Examination of the patient in the seventeenth and eighteenth centuries*

At the beginning of the seventeenth century, developments in science and technology that would create modern medicine still lay in the future – the stethoscope, bacteriology, the X-ray. The world of the seventeenth-century physician was very different. To determine the nature of illness, he relied chiefly on three techniques: the patient's statement in words which described his symptoms; the physician's observation of signs of the illness, his patient's physical appearance and behavior; and, more rarely, the physician's manual examination of the patient's body.[1] Seventeenth– and eighteenth–century physicians generally used the word "symptom" to mean any datum of clinical evidence that indicated some departure from good health. The term "sign" generally denoted a symptom that provided special information to the physician: for instance, to indicate that a certain phenomenon of illness had occurred, or even might occur. A change in the medical meaning of these words came about gradually during the nineteenth century; symptom was and is often used to designate a sensation of disease perceptible only to the patient, and sign, a mark of disease that the physician could observe. Not all physicians have maintained this distinction. James Mackenzie in his 1920 book, *Symptoms and Their Interpretation*, used the words symptoms and signs interchangeably to mean "a reaction of the tissues of the body to a noxious agent."[2] Except where specifically stated otherwise, I will follow Mackenzie and use these two terms interchangeably in this book.

The patient's narrative of the symptoms and the course of his illness, punctuated and partly directed by questions from the physician, was often the main source for the seventeenth–century physician making a diagnosis. Typical of this method is a clinical history written on July 7, 1663, by Dr. John Symcotts, an English physician with a widespread medical practice in Huntingdon and Bedfordshire. His private casebooks and letters constitute one of the few existing records of the daily medical life of a seventeenth–century English doctor. One of his patients,

Mistress Christian Tenum of Cambridge, fifty years of age, could sleep so little that for fifteen years she had scarcely two and only rarely three hours sleep each night. For twenty years she had a pulsing of the arteries and when she first lay down to rest many images of things passed before her eyes. Ringing in the ears. She felt as if a heavy burden or weight was continually pressing down upon the top of her head. She had a feeling of intense heat at the back of the head. She was usually delirious once a day. Pain in the left abdomen. In colic a concentration of wind. Weakness of the back. During her menses (which had stopped five years earlier) her face had swollen, and it was followed by several stools. Three years ago she was stricken with paralysis and from this she still has a numbness of the head. A continuous cough.

Dr. Symcotts prescribed a fluid diet and medicine that caused Mistress Tenum to void stones in her urine, after which he claimed that she was cured.[3] (Because he gave no diagnosis, it is difficult for a modern clinician to make one from the symptoms reported.)

The narrative technique permits a subjective portrait of the illness, greatly influenced and perhaps distorted by the patient's intellect and personality. In the lines quoted, Mistress Tenum is the chief witness to and interpreter of the events of her illness. She manipulates the memories of the sensations she experienced while ill, diminishing or magnifying their severity as she chooses. Her account is not an objective description of the events but a personal statement of their meaning. The listener is being drawn into the human drama of this illness. Although Dr. Symcotts cannot verify the accuracy of most of his patient's statements, he accepts the narrative at face value. He apparently does not leave his role of listener or interrogator to become a detached observer. His casebook contains no remarks suggesting that he made any effort to examine Mistress Tenum physically.

Observation of the patient was a second, highly regarded method, which seventeenth–century physicians employed to evaluate illness; it was frequently not exploited as fully as the patient's own account.[4] The physician focused upon the outward appearance of the patient's body, mainly the facial expression, posture, tongue, skin color, and manner of breathing. He also examined the appearance of the blood, urine, and stools. A third method used to judge the presence of disease – and the method least used – was the physical examination of the body. At this period the physician's only tool was his sense of touch. He used it most often to feel the pulse and estimate its quality, without determining its exact rate. He used a sense of touch somewhat less frequently to judge the body's temperature, and occasionally to detect tenderness or abnormal masses by briskly probing the tissues beneath the skin. A clinical history of another case, also reported by Symcotts, illustrates a typical combining of the techniques of narrative, observation, and physical examination:

I called on Mistress Paradine of Bedford, a linen draper, who on the 26th of that month [June, 1637] had returned from London (but this fact the messenger concealed from me). She fell ill on the journey and when she reached home on the 27th she collapsed, felt pain all over her body, could not sleep. On the 28th she vomited much and was prostrated by a very bad headache, yet she got up for the greater part of the day. Along with the vomiting she was racked by a hiccough, together with a flux of blood from the nose which was thought to be up to ten ounces.

On the 29th her stomach was disturbed, she was afflicted by a great thirst, brought up all solid foods. The hiccough grew worse, but often stopped altogether and then began again as bad as before. That night on my advice a clyster was injected which stopped the vomiting but not the hiccough.

On the evening of the 30th, when I arrived, I found her lying down, and the hiccough, which had been stopped (by the medicine sent by the Countess of Bolingbroke) was again tearing her to pieces. She was very restless, anxious, found the bed uncomfortable, could not sleep, was delirious but not quite out of her mind, for she refused nothing that was given her and heard what we were saying.

A surgeon of the name of Rowland, a resident of that town, applied dry cupping glasses to the stomach and umbilicus and left them for some time, but they had no effect on the hiccough. Her pulse was hard, deep, swift and tumid, and I thought it a bad sign that a sweat broke out over her whole body. She was very thirsty and asked for drink; we gave it to her, but the cold drinks made the hiccough, which had stopped for some time, start again. She was still unable to sleep.

On July 1st, Mr. Woodcock of Ampthill, who had arrived long after me on the previous night, accompanied me on my visit to the patient. The urine, as on the preceding days, was turbid, highly coloured, and appeared to be slightly blackish in spots. The pulse was fast, jumpy and occasionally intermitting. Mr. Woodcock wanted to let blood; I was against it, but he was importunate and I assenting only on condition that no more than five ounces was taken, it was agreed. The blood was drawn; nobody was at fault. The pulse then became weaker and frequently intermitted; advice was given about diet, medicine and other things required for the future, and everything was entrusted to Rowland.

We left the bedside and were just about to leave for breakfast when the woman made a sign to her husband to enquire about the pain in her abdomen. Straightway he urged Rowland to see what it was and to look and see if any plague bubos were

3

coming up. The latter did so and asserted most emphatically that a bubo had broken out in her groin. There was little for us to advise in this case.[5]

Mistress Paradine died several days later.

The Paradine case illustrates how the observational method of diagnosis, in contrast to the narrative technique, allows the physician to make judgments about the illness solely on the basis of his own sense impressions. Yet the use of the observational technique does not free the physician from consciousness of the patient as a person. The human form generally demands to be experienced with empathy, whether the bond it creates between people serves a practical end or not. We sympathize with the plight of Mistress Paradine because suffering is indicated by the external effects of the illness described by her physician–observer. The hiccough "tears her to pieces," she is "very restless," she looks "anxious" and "delirious." The movements of her facial muscles and body give some sense of her inner misery.

This account of Mistress Paradine's illness also reveals how seventeenth–century doctors typically approached physical examination of their patients. The doctors' examinations of Mistress Paradine were limited to feeling her pulse, which was "hard, deep, swift and tumid" one day, "fast, jumpy and occasionally intermitting" the next. Neither physician made any effort to evaluate her temperature by touching the skin. Even when the bubo was called to their attention, they noted it visually but apparently made no attempt to examine it manually. The Paradine case thus demonstrates that, in the seventeenth century, the physician would attach far less weight to the evidence obtained by his sense of touch than to the patient's narrative and to his own visual observations. The maintenance of human dignity and physical privacy placed limits on human interaction through touch, and in the seventeenth century this principle was adhered to in the relation of a physician to his patient. Only in relatively modern times have patients and physicians learned to accept physical intrusion upon the body as necessary to the diagnostic process. However, the Paradine case and the previously cited one about Mistress Tenum indicate that neither the physician nor the patient felt the same degree of inhibition in discussing the personal aspects of the patient's illness.

During the eighteenth century, no significant change took place in the methods used to evaluate illness. Case records taken from the

4

files of the Public Dispensary at Edinburgh in 1776, and published to aid medical students, show that the patient's narrative often predominated as the basis for diagnosis. One such case record is the following:

D____ M____, a man aged twenty-nine, by occupation a chair-man, admitted Feb. 7. complains of obtuse pain, and frequently also of coldness in the small of his back. It is, in general, attended with shivering. From the small of his back the pain sometimes extends across the lower part of the abdomen, and occasions, as he says, a temporary swelling there, during which his respiration is considerably affected. At other times the pain ascends along the course of the spine, and affects the muscles of his neck, to such a degree as to prevent him from moving his head. It affects also his jaws, face, and gums. In the last of these it occasions a transitory soreness, and has lossened some of his teeth.

His pulse is natural, his appetite is unimpared, and his belly loose. His urine is sometimes pale and limpid, at other times of a very high colour.

Twelve weeks ago, in coming from the harvest in England, he was attacked with a pain in the abdomen, attended with vomiting and purging. To these succeeded the pains of which he has ever since complained and by which he is now rendered very weak. He imputes his complaints to fatigue in coming home. He has taken many medicines without any relief.[6]

Here the picture of the illness is drawn chiefly from the patient's subjective experiences, and to a lesser extent from observations made by the physician, such as the appearance of the abdomen and the color of the urine. The physician notes that pain journeys extensively about the body yet he makes no effort to probe for its source manually. Physical contact is limited to feeling the pulse.

The center of medical practice in the seventeenth and eighteenth centuries was the home, either the patient's or the physician's. Institutional care in places such as hospitals was mainly for those without financial means and family, friends, or domestics to nurse them; or for the sick who hoped, having tried all else, to find help away from home. The physician's visit to the patient, usually made on horseback or by carriage and frequently over rough terrain, was both a social and medical event. He was customarily invited to dine, and if the illness was serious he might reside for several days in the patient's home. The physician's consulting room was usually in his house, although if he lived in a large community he might establish an office in town. Occasionally, if a patient required prolonged medical supervision and lived far from the doctor, he might room and board with the doctor for days, even weeks. But to spare both patients and themselves the difficulty and tedium of travel, physicians often diagnosed illness and prescribed treatment through the mails. Such a practice demonstrates the doctor's general confidence in the patient's subjective account of his symptoms, as described in a letter, as well as the doctor's willingness to forego personal observation of the patient in arriving at a diagnosis. The seventeenth–century English doctor, Symcotts, had an active diagnostic correspondence with patients,[7] as did more famous physicians such as the eighteenth–century teacher, investigator, and widely sought consultant, the Dutchman Hermann Boerhaave. Wrote one of his patients:

Sir,

I am twenty seven years old, and for about four years last past, any violent action brings on me a difficulty of breathing, which is attended with a cough and spitting, which seldom holds me above half an hour or not so long, if I can spit freely; if I drink any strong spiritous liquor late in the evening, I am awakened frequently in the night with a shortness of breathing, but mostly after malt liquors, and likewise tobacco, any slight cold always aggravates it, and likewise cold weather; when action brings it on me, it is often attended with pain in my head, it has been easier this winter, than it was foregoing ones, and I have been less subject to take cold, which advantage I fancy to have received by taking twelve or fifteen drops of *oil of sulphur per Campan* in a glass of cold water at night. In my youth I had convulsion fits, and am more subject to this shortness of breath in the winter, than in the summer. I have my health otherwise very well, and a good appetite.[8]

From this letter Boerhaave diagnosed the disorder as "convulsive asthma," and sent the patient a prescription for medicine which he was to take for six weeks.

The letter of consultation was also used by John Morgan, an American physician and a chief founder of the medical school of the University of Pennsylvania. In 1765, he declared his willingness to render "an opinion in writing on the complaints of patients at a distance from Philadelphia, whenever the history of the case is properly drawn up and transmitted to me for advice."[9]

At the beginning of the nineteenth century, physicians continued to evaluate illness in the same manner as their predecessors had done. Here is a physician in 1805 describing a typical examination: the medical attendant first "becomes acquainted with the most prominent sensations of his patient; he feels his pulse and his skin, looks at his tongue, and examines the expression of his countenance."[10] A case history written in 1806 continues in similar vein. The patient,

6

Alice Hurthwaite, aged 15, was admitted into the Dispensary on the 11th of June 1805, labouring under violent pain in the right side of the abdomen, about the middle of the external oblique muscle, accompanied with great thirst, increased heat, frequent shiverings, a quick pulse, nausea, and vomiting. The account which she gave of herself was, that she was seized suddenly with the pain on the 1st of June, and with difficulty walked a few hundred yards from the place where she was in service to her mother's cottage. Of her own accord she took some opening medicine that produced a good deal of purging, which still continues. She feels most easy when the abdominal muscles are relaxed, the knees being brought towards the chin. She does not recollect having received any injury on the abdomen, and has previously enjoyed good health. She is tall, and rather thin.[11]

In this case, although the physician gains most of his information from Alice's narrative, he comments on the shortcomings of narrative in diagnosis. Only after the patient dies does he learn that the illness was preceded by a fall from a ladder, an incident forgotten by the patient and her mother when questioned by the physician at his first visit. For him, this was "one proof, beside many others, of the great difficulty we often experience in obtaining from the poor a correct history of the predisposing causes of disease."[12] The doctor's visual observations concern Alice's shivering, vomiting, and body type. He feels her pulse and possibly her skin to evaluate her temperature, but despite the violent pain in her abdomen, refrains from making a physical examination.

The failure of doctors to examine the body in the presence of internal disease, and the reluctance of patients to allow it, were common in the early nineteenth century. One English physician related that he often found "plain and obvious diseases entirely mistaken and mistreated, for months, – even years, – merely from the practitioner's neglecting this simple but necessary measure!" Yet he went so far as to urge his colleagues to examine any part of the body in which disease was suspected freed from "every species of covering that can impede the necessary examination, – always by the hand, and often by the eye; and wherever the case is at all doubtful," acknowledging "the repugnance of our patients to the measure." He advised physicians to overcome the patient's repugnance "however great this may be, and however natural and proper we may feel it to be."[13]

A new approach to diagnosis was thus developing, stimulated by an interest in anatomical changes wrought by disease on the internal parts of the body. This anatomical perspective laid the foundation for a profound alteration in the physician's perception of disease, and in his relationship to patients, as well as his methods of diagnosis.

At the beginning of the seventeenth century, physicians largely retained the view proposed in ancient Greek medicine that health and illness depended on the condition of substances called "humors," fundamental components of the human body whose number was generally placed at four – blood, mucus, black bile, and yellow bile. Their harmonious mixture ensured health; a disturbance of their balance, either an excess or insufficiency of a humor, or a displacement or putrefaction of a humor, produced illness. Essentially there was one disease state, a humoral derangement or "distemper," but as many variants of it existed as there were patients, for the symptoms of disease depended on the individual's humoral constitution. Certain groupings of symptoms had been made by this period, and particularly conspicuous clinical conditions such as syphilis, smallpox, and plague had been named. Yet even the therapy for such acute illnesses was, as a rule, not directed at the illnesses as entities but rather at restoring harmony to the patient's body functions: "Doctors treated fevers, fluxes, and dropsies rather than particular diseases."[14]

An alternative view of illness – that different patterns of symptoms corresponded to specific disease entities – had been formulated in Greek medicine, notably by Plato.[15] The idea was advocated again in the sixteenth century by the Swiss-born physician Paracelsus, who traveled and practiced all over Europe. He argued that diseases were not merely manifestations of humoral imbalances, but were real entities which differed in material composition and arose from specific causes.[16] A disciple of Paracelsus, the Flemish doctor Jean Baptiste van Helmont, elaborated this viewpoint in the seventeenth century, as did the English physician Thomas Sydenham.

Dr. Sydenham argued that any one of a variety of circumstances could cause the humors to "become exaulted into a *substantial form* or *species*," and create disorders "coincident with their respective essences." He believed that previous generations of physicians had been wrong in considering that the symptoms of illness principally originated "either in the nature of the part which the humour has attacked, or else in the character of the humour itself anterior to its specific metamorphosis," and that "in their true nature" the symptoms of illness were determined by "the essence of the said spe-

8

cies."[17] He taught that a careful analysis of illness revealed constantly recurring patterns of symptoms, which could be used to order all illness into a finite number of distinct species, much as naturalists did in defining plant species. According to Sydenham, "Nature, in the production of disease, is uniform and consistent; so much so, that for the same disease in different persons the symptoms are for the most part the same; and the selfsame phenomena that you would observe in the sickness of a Socrates you would observe in the sickness of a simpleton."[18] Sydenham based his disease descriptions on phenomena of illness revealed by the patient's story and his own clinical observations. He was one of the first physicians to combine case histories of individual patients with a particular disorder into a disease history. Notable and representative of his efforts is his portrait of gout:

Gout attacks such old men as, after passing the best part of their life in ease and comfort, indulging freely in high living, wine, and other generous drinks, at length, from inactivity, the usual attendant of advanced life, have left off altogether the bodily exercises of their youth. . .The day before the fit the appetite is unnaturally hearty. The victim goes to bed and sleeps in good health. About two o'clock in the morning he is awakened by a severe pain in the great toe; more rarely in the heel, ankle, or instep. This pain is like that of a dislocation, and yet the parts feel as if cold water were poured over them. Then follow chills and shivers, and a little fever. The pain, which was at first moderate, becomes more intense. With its intensity the chills and shivers increase. . .The night is passed in torture, sleeplessness, turning of the part affected, and perpetual change of posture; the tossing about of the body being as incessant as the pain of the tortured joint, and being worse as the fit comes on. Hence the vain efforts, by change of posture, both in the body and the limb affected, to obtain an abatement of the pain. This comes only towards the morning. . .Next day (perhaps for the next two or three days), if the generation of the gouty matter have been abundant, the part affected is painful, getting worse towards evening and better towards morning. A few days after, the other foot swells, and suffers the same pains. . .After it has attacked each foot, the fits become irregular, both as to the time of their accession and duration. One thing, however, is constant – the pain increases at night and remits in the morning. . .In strong constitutions, where the previous attacks have been few, a fortnight is the length of an attack. With age and impaired habits gout may last two months.[19]

A number of eighteenth–century physicians continued Sydenham's efforts to classify diseases. But rather than distinguish diseases by facts obtained from bedside inquiry as Sydenham had advocated, they mainly reorganized already existing descriptive data.[20] One of the most zealous and influential classifiers of disease

9

of that period was the physician and botanist François Boissier de Sauvages. He introduced his ideas in a small volume on disease classification published in 1731, and fully developed them in a large tome, *Nosologia methodica, sistens morborum classes, genera et species* (1763). This last work announced the existence of 2,400 species of disease, divided into 10 classes, 40 orders, and 295 genera.[21] William Cullen, professor of medicine at the medical school in Edinburgh, attempted to reduce the number of disorders enumerated by this book. His 1769 treatise on disease classification deleted some categories of disturbances that Sauvages had formulated, such as sneezing, hiccough, snoring, anxiety, lassitude, stupor, itching, and coldness. Cullen defended this reduction as necessary, "unless we wish to have as many genera of disorders as there are symptoms."[22] He declared that the goal of disease classification should be to define "pathognomonics," symptoms that were "so proper to each disorder, that from them alone any one might be quickly and certainly distinguished from another."[23]

Sydenham, Sauvages, and Cullen all based their classifications upon symptoms exhibited by the living patient. They rejected any idea that disease definitions required clarification from autopsies. Sydenham was particularly critical of anatomical study; he protested that anatomical investigation diverted the attention of physicians "from history and the advantage of a diligent observation of these diseases, of their beginning, progress, and ways of cure."[24] Since for him bedside evidence was the most reliable source of medical knowledge, he believed that a physician could neglect "a scrupulous enquiry into the anatomye of the parts, as a gardner may by his art and observation, be able to ripen, meliorate and preserve his fruit without examining what kindes of juices, fibres, pores etc. are to be found in the roots, barke, or body of the tree."[25]

Yet other physicians, even during the sixteenth century, had been acquiring clinically pertinent knowledge about health and illness from autopsies. Andreas Vesalius, a professor at Padua, greatly clarified understanding of normal anatomy and raised the importance of personal observation with his *De humani corporis fabrica* (1543). Before the work of Vesalius, the study of human anatomy had been hindered not only by social and religious prohibitions against dissecting the human corpse, but also by a reverent dependence upon the anatomical work of older authorities, such as the second-century physician Galen who, because of these prohibitions, had based his descriptions of the human anatomy chiefly

10

upon observations made from dissecting animals, mainly the Barbary ape. These prohibitions were moderated toward the end of the thirteenth century. Among the moderating factors were the efforts to learn the cause of epidemic disease by opening the body of a victim, and autopsies ordered in legal proceedings when, for example, death from poison was suspected. It is in this period that we find one of the first instructors to teach anatomy from the human cadaver: Mondino de' Luzzi, professor at the University of Bologna. His manual of dissection, the *Anothomia* (circa 1316), became a standard text for the next two centuries. However, the authority of tradition continued to be strong. Although Mondino himself dissected cadavers, his book was based principally on the writings of Galen and medieval Arab physicians such as Avicenna; Mondino appears to have conducted dissections more to confirm and to memorize their views than to test them or to make discoveries. Thus Mondino described the heart, after Avicenna, as having three ventricles; and numbered the cranial nerves, after Galen, at seven. He characterized the liver as five–lobed, following a Greek idea probably derived from canine anatomy, and reported the uterus as seven–celled, following medieval tradition.[26]

During the fourteenth and fifteenth centuries physicians continued to rely on authoritative texts for anatomical knowledge; few repeated Mondino's example of personally dissecting cadavers. This is illustrated in a picture placed before the *Anothomia* in a late fifteenth–century collection of short medical treatises, the *Fasciculus medicinae* (Figure 1). It shows a professor of anatomy, presumably meant by the artist to represent Mondino, reading to his audience from behind an elaborate desk raised high above the floor. At floor level are a cadaver, some academically robed students and an assistant, sleeves rolled up. The assistant dissects while one of the students points out the structures disclosed. Here, textbook knowledge is supreme. The illustration focuses on the professor discussing the text, not on the cadaver being dissected.

Such a procedure was followed by physicians of this period not only because of their confidence in the facts described in respected texts, but also because of their prejudice against using their hands in the learning and practice of medicine. The emerging universities of thirteenth–century Europe created medical faculties in which, like the rest of the university, observation of nature was neglected and a theoretical and philosophical approach to learning was emphasized. Thus medical education had become, as the modern his-

11

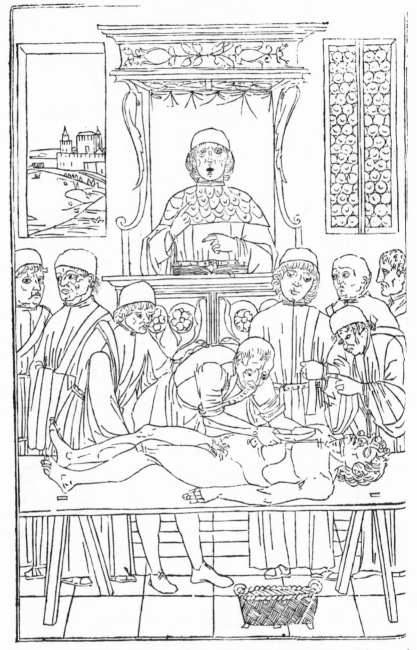

Figure 1. A dissection in the late fifteenth century. Reprinted from Johannes de Ketham, *Fasciculus medicinae*, ed. Petrus Andrea Morsanus (Venice: Johannes et Gregorius de Gregorius, 1495).

torian Charles Talbot put it, "a process of learning a set body of doctrine, and then of amplifying it and manipulating it by subtle analysis and dialectic argument."[27] Physicians who engaged in manual activities were criticized "on the assumption that the dignity of medicine could be assured only by a preoccupation with universal ideas."[28] The threat of manual work to status and, eventually, to purse made physicians shrink from it "as from a plague," Vesalius bluntly noted, "lest the rabbins [chief authorities] of medicine decry them before the ignorant mass as barbers and they acquire less wealth and honor."[29] Thus physicians generally left manual activities to others: the preparation of drugs to apothecaries, therapy involving cutting and manipulation to barbers and surgeons, and dissections to barbers.

Vesalius took a step forward. He disparaged the practice of autopsies where one person dissected the cadaver, as another described the structures supposedly uncovered by reading from a text. He likened the readers to "jackdaws aloft in their high chair, with egregious arrogance croaking things they have never investigated but merely committed to memory from the books of others, or reading what has already been described." He characterized the assistants who dissected as "so ignorant of languages that they are unable to explain their dissections to the spectators and muddle what ought to be displayed according to the instructions of the physician who, since he has never applied his hand to the dissection of the body, haughtily governs the ship from a manual. Thus everything is wrongly taught in the schools, and days are wasted in ridiculous questions so that in such confusion less is presented to the spectators than a butcher in his stall could teach a physician."[30]

The frontispiece of Vesalius' *Fabrica* reveals his different attitude toward human anatomy (Figure 2). The professor, Vesalius himself, surrounded by his students, stands next to and handles the cadaver. The role of assistants, two of whom are depicted below the dissecting table, has been reduced to sharpening knives for the anatomization. Here textbook knowledge is downgraded: the attention of the professor, students, and most of the public audience in attendance is focused on the cadaver. The *Fabrica* was a treatise that described the normal anatomy of the human body in a more detailed manner than had ever been attempted before. This required correcting some commonly accepted but inaccurate descriptions of human anatomy, principally drawn from Galen, as well as including an account of structures previously disregarded. Vesalius made

13

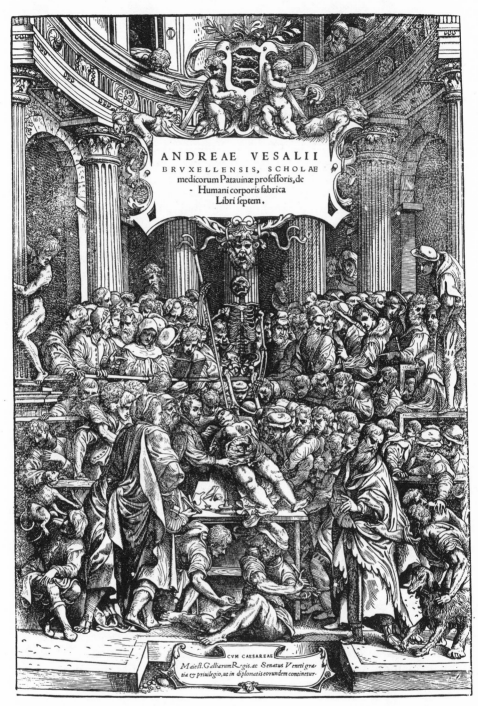

Figure 2. A dissection in the mid-sixteenth century. Reprinted from Andreas Vesalius, *De humani corporis fabrica libri septem* (Basel: 1543), frontispiece.

these corrections and additions by continual reference to the cadaver, conveyed his observations to his readers through elaborate anatomical drawings, and described explicitly a dissection technique that the readers could apply in making their own observations.

Yet the *Fabrica* was not a book that merely corrected previous anatomical errors. More important, it announced a new principle of fact finding and truth testing in anatomy: all anatomical statements and hypotheses were to be subjected to a methodical review by the dissection and observation of human cadavers, a process characterized by the historian C. D. O'Malley as "a consistent policy of doubting."[31] Accordingly, in the preface to the *Fabrica*, Vesalius disclosed that his own investigations, using the "reborn art of dissection," revealed that Galen had never dissected a human body, but "deceived by his monkeys" had committed numerous errors by seeking to infer the architecture of human anatomy from the structure of animal anatomy. Although insisting that he did not wish to appear disloyal to Galen, "the author of all good things," or seem to disregard his authority, Vesalius recognized that his work upset many physicians who, "in the conduct of a single anatomy nowadays. . .see Galen's description to have been incorrect in well over two hundred instances relating to the human structure and its use and function." To shield themselves against disillusion, some physicians zealously defended Galen. But Vesalius reported that "even they, influenced by love of truth, have little by little subsided and put more faith in their not–ineffectual eyes and reason than in Galen's writings."[32]

Before the sixteenth century, not all of Galen's anatomical observations had been wholly accepted, nor had all of the observations that contradicted Galen been wholly rejected. Yet, when the inevitable conflict arose between tradition and experience, tradition usually won. During the first half of the sixteenth century Vesalius, with a few other anatomists such as the Italian Berengario da Carpi (who wrote the first anatomical treatise that systematically used pictures to elucidate the text), advanced the science of anatomy with their original observations. More than other anatomists who were his contemporaries, Vesalius demonstrated the value of personal verification of facts. Yet it is important to keep in mind that, in working to transform medical thinking, he was not alone.[33]

The encouragement thus given to dissection multiplied observations not only of normal anatomical structures but also of the transformations they sustained when attacked by disease. One of the first physicians to codify such data was the Frenchman Jean Fernel. In the section *Pathologia*, from his 1554 treatise *Medicina*, Fernel systematically considered the symptoms of each disease in relation to their pathological causes, among which were anatomical lesions. He demonstrated changes that disease produced in the solid parts of the body, and spurred efforts for their more rigorous delineation.[34]

A plea for the performance of autopsies was made later that century by an Italian, Marcello Donati, in his *De medica historia mirabili* (1586). "Let those who interdict the opening of bodies well understand their errors," he warned. "They prevent the physicians from acquiring a knowledge which may afford the means of great relief eventually to individuals attacked by a similar disease." The community was not the only agency censured by Donati. He also indicted physicians "who, from laziness or repugnance," eschewed dissection, choosing rather to "remain in the darkness of ignorance than to scrutinize laboriously the truth."[35]

Autopsies to detect pathological changes had become common by the opening of the seventeenth century. However, during this century, no systematic classification of pathological lesions emerged. Anatomists too often focused on the rare and odd transformations of body structure caused by disease. They also tended to produce treatises in which they abundantly supplemented their own work with the anatomical observations of others – too often accepted uncritically. The most extensive and influential of these collections of autopsy data was Théophile Bonet's *Sepulchretum, sive Anatomica Practica* . . . (1679). Over 1,700 pages long, it was filled with clinical histories and reports of subsequent autopsies.[36] But it was Giovanni Battista Morgagni's 1761 treatise, *The Seats and Causes of Diseases Investigated by Anatomy*, that established the foundation of the modern understanding of disease through anatomy.[37]

Morgagni built his work on a structure of carefully selected case histories, written by himself and other physicians, about the clinical course of illness in patients; reports of pathological lesions found by physicians at autopsy; and discussion of the cases that pointed to a relation between occurrences in the living and in the dead body. The primary flaw of Bonet's work – the lack of comprehensive indexes that compared symptoms in the living with lesions in the dead – was remedied in Morgagni's work, whose central feature was its four indexes. The first, essentially a table of contents, enumerated the book's major divisions. The last was a detailed listing

16

of names and subject entries. The key indexes were the remaining two. One showed what physicians had found in living bodies, and a second enumerated observations made on the dead, "so that if any physician observe a singular, or any other symptom in a patient, and desire to know what internal injury is wont to correspond to that symptom; or if any anatomist find any particular morbid appearance in the dissection of a body, and should wish to know what symptom has preceded an injury of this kind in other bodies; the physician, by inspecting the first of these indexes, the anatomist by inspecting the second, will immediately find the observation which contains both."[38]

Employing this method, Morgagni established two premises that became fundamental to the education and practice of future generations of physicians. First, disease often leaves telltale footprints on the tissues of the body; second, study of these footprints is the best way for physicians to verify judgments made on the living, and the key to achieving clinical excellence. Prior to this point, physicians had usually sought to explain disease through hypotheses which linked the symptoms in the living patient to the character of the obscure basic forces that initiated the illness. The anatomist now supplied a clear, verifiable link in the causal chain which connected the forces initiating the illness with their symptomological expression in the patient.[39]

But Morgagni's appeal to the physician – to examine the structural changes wrought by disease on the body's inner fabric – had to contend with imbued misgivings about anatomical study expressed in the previous century by physicians such as Sydenham, doubts that were supported by a number of Morgagni's contemporaries. They argued that most anatomical defects discovered during autopsy were either the natural results of decomposition after death, or artifacts created by the therapy used before death. Furthermore, since anatomical lesions represented the effects, but not the basic causes of disease – a fact acknowledged by Morgagni – his critics failed to see why so much effort should be spent on finding and describing them. Morgagni replied that physicians who conscientiously dissected bodies, who routinely matched the lesions they found with symptoms experienced by the patient during life, could learn to distinguish disease–generated lesions from all others. Physicians who regularly checked and connected the symptoms they observed in patients during life, with the lesions they located within them after death, improved their ability to diagnose

17

disease in the living and, what was equally important, to separate curable from incurable patients. If a patient were actually suffering from a fatal disease, and the physician believed that he could be restored to health, the physician could be misled into using vigorous therapy, and thus augment the suffering or accelerate the death of the patient. In such a case, a correct diagnosis encouraged a gentle treatment, directed solely at the relief of suffering. In addition, the subsequent autopsy would demonstrate to the patient's relatives and friends the true nature of the malady, and satisfy them that sound medical care had been provided. The physician thus protected, and perhaps enhanced, his reputation.

Finally, Morgagni declared his conviction that dissection could advance knowledge about the basic origins of disease by alerting physicians to antecedent circumstances, such as hereditary or accidental events in the life of the patient, which could be "the obvious causes of anatomical alterations."[40] However, Morgagni advised physicians to focus their attention on the proximate generators of illness – the anatomical lesions – "which not only provoke the maladies, but are also responsible for their intrinsic differences."[41] Like his critics he refused to speculate about the ultimate physical causes of health and disease, since they were inaccessible to the senses and rested "in hidden forms of invisible particles."[42]

The anatomical viewpoint advocated by Morgagni achieved growing acceptance, as was evidenced by the excellent reception and brisk sale of a treatise published in 1793 by the Scotsman Matthew Baillie, *The Morbid Anatomy of Some of the Most Important Parts of the Human Body*. Baillie wrote his book some thirty years after Morgagni's to correct certain defects in the latter's work that tended to discourage medical practitioners from consulting or purchasing it: disease descriptions whose clarity suffered from excessive generalization and irrelevant discussion, and a length too long and an expense too great to suit the limited time and lean purse of many physicians.[43]

A significant conceptual advance in the interpretation of anatomical changes caused by disease followed in 1801. Whereas Morgagni and Baillie thought of the body's organs as the units to consider in discussing the effects of disease, the French physician Marie–François–Xavier Bichat, in his *General Anatomy, Applied to Physiology and Medicine*, demonstrated that grossly visible biological sub-

18

stances, which he called "tissues," and classified into 21 types, were the building blocks of organs. Bichat understood disease as a local injury to one of an organ's several tissues, rather than as a general impairment of the entire organ. This theory allowed two classes of disease symptoms to be distinguished: those characteristic of the disturbed tissue, and those characteristic of the organ in which the diseased tissue lay. Bichat stressed the message so central to Morgagni's work, that observation of symptoms in the living patients without study of their effects on the anatomy in the dead was folly. "You may take notes, for twenty years, from morning to night at the bedside of the sick. . .and all will be to you only a confusion of symptoms, which, not being united in one point, will necessarily present only a train of incoherent phenomena. Open a few bodies, this obscurity will soon disappear, which observation alone would never have been able to have dissipated."[44]

By adopting a theory of the anatomical localization of pathology, physicians came to accept the surgeons' approach to disease. In making diagnoses, for several centuries before Morgagni's treatise appeared, surgeons had correlated their clinical findings with structural changes in the body. They could not operate without visualizing the anatomical change responsible for the disorder. Even physicians who doubted that a knowledge of anatomy was essential to their own practice believed it was essential for surgeons. Thus, during the eighteenth century, the anatomical orientation of medicine was aided, at least in part, by an increasing convergence of medicine and surgery, pathological anatomy being cultivated by both disciplines.[45] The physician's subsequent adoption of a manual and instrumental approach to practice, which was at the center of surgery, probably furthered the significant rapprochement between the two disciplines that occurred in the latter part of the nineteenth century.

The practice of dissecting bodies to find physical evidence of disease began to transform some eighteenth–century physicians from word–oriented, theory–bound scholastics to touch–oriented, observation–bound scientists. Yet, despite Morgagni's classification of disease through dissection, which involved an aggressive manipulation of the body and linked the characteristic lesions found after death to specific diseases in the living, he did not take the further step of advocating an analogous physical examination of the living patient; he continued to rely chiefly on the patient's narrative, and on a passive observation of symptoms.

In 1761, the year that Morgagni's *The Seats and Causes of Diseases* appeared, a Viennese physician Leopold Auenbrugger published a small monograph, the *Inventum novum.*[46] It described a method of examination he called "percussion" – striking the body with the fingers to produce sounds indicating the vitality of underlying organs. Auenbrugger believed his method would revolutionize the diagnosis of chest disease, by giving physicians a trustworthy alternative to their accustomed methods. Since he doubted the reliability of symptoms related by patients, which he criticized as inconstant and untrustworthy, and external signs of illness observed by physicians, he drew attention to the difficulty of separating diseases with such evidence. For Auenbrugger the morbid sound *he* elicited from the body, not the patient's thoughts or his physical appearance, was the most dependable index of the nature and course of chest disease. He proudly proclaimed his ability to diagnose disease "by the testimony of my own senses."[47] In Auenbrugger's work, the central medical objective was to examine the character of the sounds produced by the activity of the physician. He advocated a technique that removed the personality and physical appearance of the patient from their earlier central place in the evaluation of illness.

Just as Morgagni concentrated on identifying disease–produced alterations of internal structure in the dead body, Auenbrugger searched for such altered structures in the living. The two men were equally concerned with finding *objective* evidence of disease, and both were convinced that understanding the relation of a specific structural change to a specific illness was the key to learning medicine.

Auenbrugger's work was slow to attract the attention it deserved from his medical contemporaries. For example, Anton de Haen and Gerard van Swieten, leading figures in Viennese medicine, did not mention his work in their writings although much of it had been carried out in hospital wards overseen by them, and Auenbrugger had praised van Swieten in the preface of his book. The reception of percussion outside of Vienna was no better. The Scot William Cullen in his widely read and authoritative eighteenth–century text, *First Lines of the Practice of Physic*, noted the existence of percussion but says he never used it. Although translated into French in 1770, Auenbrugger's work was practically unknown in France until its publication in a new translation with commentary by Jean–Nicolas Corvisart in 1808.[48]

There are several possible reasons for the neglect of percussion in the eighteenth century. Auenbrugger's treatise was too brief (only 95 pages in the original) to portray the specific differences in the percussive sounds that he claimed would allow physicians to discriminate among diseases. The delicate variation in sound that had to be distinguished to apply this technique was an obstacle to the learner, who required extensive explanations and examples to appreciate the shades of differences among the various possible sounds. Auenbrugger did not provide such aids. In his treatise terse, vague descriptions of complex phenomena abounded, such as: "If a sonorous part of the chest, struck with the same intensity, yields a sound duller than natural, disease exists in that part."[49] What did he mean by "sonorous," and by "natural"? At what intensity should the chest be thumped? How to determine a standard measure of intensity? What constituted a normal sound and what degree of dullness was needed to indicate pathology? For Auenbrugger, these inexact phrases had a meaning gained from his seven years of experience in developing percussion but the meanings were not apparent to others. His qualitative terminology also led to confusion between his technique and another diagnostic method called "succussion." First mentioned by Hippocrates and used sparingly throughout the following centuries, it consisted of physically shaking a patient and listening for sounds that told whether fluid existed in the chest. Some physicians believed percussion to be only a variation of this procedure.[50]

Use of percussion also required that the physician be able to infer the nature of the internal lesion from the character of the sound created by striking the chest; he thus had to transform auditory patterns quickly into their visual analogues, a concept slow to find acceptance. Many doctors had not adopted the view that disease was basically a localized phenomenon, and were thus not persuaded that it was necessary to dissect cadavers or look for an association between symptoms in the living and lesions in the dead.[51] Furthermore, Auenbrugger did little to convert doctors to his point of view. He had carried out autopsies to perfect his technique, yet in his treatise he did not explicitly discuss their importance. He gave the reader only occasional and very brief accounts of the specific conditions found in the chest after death as they related to the percussive tones heard in the living body.

Many physicians in Auenbrugger's time were still prejudiced against engaging in manual activities. The physical intimacy

21

required by percussion threatened to undermine the professional and social standing of the physician, whose philosophical bent and intellectual training often made the application of a manual method of diagnosis beneath his dignity,[52] or placed him in a class with the surgeon. The latter's largely apprenticeship training and empirical learning, lack of academic degree, and craftsmanlike approach to illness through manual techniques and tools had allowed the physician – educated as he was with the gentry in the university and learned in the theoretical knowledge of medicine – to assert a claim to social and medical superiority over the surgeon.

The adoption of percussion was also delayed because Auenbrugger himself proved a poor advocate. He balked at publicizing or even defending his method, convinced that all competent physicians would appreciate its merits without prodding. He stated in a provocative tone, which may have offended his colleagues and other physicians, the belief that his innovative work would stir "envy" and "malice" in critics, and so refused to "every one who is actuated by such motives as these, all explanation of my doctrines."[53]

In the seventeenth century, the physician principally used verbal and visual techniques to make a diagnosis. He listened to the patient's description of his symptoms, and observed his appearance and that of his body fluids. In the eighteenth century, the physician began increasingly to use manual techniques. Morgagni and his successors dissected the dead body to find the pathological lesions left by disease, which they correlated with symptoms the patient had described. Auenbrugger introduced percussion, the manipulation of the living body, to find signs of disease, whose traces might later be visible at autopsy. Together, Morgagni and Auenbrugger and their followers prepared the way for a key figure in medicine, who would alter the nature of clinical diagnosis and hence of medical practice by publishing a new treatise on medical diagnosis.

2 The stethoscope and the detection of pathology by sound

In 1819, a young French physician, René–Théophile–Hyacinthe Laennec, published his *On Mediate Auscultation*, which contained the most numerous and detailed accounts yet written of pathological lesions found in the chest at autopsy. The innovative aspect of the work lay in its account of a new technique – mediate auscultation (in some ways resembling Auenbrugger's percussion) – which made it possible for the physician to detect chest disease in living patients by studying the character of the sounds the damaged tissues produced.

Hippocrates was the first to describe the basic aspect of auscultation in his *De Morbis:* "You shall know by this that the chest contains water and not pus, if in applying the ear during a certain time on the side, you perceive a noise like that of boiling vinegar."[1] Physicians after Hippocrates largely ignored the ideas suggested by this passage, but reported occasionally on the generation of sounds by the organs within the body. In the early 1600s, for example, William Harvey wrote in *De Motu Cordis* of sonorous notes he had heard in the chest, which accompanied each pulsation of the heart.[2] Robert Hooke speculated, in a remarkable statement written later that century, that great medical benefits might follow from examining the character of sounds produced by the body's organs:

There may be also a Possibility of discovering the Internal Motions and Actions of Bodies by the sound they make, who knows but that as in a Watch we may hear the beating of the Balance, and the running of the Wheels, and the striking of the Hammers, and the grating of the Teeth, and Multitudes of other Noises; who knows, I say, but that it may be possible to discover the Motions of the Internal Parts of Bodies, whether Animal, Vegetable, or Mineral, by the sound they make, that one may discover the Works perform'd in the severals Offices and Shops of a Man's Body, and thereby discover what Instrument or Engine is out of order, what Works are going on at several Times, and lies still at others, and the like. . .I

23

have been able to hear very plainly the beating of a Man's Heart, and 'tis common to hear the Motion of Wind to and fro in the Guts, and other small Vessels, the stopping of the Lungs is easily discover'd by the Wheesing, the Stopping of the Head, by the humming and whistling Noises, the fliping to and fro of the Joynts in many cases, by crackling, and the like; . . .and so to their becoming sensible they require either that their Motions be increased, or that the Organ be made more nice and powerful to sensate and distinguish them as they are. . .for the doing of both which I think it not impossible but that in many cases there may be Helps found.[3]

Harvey and Hooke, like Hippocrates, did not systematically explore the diagnostic possibilities of these acoustic phenomena, nor did they persuade other physicians to do so. In the eighteenth century, when physicians encountered pathological noises emanating from the body, they too dismissed the event as a curiosity. Typical was James Douglass, who in 1715 thought it "almost incredible" that the heartbeat of one of his patients could make "such a Noise in his Breast, as plainly could be heard at some Distance from his Bed-side."[4] Even the New England physician Edward Augustus Holyoke did not know what to make of the patient with a tumor in the chest who asked him: "What could occasion that blubbering noise (as he expressed himself) in the sore? Upon which, applying my ear near to the part where he perceived the noise, I plainly heard a whizzing, and he termed it, a blubbering noise at every breath, exactly resembling such as arises from the running of air through a small orifice." Dr. Holyoke explained the sound by postulating the development of a passage between the tumor and the lungs, but he drew no wider conclusions from the episode.[5]

Early in his medical career Laennec came upon the Hippocratic reference to acoustic phenomena in disease. But he dismissed it as valueless because he believed that what Hippocrates heard was simple respiration: "At the time I considered it, as it indeed is, one of the mistakes of that great man, and had altogether forgotten it."[6] Laennec also noted remarks on acoustic phenomena from his teacher J. N. Corvisart, who discussed the possibility of using sounds emanating from internal organs to detect disease, only to dismiss the notion: "Some authors assert that they could hear, in certain diseases of the heart, the noise produced by the violent strokes of this organ, even at a small distance from the patient's bed. I have never had an opportunity, I repeat it, of ascertaining these unquestionably rare observations; I have barely heard these strokes by applying my ear close to the patient's thorax."[7] More important for Laennec however than the discussions by Hippocrates or Corvisart was the example of his colleague Gaspard Bayle, who applied his ear to the patient's chest. His efforts induced Laennec to try the procedure in diagnosis, but he used it sparingly because he found it inconvenient and distasteful to move his ear over the patient's chest, and the procedure often embarrassed the patient.

These were the events leading to the notable day in 1816 at the Necker Hospital in Paris when Laennec, then 35, examined a young woman who had a baffling heart disorder. To diagnose her illness he tried to use percussion and palpation (pressing the hand upon the body to detect internal abnormalities): the patient's obesity thwarted both techniques. He then thought of placing his ear to her chest to listen to the heart, but the patient's youth and sex restrained him. Then a fact in acoustics flashed through Laennec's mind. He remembered that sound traveling through solid bodies becomes augmented. Rolling some sheets of paper into a cylinder, he placed one end on the patient's chest and the other next to his ear. Clear and distinct heart sounds emerged. "From this moment," wrote Laennec, "I imagined that the circumstance might furnish means for enabling us to ascertain the character, not only of the action of the heart, but of every species of sound produced by the motion of all the thoracic viscera."[8] After experimenting with different materials, he finally constructed an instrument to be used for this effort from a rounded piece of wood, one foot in length and 1½ in. in diameter, longitudinally perforated down the center to enhance its sound–carrying properties, and separable in two parts for convenient carrying. Laennec called his instrument by either of two names: the "cylinder," suggested by its shape; the "stethoscope" from the Greek words for "chest" and "I view," which became accepted usage.[9] With this instrument, Laennec examined the character of sounds emanating from the chests of healthy and of ill patients, most of which he could relate to anatomical faults he found by dissecting their bodies after death. Linking symptoms during life with findings at autopsy—the cornerstone of Morgagni's work – was also of paramount importance for Laennec, who believed anatomical lesions to be "the least variable and most positive of the phenomena of local disease."[10] The result was his 1819 treatise, *On Mediate Auscultation*. This title distinguished auscultation mediated by an object, such as the stethoscope, from immediate auscultation in which nothing was interposed between the ear of the physician and the patient's body (Figure 3).

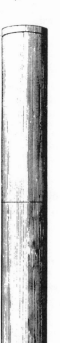
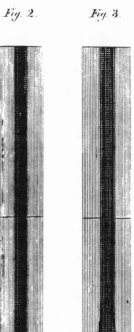
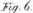
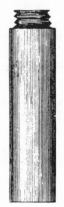
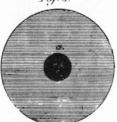

Figure 3. Laennec's stethoscope (1819). This illustration shows:
1. An exterior view of the stethoscope. The physician first sets the top end on the patient's body, then lays his ear against the other end;
2. A longitudinal section showing the hollow central bore. Insertion of the stopper improves the transmission of certain sounds, such as those made by the heart;
3. A longitudinal section with the stopper removed;
4. The stopper. Its funnel–shaped lower portion is perforated in the center so that the whole instrument resembles a hollow tube;
5. One half of the stethoscope revealing the screw that holds the two parts together;
6. The transverse section.
Reprinted from R.T.H. Laennec, *A Treatise on the Diseases of the Chest* (1821), Plate VIII.

Ailments of the chest usually manifested but a small number of symptoms that the patient could feel and discuss, or the physician could outwardly observe: mainly coughing, shortness of breath, and expectoration. In his treatise, Laennec declared them totally unreliable symptoms by which to discriminate illness. They could differ in character in the same disease, and were often similar in different diseases. Fundamentally distrustful of the patient's narrative and obvious symptoms, he also criticized previous methods of physical examination used to analyze chest disorders. He granted that, through percussion, infirmities could be found that earlier had been detectable only from uncertain narrative and observational clues. Yet percussion was useless for fat people whose chests could not be made to resonate, inaccurate when disease in both lungs made it impossible to comparatively differentiate percussive sounds – a key basis of diagnosis with the technique – and unavailing when disease existed far from the body's surface, for example in the center of the lungs. Percussion could show the presence of fluid in the chest, but could not distinguish the kind of fluid; it disclosed no sign of heart disease until the organ was very enlarged and thereby irrevocably damaged; and it failed to reveal dilation of large blood vessels in the chest until they were manifest to the eye or touch. Finally, the difficulty of executing percussion discouraged its use and encouraged error. Laennec asserted that, employed alone, percussion was either useless or misleading. His view of tactile probing of the body, or palpation, was no better: the evidence it produced was vague and uncertain. He also found fault with the technique of applying the ear directly to the body to listen for sounds (immediate auscultation): this procedure was indelicate and could cause postural discomfort for both patient and physician. As for pulse feeling, an old and popular means of ferreting out disease, Laennec attributed its popularity to ease of performance, which inconvenienced neither patient nor doctor, and to the numerous interpretations of illness that even the most unlearned physician could formulate from its variation. He condemned it as providing unreliable clinical evidence. Yet Laennec declared that all of these diagnostic techniques, especially percussion, although often of little or no value when applied alone, acquired merit when used in conjunction with the stethoscope.[11]

The magnitude of Laennec's achievement becomes clear when we compare his *On Mediate Auscultation* with Auenbrugger's the *Inventum novum*. Laennec characterized this monograph as a "simple exposition of new means of diagnosis,"[12] and correctly. As a mere outline of a method, Auenbrugger's book did not comment extensively on the new signs of disease it revealed, or on the nature of the anatomical lesions it located. In contrast, Laennec described in detail the attributes and relations of the signs and lesions uncovered by his method, not only at different stages of a disease, but also in people with differing physical makeups. Whereas Auenbrugger's text filled but 95 pages, Laennec's consumed 928 pages. In his annotated 1808 translation into French of Auenbrugger's treatise, Corvisart had sought to overcome the defects of the original text by adding detailed comments on the quality of the sounds generated by percussion and the anatomical flaws that produced them.[13] His efforts had encouraged a number of Frenchmen to use percussion before Laennec's discovery. But the method generally failed to attract attention in England or in the United States where percussion, a physician noted in 1836, "was hardly known. . .as is manifested from the circumstance of its not being mentioned in our textbooks or treatises, until the discoveries of Laennec."[14]

Mediate auscultation succeeded where percussion had failed in eventually drawing the attention of a wide audience of physicians to the internal evidence of disease, and to the physical methods of diagnosis that disclosed it. Its success would result from the strong advocacy of Laennec and his disciples, combined with a technique that delivered accurate signs, was not excessively difficult to learn, capitalized on the growing interest of physicians in the anatomical localization of pathology, and alleviated antipathy of close physical contact between doctor and patient by placing an instrument between them. Laennec devised a method in which nonverbal sounds became the signals of disease and a new instrument, the stethoscope, became essential to broadcast their presence.

One of Laennec's case histories illustrates the profound change his new technique was to have on the physician's perception of illness:

Case No. xxxvi. Phthisis Pulmonalis. – *Tuberculous cavity partly converted into fistula, producing the metallick tinkling.* A woman, 50 years of age, who had been affected with cough and expectoration for several years, and which had got much worse within a few months past, came to the Hospital on the 13th April, having, for the first time, been obliged to desist from her ordinary occupation. She looked much older than she was, and was very thin. The pulse was quick, skin slightly hot, and the expectoration, which was in moderate quantity, consisted of thick yellow sputa intermixed with much transparent ropy mucus.

The stethoscope, applied to the anterior and upper part of the right side, and to the right axilla, detected distinct pectoriloquism [clear transmission of the patient's voice]; and, in the same places, when the patient coughed or spoke, and still more during respiration, there was heard a tinkling, like that of a small bell which has just stopped ringing, or of a gnat buzzing within a porcelain vase. A mucous rattle, or strong guggling, existed in the same points; and all these phenomena were distinctly perceptible over the whole space from the top of the shoulder to the fourth rib, – being, only, more distinct anteriorly and under the axilla than behind. The murmur of respiration was sufficiently distinct over the greater part of the chest, except at the roots of the right lung and the top of the left. The Hippocratic succussion afforded no result. From these various signs I made the following diagnosis: *Vast tuberculous cavity occupying the whole of the superior lobe of the right lung, and containing a small quantity of fluid; tubercles, especially at the top of the left and root of the right lung.*[15]

The patient died of her illness six weeks after the diagnosis was made.

This case history bears the imprint of a new medical era: the account is dominated by the physical hallmarks of the illness and the internal alterations they denote.

Between 1819 and 1850 prolonged debate ensued, which finally established physical examination as the keystone of diagnosis and transformed the work of the doctor and his relation with patients. Auscultation soon became the center of medical discussion. Laennec argued that the techniques of physical examination (notably auscultation, palpation, and percussion) were superior to traditional methods of questioning patients and observing exteriorized symptoms; he also claimed that auscultation was the polestar that guided physicians in evaluating other physical evidence of chest disease. Accordingly, physicians who defended the worth of the older methods sought to attack the shortcomings of auscultation, and doctors partial to the techniques of physical examination had to defend the merits of auscultation.[16] But Laennec's premature death in 1826, just after he had completed a second and considerably enlarged version of his treatise, left to his followers the task of converting the medical world at large to his views. They marshaled all possible anatomical, experimental, and bedside evidence to their cause.

Laennec had confirmed the diagnostic value of the sounds he heard through the stethoscope by demonstrating that the anatomic lesions they predicted consistently appeared in the cadaver. These predictions were the basis of Laennec's confidence in his technique. For example, Laennec found that when the patient's voice seemed to come directly from his chest to the ear of the examining physician using a stethoscope, this sound (which he called "pectoriloquy") denoted the presence of tuberculosis. His confidence in this sign and his understanding of its cause (tuberculosis excavations in the lung) were the products of dissection: "In upwards of two hundred instances of consumptive subjects, whose bodies I have examined after having ascertained, during life, the condition of their lungs as indicated by the cylinder [stethoscope], I have not met with a single instance in which ulcerous excavations did not exist in those points of the lung over which the phenomenon of pectoriloquism had shown itself distinctly."[17]

Laennec's followers, like the Irish physician Robert Graves, also believed that anatomical lesions were the most reliable indications of disease, "for being immediately connected, as effects, *with* the primary cause, they prove the most useful of all symptoms, in enabling us to ascertain the seat and progress of diseased action."[18] The elevation of the auscultatory sound to a level of concrete reality occurred only because of the close demonstrable correspondence between the sound and the visible lesion disclosed at autopsy. Successful auscultation required the physician to transform the sound he heard into a picture he could visualize. One metaphor that recurred regularly in the medical literature between 1820 and 1850 was "seeing" disease by listening through the stethoscope: "We anatomise by auscultation (if I may say so), while the patient is yet alive," proclaimed a doctor, for whom the ear became an eye through auscultation.[19] It is "a window in the breast through which we can see the precise state of things within," insisted another.[20]

Auscultatory sounds also proved more reliable as signs of disease because their causal connection with anatomical lesions could be confirmed through laboratory experiments, whereas the link between narrative and exteriorized signs and anatomical defects could not be so demonstrated. Auscultatory sounds could be demonstrated in the laboratory "with all the precision attainable in some of the higher branches of physics. We can imitate a great number of them in the dead body, and even out of the body, so as to have the most certain proof of the truth of our conclusions; and the result is, that our knowledge of this class of diseases [disorders of the chest], instead of being, as it was five–and–twenty years ago, more imperfect than of any other, has attained a degree of certainty and precision which the most sanguine man could not then imagine, and which fully entitles it to be compared with that which we possess of the more exact sciences."[21]

The experimental evidence is well illustrated by the work of another French physician François Magendie. He showed that in the animal body, as in the external material world, sound comprehended simple physical phenomena. To exhibit the conditions that accounted for the murmurs arising in arteries, he forced water through tubes of different sizes and compared the sounds produced with those heard in the body: "The reasoning is not indeed rigorously strict or demonstrative, but it is the nearest approach that we can make to an explanation in the present state of the science."[22] The existence of physical principles, which explained the mechanisms of the sounds produced by the body's organs, bore witness to the superiority claimed for auscultatory signs. Physicians venerated such evidence. It brought them close to a dream of that period: to be able to base medical practice on scientific law.

Supporters of auscultation also used bedside evidence to prove its pre-eminence over the older signs of disease. For example, patients who suffered from either of two lung diseases, pleurisy or consumption, might display to observers the same external signs: cough, fever, expectoration of pus, emaciation, night sweats, and diarrhea. Yet the two diseases could be distinguished by the distinctive internal sounds each produced in the chest, which were only apparent to the physician who applied his stethoscope.[23]

The growing disenchantment of many physicians with the reliability of external signs was matched by their skepticism about the reliability of the patient's testimony. Sometimes misrepresentations resulted from the patient's "prejudice or ignorance."[24] Physicians also encountered situations where patients willfully distorted the facts of their ailment. These problems vanished when the stethoscope was used. Auscultatory sounds were "independent of the caprice or ignorance of the patient," who was unable "to simulate or to conceal, to exaggerate or to lessen them."[25] In the late 1820s when one physician, unconvinced of the superiority of physical diagnosis, challenged an auscultator, Dr. James Hope, to test the matter, a public trial of the old and new schools of diagnosis ensued. At St. George's Hospital, London, each physician examined the same patient, and each applied only his own techniques. Autopsy subsequently affirmed the correctness of the auscultator's diagnosis, and silenced the critic.[26]

31

But despite the clear superiority of auscultation in diagnosing chest disorders, the old techniques still had their supporters, who justified their adherence to the old ways with reasons essentially typical of those which have given traditional practices in medicine considerable staying power. As generally happens when faced with a new technical advance, some physicians were reluctant to abandon techniques that had cost them so many long hours to learn; others recognized in themselves certain physical limitations such as poor hearing, or harbored the vague fear of being unable to master the new technique. Still others disliked abandoning familiar habits, giving up the role of master, and beginning over again as student. Some physicians reiterated Laennec's conviction that by fostering a more analytic attitude toward diagnosis than had existed in the past, auscultation improved the skill with which the older signs of disease were evaluated. A number of physicians who did adopt auscultation at the same time continued to use the old techniques, because they seemed to illuminate their understanding of chest disease. These physicians warned their colleagues further that physical signs must be tested and confirmed against the history and outer symptoms exhibited by the patient.[27]

Perhaps the most notable expositor of this viewpoint was the French physician Pierre Louis. He initiated a method of clinical teaching and diagnosis based upon precise observation, collection, and statistical comparison of all indications of illness. For Louis, the omission of any observation meant that the physician's understanding of illness might be false or incomplete. Commencing with queries on age, profession, nutrition, and previous diseases, Louis carefully questioned the patient about the sensations he experienced, what events had occurred, and what his own opinions were of his illness. With Louis, the patient's narrative assumed renewed importance in diagnosis. But under him, it became a wholly different clinical instrument, as he insisted that the physician must direct the unfolding of the patient's story, although he must not question in a way that invited a particular answer; the technique followed in questioning the patient, like that used to examine a patient physically, must be carefully chosen.

How could physicians check the diagnostic significance of the narrative and of external signs of illness, when their lack of specificity produced less satisfactory correlations with autopsy findings than correlations based upon techniques such as auscultation and

32

percussion? Louis addressed this problem by counting the frequency with which every symptom of an illness occurred in many individual cases. He could then know which manifestations of a given illness were especially characteristic of it, and which were not. He advised that if physicians wished "to appreciate the value of symptoms, to know the progress and duration of diseases, to assign their degree of gravity, their relative frequency, the influence of medical constitutions upon their development, to enlighten ourselves as to the value of therapeutical agents, or the causes of disease," that it was "indispensable to count."[28] Louis objectified each footprint of disease by numeration. For him, all signs had equal merit, the criteria for their excellence being the care with which they were observed and described, and their statistical correlation with a particular disease, checked when possible by the autopsy. His exacting method of observation and numerical comparison was too difficult to be used by most physicians, who could not give it the necessary time and labor. Yet Louis's belief that narrative and exteriorized evidence could be as objective as the evidence of auscultation or percussion, given a purposeful method of elicitation, was the strongest support raised in the second quarter of the nineteenth century in favor of the older techniques of diagnosis.

While many auscultators in this same period questioned the merits of the time–honored diagnostic methods, they also had to defend their own procedure as a general method. A central point of contention was the value of precise diagnosis, given the still impoverished state of medical therapy. Auscultators claimed that by discovering disease in its earliest stages, by converting suspicion into certainty, illness could be treated with a vigor and success not possible when doctors depended on the traditional, inexact means of diagnosis. Furthermore, even when the disease was incurable, an accurate diagnosis enhanced the physician's reputation and the confidence of patients in him, spared patient and family the pain and possible financial ruin that might occur when physicians mistook one disease for another, and allowed the patient time to prepare for his death. "Is it nothing to abstain from torturing a patient with not alone inefficient, but positively injurious means?" asked the English physician William Corrigan. "Is it nothing to foretell, and thus in some measure take from, the approaching calamity? Is it nothing, instead of giving delusive hope, to prepare the individual himself for his last great change, and that, in all probability, to be sudden?

33

Are all these matters of little consideration?"[29] Yet some practitioners insisted that by confirming the presence of an incurable disease, leaving no room for hope, auscultation paralyzed the physician's will to heal. "How sad is this auscultation?" wrote a young doctor to his physician father, "these positive physical signs; which, though in themselves not enough, yet put the seal of certitude upon what before was doubtful; destroy the plausibility of many a willing interpretation of other symptoms; and leave us to fold our hands and await the event."[30]

A greater threat still to auscultation was its overzealous supporters,[31] who attributed powers to the technique which it in fact did not possess; they subdivided the sounds heard to an extreme degree and attached an invariable significance to each. Accordingly, when more careful physicians tried to put auscultation to the test in practice, they became disillusioned by its results. To raise the status of auscultation, its partisans excessively disparaged the older diagnostic methods, sanctioned in the past, and thereby additionally jeopardized the spread of auscultation. These problems led Oliver Wendell Holmes, Harvard's professor of anatomy, to make the overzealous auscultator the subject of a comic ballad, "The Stethoscope Song." It is a tale of a physician, just returned from medical studies in Paris, who made a number of false diagnoses because several insects (unnoticed) were nesting in his stethoscope:

> There was a young man in Boston town
> He bought him a STETHOSCOPE nice and new,
> All mounted and finished and polished down,
> With an ivory cap and a stopper too.
>
> It happened a spider within did crawl,
> And spun him a web of ample size,
> Wherein there chanced one day to fall
> A couple of very imprudent flies.
>
> The first was a bottle-fly, big and blue,
> The second was smaller, and thin and long;
> So there was a concert between the two,
> Like an octave flute and a tavern gong.
>
> Now being from Paris but recently,
> This fine young man would show his skill;
> And so they gave him, his hand to try,
> A hospital patient extremely ill.

There was an old lady had long been sick,
    And what was the matter none did know;
Her pulse was slow, though her tongue was quick;
    To her this knowing youth must go.

Now, when the stethoscope came out,
    The flies began to buzz and whiz; –
O ho! the matter is clear, no doubt;
    An *aneurism* there plainly is.

Now, when the neighbouring doctors found
    A case so rare had been descried,
They every day her ribs did pound
    In squads of twenty; so she died.

Then six young damsels, slight and frail,
    Received this kind young doctor's cares;
They all were getting slim and pale,
    And short of breath on mounting stairs.

So fast their little hearts did bound,
    The frightened insects buzzed the more;
So over all their chests he found
    The *râle sifflant*, and *râle sonore*.

He shook his head; – there's grave disease; –
    I greatly fear you all must die;
A slight *post-mortem*, if you please,
    Surviving friends would gratify.

The six young damsels wept aloud,
    Which so prevailed on six young men,
That each his honest love avowed,
    Whereat they all got well again.

This poor young man was all aghast;
    The price of stethoscopes came down;
And so he was reduced at last
    To practise in a country town.

Now use your ears, all you that can,
    But don't forget to mind your eyes,
Or you may be cheated, like this young man,
    By a couple of silly, abnormal flies.[32]

Laennec must shoulder at least some of the blame for his followers' rashness. For he attached too much importance to auscultation, too little to facts obtained from the patient's narrative and his

visible symptoms. Laennec's originality and perceptivity for a time also had the effect of discouraging further research in auscultation; during the twenty years following the first edition of *On Mediate Auscultation*, few novel stethoscopic signs of disease were discovered. Even when Laennec's disciples found errors in his work, they hesitated to challenge his word. One of them acknowledged that it would "have seemed a sort of heresy. . .to question the accuracy of what the great discoverer had pronounced to be true, to look beyond the secrets he had chosen to reveal."[33] Laennec's own remarkable acoustic perception and long practice with auscultation also created difficulties for his followers. It is certain, from commentaries on Laennec's observations, that he heard and described differences in sound that most physicians could not distinguish, yet failed to recognize his advantage. This is illustrated in a passage from Laennec's treatise and the comments on it by his translator and disciple John Forbes.

Laennec:
The peculiar and distinctive character of these phenomena [the physical signs of pneumonia], when profound or superficial, can easily be ascertained by a person of only moderate experience. I have known pupils, who had practised auscultation only three months, make the distinction without hesitation.
Forbes:
I can hardly agree with our author as to the certainty of detecting all the preceding varieties of partial pneumonia by the stethoscope. His tact and experience were certainly matchless; and no doubt he did what few of his followers can accomplish. At all events, I think *the student* ought hardly to expect to compass so minute a diagnosis; as failure might weaken his confidence in the unquestioned and unquestionable powers of the instrument.[34]

Patients were sometimes embarrassed and frightened by the assault on their bodies made by the stethoscopic examination. Some thought, when the stethoscope appeared in the doctor's hand, that an operation would ensue, for patients associated instruments with the surgeon, not with the physician. Yet they were amazed at the ability of the physician who used the stethoscope to learn about the inner structure of the living body, from sounds inaudible to the patient. Chest diseases could no longer be concealed – the physician with a stethoscope could, in a sense, autopsy the patient while still alive. As a result, popular sentiment in favor of the stethoscope became so strong that, even in the late 1820s, practitioners who refused to use the instrument (and therefore the technique it represented) placed their professional reputation in jeopardy. An

English doctor who signed himself "One of the New School" declared that physicians who undervalued the stethoscope were not worthy of public patronage, and cautioned, "We now know who the physicians are that duly appreciate this inestimable discovery, and who are really deserving of the public support. Doubtless they will receive it, for John Bull is attached to the good things of this life. . .Those physicians who 'close their ears to the voice of the charmer,' will be as regularly shewn up, as in times past, and in the columns of John Bull, were those of the clergy who persisted in praying for Queen Caroline."[35] In such a climate of opinion, some doctors, unable to distinguish a wheeze from a murmur, adopted the stethoscope for the sake of public appearance. A case was described of a pretender who assumed a look of great wisdom, applied the wrong end of the stethoscope to his ear, held the other end above the patient's chest, and reported hearing a respiratory murmur. What he really heard was the noise of a hackney coach passing in the street below.[36]

Although Laennec had striven mightily to wed the performance of auscultation to the stethoscope, within a few years, a number of physicians declared that auscultation with the instrument held no superiority over auscultation with the unaided ear and was inferior to it in many circumstances. In the second (1826) edition of his treatise, even Laennec acknowledged that some physicians preferred to auscultate without the stethoscope.[37] Several factors favored the use of the unaided ear rather than the stethoscope. Learning to use the stethoscope required more practice and more time than employing the naked ear alone. For this reason, some French physicians gave up the use of the stethoscope.[38]

The inconvenience of carrying the instrument also stirred opposition. Some ingenious physicians adopted the expedient of transporting it crosswise inside their top hats. But even this could be troublesome. One Edinburgh medical student was accused of possessing a dangerous weapon when his stethoscope fell from his top hat during a snowball fight.[39] Physicians worried too that listening to the chests of patients through a wooden tube, "as if the disease within were a living being that could communicate its condition," might make them appear foolish in the eyes of the patients.[40] Another deterrent was that as auscultation, like surgery, required the use of the hands and an instrument, some physicians feared that using the stethoscope would cause them to be classed with surgeons, as mere craftsmen. One practitioner explained that

37

physicians had long "reprobated that branch of medicine which is denominated 'surgery,' as the *'instrumental'* branch of the science – the chirurgical, the manipulating department, – and affecting to despise all mechanical contrivances, the M.D.s, both Dubs and Regulars, have rejected every species of chirurgical instrument, from the lancet down to that dexterous finger of Sir Astley Cooper which forced its way to the aorta of a suffering being who ended his existence in Guy's hospital."[41]

By the 1840s, the medical literature in England and the United States was reflecting the general belief that Laennec had exaggerated the advantages of the stethoscope, and that the naked ear did just as well. The mystical properties of the tube were vanishing – it was now appreciated as merely a good conductor of sound.

The effects of the stethoscope on physicians were analogous to the effects of printing on Western culture. Print and the reproducible book had created a new private world for man. He could isolate himself with the book and ponder its messages. As the sociologist David Riesman comments: "As long as the spoken or sung word monopolizes the symbolic environment, it is particularly impressive; but once books enter that environment it can never be quite the same again – books are, so to speak, the gunpowder of the mind. Books bring with them detachment and a critical attitude that is not possible in an oral tradition."[42] Similarly, auscultation helped to create the objective physician, who could move away from involvement with the patient's experiences and sensations, to a more detached relation, less with the patient but more with the sounds from within the body. Undistracted by the motives and beliefs of the patient, the auscultator could make a diagnosis from sounds that he alone heard emanating from body organs, sounds that he believed to be objective, bias–free representations of the disease process.

By the 1850s, physical examination of the patient and the use of mechanical aids, such as the stethoscope in diagnosis, had gained general acceptance in Great Britain as in the United States: "We have no longer gravely to discuss whether there be advantages or not in the use of the eye and the ear, as some seem to have doubted who have questioned the value of the aids to these senses in the study of disease," declared the English physician William Gull. "He must have taken the wrong path who asks 'Is the microscope of use? Is the stethoscope of use?' "[43] But whereas auscultation was comfortably established in medical textbooks as an accepted diagnostic technique, challenges were appearing to the widely held notion that most diseases of the heart and lungs generated specific sounds that identified them. The endless subdivision of tones that Laennec and his successors had described proved confusing to many doctors. The explicit meaning of a given sound was often unclearly communicated by the term used to describe it, and a particular phrase was sometimes used to convey several different meanings. "Ask a dozen physicians what they mean by muco-crepitant râle," suggested the clinician William Markham, "and I very much doubt whether any two will give the same account of it."[44] This perplexity demonstrated that auscultation was not as objective a technique as Laennec had portrayed it in his treatise. Accordingly, asked Markham, "Is it not reasonable to suppose, that our *principia* must be somewhere faulty?"[45]

Only gradually did physicians conclude that no single man could encompass all of auscultation, and that the subject required more exploration than Laennec had given it. Among those who did was Josef Skoda, who taught and practiced medicine in Vienna and was the leading figure in the German school of auscultation. Although his authoritative book on percussion and auscultation was printed in 1839, his research was largely disregarded in Great Britain and the United States until the 1850s. One reason was the current English fashion of ignoring the works of German writers, from patriotic sentiment, as if some "national inaccuracy appertained to all of them."[46] Some also viewed Skoda's writings as excessively theoretical, even fictive. But when his works were translated, they exerted an extensive influence in these English–speaking countries.

Skoda submitted Laennec's teaching to searching criticism. Using experiments, he traced many of the sounds heard in auscultation and percussion to their physical origins, and demonstrated that each sound was characteristic of a specific physical alteration that could have been produced by any one of several causes, but was not necessarily distinctive of a specific disorder. Accordingly, he disagreed with many of the specific signs of disease and the causal explanations Laennec advanced for them. Laennec believed that the sound he called pectoriloquy, produced by cavities in the lungs found in tuberculosis, was a signpost of the illness, often present when all other signs of tuberculosis were absent. He distinguished pectoriloquy from bronchophony, the sound that the voice made when resonating in a bronchial tube. In bronchophony, the sound that reached the auscultator's ear was diffuse and not as direct as in pectoriloquy. Skoda could not reliably distinguish pectoriloquy from bronchophony in the living patient: "I consider it certain that the perfect or imperfect passage of the [patient's] voice through the stethoscope, does not enable us to decide upon the presence or absence of a cavity in the lungs; and, consequently, that attempts to draw a distinction between pectoriloquy and bronchophony are useless, and can only be productive of error."[47]

Skoda also tested the signs of percussion by experiment. He found, for example, that the different sounds produced by percussing the body over organs such as the heart and lungs did not depend on special properties of those organs, but on variations in the quantity, distribution, and tension of the air surrounding them and the force of the percussion stroke. "There is no such thing as a liver–, spleen–, heart–, lung–, or stomach–sound," Skoda declared.[48] By the 1870s many physicians subscribed to Skoda's system of classifying the sounds of auscultation and percussion according to their physical cause. They believed, with Skoda, that pathognomonic physical signs were "exceedingly rare," that no disease had "one or more individual signs like labels. . .always associated with it and no other," and that physical signs represented "merely physical conditions which may be common to several diseases."[49]

As for the stethoscope itself, during the second half of the nineteenth century, Laennec's original instrument encountered increasing criticism and competition from newly modified forms.[50] Physicians maintained that the wooden tube caused discomfort to both patient and auscultator, and that its ability to augment sound was about that of a low–power microscope to magnify sight. Its short length and inflexibility required patients to change position repeatedly while being auscultated, and to bear the sometimes painful pressure of the rigid instrument on their bodies. Thus at the medical school in Edinburgh, novice physicians were even denied permission to practice upon patients with the wooden stethoscope. A physician who used the rigid stethoscope was also forced to bend over the patient and to place his head directly over the patient's chest, a posture difficult to maintain, especially for obese doctors.

To remedy some of these faults, monaural, flexible stethoscopes were designed. The first model was constructed by the Edinburgh physician Nicholas Comins in 1829, in the form of two rigid tubes united by a joint that permitted the instrument to be twisted at any angle. In the 1830s and 1840s, other monaural stethoscopes appeared, made of pliant tubing. These instruments could be applied to the body without requiring the patient to alter his posture frequently, and without exerting much pressure. They also kept the physician sufficiently distant to alleviate his fear of contracting an illness from the patient, and to stimulate his confidence that the stethoscope could be applied to ladies "in the highest ranks of society without offending fastidious delicacy."[51] Some women, unwilling to permit the rigid stethoscope to be used on them, did not object to the use of a long, flexible tube that kept the physician at a suitable distance.

To combine the benefits of pliancy and improved acoustical properties, Dr. Arthur Leared in 1851 designed a binaural instrument consisting of a small, rigid chest piece connected with two flexible gutta–percha pipes that passed to the auscultator's ears. "As certain nebulae are resolved into stars by powerful telescopes," he wrote, "so specific chest sounds, obscure from their lowness, may be determined by the double stethoscope."[52] The concept of a binaural stethoscope had occurred earlier. In 1829, Comins had suggested that such an instrument might be useful in practice, but it is unclear whether he ever built one. Charles J. B. Williams fashioned a binaural stethoscope sometime in the mid-1840s, but it was rigid, awkward to use, and never came into general use.[53]

Another flexible instrument, invented by S. Scott Alison in the 1860s (Figure 4), enabled auscultators to compare sounds generated in separate parts of the chest. Called the differential stethoscope, it had two pliant tubes made of metal wire, each with its own chest piece and separately attached to each ear. Alison's instrument, whose two individual hearing tubes allowed consecutive or simultaneous listening to tones from two parts of the chest, received acclaim for its ability to give physicians new combinations of sounds to interpret.[54]

Professor David Hughes and Dr. Benjamin Ward Richardson carried the amplification of stethoscopic sounds even further when in 1878 they announced experiments, using Richardson's recently invented microphone, to amplify heart and lung sounds. Physicians commenting on their work believed that as the microphone made even the steps of a fly audible at a great distance, it could easily render any movement within the human body acutely perceptible to the hearing.[55]

Some physicians believed that the new instrument would significantly advance auscultation, but their confidence was premature.

41

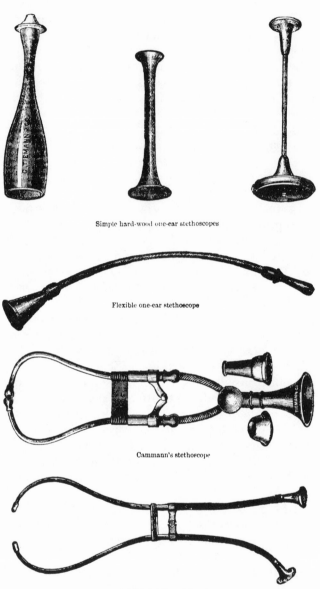

Simple hard-wood one-ear stethoscopes

Flexible one-ear stethoscope

Cammann's stethoscope

Allison's differential stethoscope

Figure 4. Stethoscopes designed in the nineteenth century. Reprinted from Paul Guttman, *A Handbook of Physical Diagnosis* (1880), p. 93.

Although the microphone could broadcast sounds made by the heart and lungs, the tones lacked the clarity possible with the simple stethoscope. Soon amplification itself came under attack, as critics charged that it distorted familiar acoustic signs, so that the technique of auscultation had to be relearned. The situation became more confusing when the attempt to make the instrument more portable produced still other versions of the stethoscope. One doctor commented that "if a striking and compendious illustration were required of the way in which man will, on some occasions, abdicate his reason, I think a table covered with the different forms of stethoscopes would excellently furnish it."[56] Was the form of the stethoscope the crucial element in auscultation, critics asked, or were a well–trained ear and prescient understanding the prerequisites upon which successful auscultation depended? Many physicians agreed with James Pollock: "It is truly to the tact of the observer, and not to the medium applied to the chest, that we owe precision in auscultation."[57]

Thus, in spite of these advances in technological aids, the skill and perception of the physician himself were still regarded as more crucial elements in auscultation than the instruments he used to practice it. Accordingly, the more convenient binaural stethoscope after the design by Leared (essentially the one in use today), did not displace the more cumbersome, monaural stethoscope until the 1890s. The sounds transmitted by the Laennec model seemed sufficiently accurate and carried meanings well enough understood by physicians to produce satisfactory diagnoses.

The stethoscope focused the attention of physicians on a new class of disease signs – the sounds produced by defective structures in the body. So precisely did these sounds seem to denote the character and progress of chest disease that older techniques of diagnosis were given less weight. A model of disease, deduced from these sounds and from the assorted lesions in the body found at autopsy, largely replaced the model constructed from the patients' subjective impressions and the physicians' own visual observations of the patient. The physician's withdrawal from such person–centered signs of illness was increased by the fact that the auscultatory process required the physician to isolate himself in a world of sounds, inaudible to the patient. Moreover, the growing success with which disease could be diagnosed through auscultation encouraged the physician to favor techniques that would yield data independent of the opinions and appearance of the patient.

In the second half of the nineteenth century, new methods of diagnosis were to appear, greatly extending the power of senses other than hearing, and bringing the doctor into contact with the most recondite structures and functions of the body. The vanguard comprised four sets of techniques: one visually probed gross anatomical structures; a second revealed the imperceptible cellular components of biological life; a third analyzed the functions of organs and gave the results in the form of graphs and numbers; and a fourth disclosed the composition of the solids and fluids of the body, by means of chemistry.

3 Visual technology and the anatomization of the living

The characterization of the stethoscope as an instrument for "seeing" into the chest revealed a specific desire physicians had developed during the era of auscultation – to inspect the architecture of the internal organs during life with the ease and clarity possible after death. This ambition was to inspire inventions which actually allowed physicians to visually penetrate the body's opaque skin cover and dark passages, beginning with an instrument for seeing into the human eye.

Until the early nineteenth century, the blackness which concealed the structures within the eyes of humans and animals was generally ascribed to the absorption of entering light by the eye's lining. Observers had occasionally reported seeing a transient luminescence in the eyes of animals in the dark. Its origin was puzzling and was attributed to various causes, such as the emission of stored light or the generation of electricity by structures within the eye. In 1810, the French scientist Bénédict Prévost demonstrated this luminosity never occurred in complete darkness but was created solely by the reflection of external light from the eye. How this happened remained a mystery.

In his 1823 treatise on the physiology of vision, the Czech scientist Jan Purkyně tells of inspecting a dog's eye to learn about this "shine." He conducted the examination while wearing his spectacles, whose lenses were concave. When he viewed the dog's eye from a certain direction, the light from a nearby candle seemed to be thrown back from the dog's eye into his own. He found that the candle's light was being reflected from the surface of his spectacles into the dog's eye. When he repeated the experiment with humans, the same result occurred, "indeed, the whole of the pupil lit up in a beautiful orange color." (It is uncertain whether he ever saw the optic nerve and blood vessels on the inner surface of the eye, which is possible with this technique.) Purkyně thus discovered a method of reflecting light into and illuminating the eye through an arrange-

45

ment of a lens and a light source. He urged practitioners not to spurn "the painstaking inquiry of physiologists" and to exploit this method for "ocular diagnosis."[1] Yet he himself did not publicize the technique or appear to pursue this line of inquiry further. His work on this subject went virtually unnoticed at the time.

Other investigators of the period were attracted to the problem of reconnoitering the eye's interior. In 1846 the English physician William Cumming found that the eye could be made to appear luminous if the subject were put in a darkened room, a light placed at some distance in the background, and the observer stood in a nearly direct line between subject and light. Cumming thought the character of the luminescence, or its absence, could be valuable signs of eye disorders. In 1847, Ernst Brücke, a Viennese physiologist, conducted experiments similar to those of Cumming. But these investigators could not see the structure of the inner eye, only a diffuse appearance of light which covered the whole pupil.

Then in 1850, the German physician and scientist Hermann von Helmholtz was preparing lectures to discuss the work of Cumming and Brücke and try to explain their observations (Helmholtz seemed unaware of Purkyně's work at this time). He decided to apply the principles of optics to analyze the path taken by the light rays in the experiments they described. He found that when light was emitted from the eye's pupil, it traveled in the same course it took when it entered the pupil. It came to him why Cumming and Brücke, who had made the eyes of a subject shine, could not delineate its interior structures – they had not placed their eye at the light's point of origin. To overcome this problem, an instrument was needed which would allow an observer to position his eye in a line with the rays of light entering and leaving the eye of the subject. Helmholtz labored for eight days to arrive at a solution. He stationed a lamp at the side of the examiner and subject, who were facing each other. A glass plate, mounted on his instrument and acting as a mirror, was held at an oblique angle between examiner and subject and cast light from the lamp into the subject's eye. These light rays were reflected from the back of the subject's eye to the glass plate, which reflected a portion of them back to the light source. But the glass plate was transparent enough for the rest of the rays to pass through to the eye of the observer. The subject's eye being illuminated, the observer had only to select an appropriately curved concave lens to focus the rays, and place it behind the glass plate, to transform the diffusely lit pupil into a clear picture of the retina with all of its anatomical details (Figure 5). Helmholtz noted that as far as he knew, he was the first person to explain the connection between the direction of rays entering and leaving the eye, and thus to discover the reason for the black appearance of the pupil and the principles of constructing an instrument to see into the eye: "All that was original with me in the matter was that I went to ask how the optic images could be produced by the light coming back from the illuminated eye. All my predecessors had failed to put this question to themselves."[2] He described his device, which he called the ophthalmoscope, to the Physical Society of Berlin in 1850 and published an account of it in an 1851 monograph, *Description of an Ophthalmoscope for the Investigation of the Retina in the Living Eye.*

The instrument gained rapid popularity. The delicacy and beauty of the eye's interior, "this spectacle of the red vessels on the transparent white ground," fascinated physicians.[3] The instrument made obsolete the definition of unexplained blindness as a condition in which "the patient sees nothing and the surgeon likewise nothing."[4] The ophthalmoscope exposed causes of eye disorders in the living that previously could be seen only during autopsy of the dead. The doubts physicians harbored about their ability to judge the character of structural changes in the eye just from the patient's verbal account of his symptoms were replaced by the certainties of direct sensory perception: physicians could evaluate the pathology firsthand. Detection of astigmatism in a patient who could not read, or of feigned nearsightedness in recruits hoping to escape military service, now became possible without interrogating the patient.[5]

Before the ophthalmoscope's invention, scientists and physicians often judged a person's vision by having him identify items from varying distances. The fitting of spectacles, invented in the fourteenth century, particularly required some well–defined test object to evaluate vision. For people who could read, the distance at which they perceived the words in a prayer book was a commonly used test; for the illiterate, a line of mustard seeds was employed. Nineteenth–century physicians were using geometric designs and small pictures of familiar things, such as birds and guns. An important advance in testing eyesight was the formula developed by the nineteenth–century Dutch ophthalmologist Cornelius Donders, and modified in 1862 by the German doctor Franciscus Snellen. It expressed visual acuity in numbers based upon the size of the test objects and the distance the patient stood from them.[6] Thus the

47

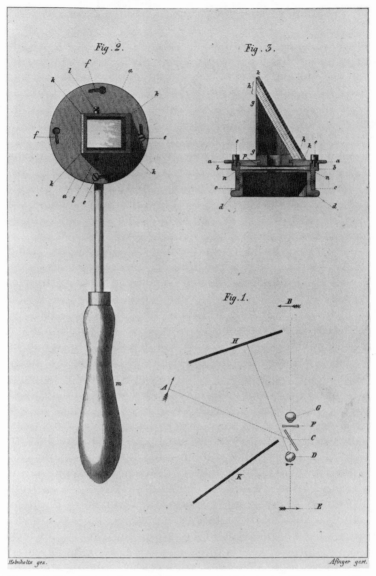

Figure 5. The Helmholtz ophthalmoscope (1851). In this illustration, Fig. 1 shows how light rays travel through the ophthalmoscope. *A* is the light source, *C* the plate composed of three separate pieces of glass set close together, *D* the subject's eye, and *F* the concave lens. Fig. 2 is a view of the side of the instrument facing the subject. Fig. 3 is a horizontal cross-section which shows the placement of the glass plate, *hh*, and the concave lens, *nn*. Reprinted from H. Helmholtz, *Beschreibung eines Augen–Spiegels zur Untersuchung der Netzhaut im Lebenden Auge* (Berlin: A. Förstner'sche, 1851).

doctor could now quantify his patient's subjective visual sensations. Although quantification improved the precision with which the patient's testimony could be expressed, inadequate intelligence or pretense on his part could still influence the outcome. The instruments invented by Helmholtz allowed physicians to evaluate sight even without the patient's full cooperation. Four years after developing the ophthalmoscope, Helmholtz published a description of the ophthalmometer, which measured the curvature of the eye's cornea and further aided doctors in testing vision. Although the instrument was accurate, the need to make from fifteen to twenty readings on a single patient, then do mathematical calculations, prevented its adoption until the late 1880s, when it was simplified.[7]

In 1894 the American Medical Association, in a report on the fitting of eyeglasses presented at its annual meeting, advocated that vision testing begin with an objective examination with the ophthalmoscope, opthalmometer, and several other instruments; continue by application of patient–centered, subjective methods employing geometric figures or numbers and trial glasses; and conclude with a comparison of the subjective and objective findings.[8] Physicians who delivered other papers on vision testing at this meeting praised the subjective techniques as the most satisfactory agents to detect minute changes in the vision of an intelligent, cooperative patient. But they devoted more attention to the objective techniques that reduced the physician's dependence "on the faltering judgment of the untrained patient, substituting therefor the skill of the expert who, reasoning from scientific data, is thus able to fit glasses in less time and more accurately with consequent satisfaction to himself and his patient."[9]

By facilitating accurate diagnosis, the ophthalmoscope also transformed the ease of therapy. Once an eye disorder was accurately identified, the chance for amelioration or cure improved. But if a disease were not sharply delineated, the wrong treatment might often be applied. This occurred particularly in the therapy used for dark, floating spots before the eye (*muscae volitantes*). To its supposed alarming causes physicians could match equally numerous, deplorable remedies: "Visions of cupping, bleeding, leeching, and purging, rise in ghastly array! Setons and blisters, fell caustics and rank poisons follow on, swelling the list in horrible numbers! Turn we away from the unhappy picture, and behold the brighter side! These formidable *muscae*," the ophthalmoscope demonstrated,

49

usually did not denote grave disease and were "brought to their proper sphere."[10] The instrument further changed the physician's concept of the prevalence and curability of eye diseases by demonstrating that some disorders, formerly supposed incurable because they had been detectable only at an advanced stage, in fact were susceptible to treatment when discovered earlier. Although most often the ophthalmoscope uncovered diseases whose cure was not hastened merely by recognition, it did permit the alert physician to ally himself more closely with a vital moral principle of medical practice, announced in the Hippocratic writings and passed on to successive generations of doctors; to help, or at least not to harm.[11]

Opposition to the ophthalmoscope nevertheless arose because of the fear (largely unfounded) that the concentrated light it projected would damage the eye. Antagonists accused the instrument's users of generating disease in their very search for it. They urged a return to a method of diagnosis that used the safely elicited, subjective complaints of the patient, rather than risk blinding the patient merely so that the physician himself could locate objective signs of disease.[12] Disappointed purchasers who expected to be able to instantly explore the eye with the ophthalmoscope also created enmity. Some were slow to recognize that inexperience with the procedural aspects of the eye examination, such as focusing the artificial light necessary for illumination and positioning the patient properly, as well as an incomplete knowledge of the pathological expressions of visual disorders, could prevent the novice from seeing the tracks of even the most serious eye disease. In addition the reaction of some patients hampered the adoption of the instrument; a number became alarmed during the examination, first at being ushered into a darkened room, then at having reflectors and lenses project a powerful light into their eyes.[13]

Supporters of the ophthalmoscope believed that some of these criticisms were diversions meant to hide an unwillingness to expend time and labor on its mastery. Yet it was difficult sometimes for doctors who had left school and were engaged in busy practice to master its use. Supporters placed the ophthalmoscope first among techniques developed to painlessly "autopsy" the living patient, ahead even of the stethoscope, because they believed visual information superior to any other form of data.[14] The number and complexity of eye diseases revealed by the ophthalmoscope motivated a number of physicians to specialize solely in disorders of vision. General practitioners, too, found that alterations in the eye's structure could provide important evidence of disease established in other parts of the body such as the brain, kidney, and heart, and by the 1870s they began to incorporate the ophthalmoscope into their small but increasing armory of medical instruments.[15]

The larynx was the next internal organ to have its architecture illuminated by visual technology. The efforts that led eventually to the successful construction of an appropriate instrument began when Philipp Bozzini published in Germany his 1807 pamphlet, "The Light Conductor or Description of a Simple Device and Its Use for the Illumination of the Inner Cavities and Interstices of the Living Animal Body."[16] While studying the forces which produced movement in the internal organs of the body, Bozzini had become excited at the thought of designing an instrument that would allow him to actually observe the organs. He constructed a device having a light source and tubes containing mirrors, which carried the rays of light into the body cavities and then reflected the image back to the observer. Bozzini believed that seeing the motions and forms of internal organs was essential to learning their character, and declared moreover that biological concepts based upon nonvisual evidence were uncertain and erroneous.

Public excitement followed the revelation that this invention would enable physicians to inspect the inlets of the body and the internal organs themselves, but the Faculty of Physicians in Vienna proclaimed in an 1807 report that "premature conclusions were likely to be arrived at concerning the instrument. . .Only very small and unimportant parts of the body could be examined. . .[and] the illuminated spot was so small – its diameter being never more than an inch – that if a person did not know beforehand exactly what he was to look at, he would not generally be able to tell what part of the body was presented to view."[17] Nevertheless, Bozzini's work drew the attention of his contemporaries to the feasibility of seeing into the body. Although he did not attempt to examine the larynx, Bozzini believed, correctly, that his invention could be adapted for this task. He had recognized the importance of two essentials required to survey the voice box: strong illumination, and a mirror to reflect the structures revealed back to the observer's eye.

From the 1820s through the 1840s, several physicians attempted to see the organ of voice with apparatus they had designed. Their devices had the advantage of being good ideas but failed to stir the

51

interest of most doctors, being cumbersome to use, and unsuitable to apply in overcast weather because they depended on sunlight for illumination.[18]

An important advance occurred in 1855 when Manuel Garcia, a London singing teacher, published an account of the motion of the vocal cords during breathing and speaking, based upon research he conducted entirely on himself as subject.[19] His technique required the observer to hold a mirror in one hand, which was then placed at the back of his throat to catch the image of the larynx. This image, in turn, was cast onto a second mirror, used to reflect sunlight into the mouth, and held in the other hand. Most physicians regarded this procedure with incredulity, and ignored it.

But two years later, Johann Czermak, a Polish professor of physiology, repeated Garcia's experiments, using an instrument borrowed from its designer, Dr. Ludwig Türck. Like previous contrivances to view the larynx, Türck's instrument required sunlight to illuminate its field and made the physician a captive of the weather, but in Czermak's hands it was transformed. He substituted artificial light for the glow of the sun, and used a large mirror attached to the examiner's head to reflect light into the throat, thus freeing the hand that before had held the mirror. Czermak promptly wrote an essay on his work, in which he urged the use of his redesigned instrument to inspect the larynx and other parts of the throat, as well as the nose.[20] The originality of his new instrument was matched by the intensity with which he publicized the laryngoscope, as he called it. His brilliant public demonstrations delighted and astonished the European medical public. Endowed with a large throat, and self-trained to tolerate the contact of a mirror against the usually sensitive surface of the palate, Czermak was a master at exhibiting the structure of the larynx to an audience. Some doctors who witnessed the vocal cords moving, and beheld the transformation of motion into sound, thought the sight one of the most interesting and instructive in medicine. After observing a demonstration of the laryngoscope one doctor wrote: "I little dreamt of the possibility of actually being able to *see* thus far down the larynx. There was no disbelieving the evidence of one's senses, but it was some time before I could certainly realize in my mind the fact of having seen, from the mouth, the bifurcation of the trachea in a living and healthy person."[21]

The previous hallmark of laryngeal disorder had been symptoms based on sound – notably chronic hoarseness, cough, noise accompanying breathing, and the inability to speak audibly. But with the revelations of the laryngoscope, the voice box ceased to be an internal organ to physicians, and the cardinal signs of its breakdown became expressed in visual terms which were more precise than the older indices based on sound. Cases like the following demonstrated this:

Richard P_____, aged fourteen, formerly a worker in the sheds of the Great Northern Railway Company, Peterborough, first seen by me on the 12th of August, 1861; presents an anxious aspect; face pale, and bathed with perspiration; lips livid; pupils somewhat contracted; hands cold; he respires with the greatest difficulty, all the accessory muscles being thrown into violent action, and each inspiratory act being accompanied by a loud laryngeal murmur. . .On inquiry, I learned that for eight years the boy has been very hoarse, never during the last six years speaking above a whisper. His breath has been rather short for about the same period. For about eighteen months he has been quite disabled from doing any hard work, on account of the distressed breathing induced by exertion; gave up work altogether about six month ago, and for three months has been unable to move across the room or exert himself in the least. When he sleeps, he makes so much noise in breathing that he is heard in the neighbouring cottages. His appetite is good, but he becomes daily weaker and weaker. . .He has been treated at various intervals by different medical men. For about a week he has seemed in the same imminent danger as to-day. A laryngoscopic examination at once reveals the source of the dyspnoea [shortness of breath]. . .Immediately above the anterior attachment of the right vocal cord, is a polypoid growth, presenting an irregular mulberry surface, which, being about the size of the tip of the little finger, and some ten lines long, acts as a valve.[22]

The physician severed the tumor with a wire loop, thus immediately relieving the patient's symptoms, and later declared that without the laryngoscope he could not have diagnosed or successfully treated the patient.

Some physicians believed that advocates of the laryngoscope for diagnosis displayed too little caution and reserve, that more time was needed before its value could be properly assessed. Resenting its elevation over other diagnostic modalities, they were not ready to discard the older signs – still sufficiently reliable, they thought, to determine the nature of many laryngeal disorders, and essential in cases when good laryngoscopic examination was difficult or impossible to conduct, as when treating children.[23]

Critics offered the caution that placing the voice box so completely within the doctor's reach increased his temptation to be meddlesome. They warned, too, that visual demonstration of lesions on the larynx could lead physicians to perceive illness as a localized occurrence, and to forget that a diseased larynx could be an effect of a generalized disorder of the body, which required a plan of treatment different from that of a circumscribed lesion. Advocates responded that by facilitating the removal of growths, and by improving diagnostic accuracy, the laryngoscope prevented inappropriate treatment, as had been the case previously before accurate diagnosis. Critics also complained that the sight of the lamps and mirrors used in the laryngoscopic examination could provoke anxiety in patients; that the examination itself could traumatize patients, who cried and sometimes moved so much that investigation was impossible. But the instrument's supporters denied that apprehensiveness or trauma would occur if the apparatus for the examination were not prominently displayed and if the procedure was conducted carefully. One physician told of his conversion to the laryngoscope by Czermak himself. "Thinking that the introduction of the speculum into the throat must be very disagreeable, and productive of [an] inclination to vomit, I requested the Professor [Czermak] to examine my chordae vocales. In consequence, I can bear testimony to the very slight amount of inconvenience occasioned by the *skilful* introduction of the mirror."[24]

Learning to apply the laryngoscope correctly demanded considerable practice, tact, and dexterity. The disputes stirred by the laryngoscope – like those that plagued the stethoscope – arose partly from the unique dexterity with which the innovators of an instrument applied it, a skill that learners found difficult to emulate. The observations that Garcia and Czermak made themselves, with their unusual ability to exhibit the larynx, were sometimes disparaged because other physicians could not repeat them. Experienced physicians had constantly to remind beginners that practice was needed before objects revealed through the laryngoscope could be discerned, that to notice an object required a certain mental attitude and orientation: "The part may be visible, and yet not seen by an unskilled observer; so that the beginner need not wonder if he cannot see all that even ought to be seen, in his first views of the larynx. For this very reason it is equally difficult to show to another, either on oneself or in a patient, what he ought to see."[25]

Despite these difficulties, by the 1860s the laryngoscope's value was widely recognized in medical circles in England, Europe, and the United States.[26] As a simple instrument, price posed no obstacle to its adoption; it could be purchased at a small expense commercially, or the physician might even construct a laryngoscope himself.[27] Physicians who used it discovered pathological conditions which they previously had missed. Many physicians looked upon the external signs of laryngeal disease which they could observe with their unaided senses, and the history of his illness as described by the patient, as allowing them only "to form a shrewd guess as to the nature of the individual disease," a guess that was "often wrong."[28] With the discovery of the laryngoscope the doubts "inseparable from a symptomatic diagnosis" were supplanted by "precise results which a distinct view of the affected parts must afford."[29]

Before the invention of the ophthalmoscope and laryngoscope, internal disorders in patients were not visible to the eye, unless the body's surface were violated through surgery. Vision now competed with sound as the doctor's main sensory probe of the human interior. Laennec had listened for disease; Helmholtz and Czermak looked for it. Each could do so without recourse to the patient's appearance or testimony. The ophthalmoscope and laryngoscope, invented to detect gross structural changes in the body, also represented a continuation of the anatomic tradition to which the stethoscope adhered. This sustained the tendency of doctors to regard illness in terms of discrete, picturable lesions, as a disturbance of one part of the body more than of the person himself.

The benefits that the ophthalmoscope and laryngoscope conferred on medicine stimulated the development of devices to explore other body cavities that could be made accessible to view through natural anatomical channels. At the start of the 1860s, contrivances appeared that illuminated the urinary bladder, rectum, and stomach.[30] Even the inspection of the vagina through a round metal speculum, having origins in ancient Greek medicine, began to be accepted. In the first half of the nineteenth century, physicians had been reluctant to risk offending feminine delicacy by using the speculum. They depended mainly on the patient's description of her symptoms and on palpation of the abdomen to make a gynecological diagnosis. Advocates of the speculum now began to surmount the fierce opposition by critics who labeled its use immoral and offensive, so that it gradually became an acceptable feature of gynecologic practice. As one doctor wrote: "There is an old and trite saying that 'seeing is believing'; and, in a realistic age like the present, it might almost be said that not seeing is not believing."[31]

For stronger illumination of the body cavities, inventors in the 1870s began to design scopes whose light was generated by electrically powered incandescent lamps, but these instruments were heavy, delicate, and expensive. Thomas Edison's 1881 carbon–filament lamp transformed the situation by producing three times as much brightness, less heat, and eliminating the water-based cooling device required by the old lighting. The lamp encouraged the manufacture of a wide variety of visual scopes, each specially constructed to light a different channel of the body. Scientists, including Edison, were also able to introduce light into the stomach and the sinuses of the head, a light brilliant enough to outline their shape and contents through dense covering tissues. But technical difficulties and the insufficient distinctness of the structures illuminated halted these visual efforts for a time.

The emphasis on vision posed a threat to the diagnostic use of the other senses, and exasperated some physicians. They spoke out particularly against the visual instruments being developed to detect the common disorder of stones in the bladder, and advocated instead the time–honored method of inserting a probe into the organ to feel the objects.[32] Such objections failed to undermine the widely held belief within medicine that the most significant advances in diagnosis would come from new ways of visualizing pathology.[33] This disposition among physicians was strengthened by the great popularity accorded to a major technological innovation of the nineteenth century – photography.

Through research involving optics and chemistry a number of investigators, notably Joseph Nicephore Niepce, Louis J. M. Daguerre, and William H. Fox Talbot, developed techniques to fix visual images onto solid matter and by the fifth decade of the century had created the science of photography. In the 1850s a number of physicians were discussing the possibility of using photographs in medicine as an objective record, to eliminate arguments engendered by conflicts between different subjective evaluations of disease phenomena. The English medical journal, *Lancet*, called photography the "Art of Truth."[34] It checked the personal biases of an observer which often distorted representation of an illness depicted only through words and drawings. Surgeons occasionally made photographs of unusual bone deformities; one hospital even employed a photographer to take pictures of patients before and after a surgical operation, which could be incorporated into their records as evidence of therapeutic changes. Anatomists also used photographs to study the body.

Because of such advantages, some physicians expected the photograph to become an integral part of medicine in the 1850s. But such hopes were premature. One reason for the neglect of this new tool was the long exposures and elaborate paraphernalia required by the collodion process used to prepare the photographic plate for picture-taking. The development of the dry–plate process in the early 1870s, which simplified preparation and shortened exposure times, encouraged the general use of photography. The physicians' special interest in photography reemerged in the 1880s under the stimulus of several events; the photographs of birds and men in motion by Eadweard Muybridge[35] led some physicians to apply his techniques to study body movements produced by nervous disorders; and the photographing of the organisms revealed through the microscope became a major factor in the development of bacteriology. Also significant was the production by Francis Galton of composite portraits of tubercular patients to demonstrate the error of the centuries–old belief that persons who possessed narrow and ovoid facial characteristics were especially liable to the disease.[36] Galton made his composite portraits by casting the images of several negatives in succession upon a photographic plate held in a special camera, which allowed the operator to bring the various images into exactly similar relation. The composites in turn could be exposed to another plate, resulting in photographs incorporating a larger number of individual images. Galton spoke of composite portraits as pictorial averages. Like numerical averages, they were less liable to be influenced by the predilections of the operator and were a unique transformation of mathematical technique into visual form.

Medical interest in photography continued in the 1890s. It was thought that verbal statement was unable to match the descriptive record of a good photograph. And the sensitive photograph could reveal aspects of visual events which the human eye failed to perceive. Medical students were urged to sharpen their powers of clinical observation by studying photographic depictions of illness; a picture was recommended as a means of capturing the events in hospital wards, operating theaters, autopsy rooms, and laboratories. But there were deterrents to the use of photography. The technique still required considerable equipment, extra personnel, and hence additional expense. Some hospital administrators objected to photographing patients without their permission, and insisted that consent had to be obtained from relatives or friends if the patient could not give it. The foreshortening of photographed objects produced distortions that led many physicians to question the picture's accuracy.[37] Although photography was not widely used in clinical medicine of the 1890s, the experience many physicians had with it in private and professional life, and the value placed on the visual representation of pathology, were important factors in their reaction to the invention of the transcendent instrument of visualization in medicine – the X-ray.

Late in the nineteenth century, a group of scientists was conducting experiments in which they discharged electric currents through air in a partially evacuated (Crookes) tube, inside of which stood a negative and positive electrode. The observers could watch the behavior of the stream of particles produced, called cathode rays (later identified as electrons). To overcome the limitations placed on studying cathode rays, which were thought unable to penetrate the glass of the Crookes tube, the German physicist Philipp Lenard designed a tube with a very thin aluminum window through which, as Heinrich Hertz had demonstrated, the rays could pass, and flow a few centimeters into the outer air before being dissipated. Their exit was often detected by fluorescence of a paper saturated with a barium platinocyanide compound. In some of his experiments, Lenard covered his aluminum–windowed tube with opaque material, which prevented visible light from the tube penetrating to the outside and obscuring the fluorescent signals.

Wilhelm Roentgen, a professor of physics and director of the physics institute at the University of Würzburg in Bavaria, became interested in cathode rays in the spring of 1894 and repeated some of Lenard's experiments. After several months he broke off his research. He resumed it in the fall of 1895 and at some point during this time, as described in the generally accepted account of the X-ray's discovery, Roentgen had an idea. Perhaps cathode rays did penetrate the glass of ordinary Crookes tubes, but had been undetected by previous experimenters because the luminescence the rays could produce on a fluorescent screen was obscured by light generated within the tube itself. Roentgen tested his idea on the afternoon of November 8, 1895. He covered an ordinary Crookes tube with black cardboard, darkened the room, and, before setting

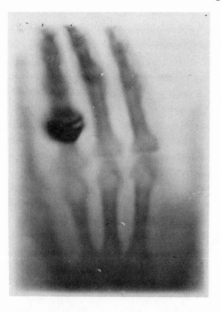

Figure 6. The first X-ray of a human being: Frau Roentgen's hand (1895). Reproduced by kind permission of the Francis A. Countway Library of Medicine, Boston.

up the fluorescent screen, discharged the tube to make sure its light did not pass beyond the covering. To his surprise the screen, lying on a bench about a yard from the tube, emitted a faint glow. Astonished, he again discharged the tube – the phenomenon appeared once more. He repeated the experiment with the screen at ever greater distances – with the same result. Since he knew cathode rays had never been reported to travel more than several centimeters through air, he thought it likely that some other kind of radiation was at work.[38]

In succeeding weeks he conducted more experiments, which confirmed that these emanations were not cathode rays. The experiments that Roentgen wrote about disclosed that the new radiation could penetrate solid objects – in general the lower the density the better. Thus they easily passed through a 1,000–page book, a double pack of cards, wood, and hard rubber. They did not easily pass through more dense substances, such as lead or bone: "If the hand be held before the fluorescent screen," wrote Roentgen, "the shadow shows the bones darkly with only faint outlines of the surrounding tissues."[39] He found that these phenomena could be captured on photographic plates as well as on fluorescent screens, and demonstrated this by producing, along with pictures of inanimate objects, a bony portrait of his wife's hand (Figure 6). Roentgen

59

disclosed his discovery of a "new kind of rays," which penetrated opaque substances, to the Physico-Medical Society of Würzburg on December 28, 1895, in a paper he sent to the society for publication in its *Proceedings*. Although publication was swift, to aid the appraisal of his discovery Roentgen, on New Year's Day, 1896, sent reprints of the article to a number of well-known physicists, accompanied by X-ray prints.

Interest immediately focused on the fact that the X-rays, as Roentgen named them because he did not know their composition, could reveal the skeleton within its case of flesh. The picture of Frau Roentgen's hand, taken to illustrate the rays' powers, was soon displayed in newspapers and scientific publications all over Europe and the United States. "The realism of this weird picture," reported *Popular Science Monthly*, "simply fascinated all who beheld it."[40] "Hidden Solids Revealed,"[41] proclaimed the *New York Times*; "A Photographic Discovery Which Seems Almost Uncanny,"[42] announced the *St. Louis Post-Dispatch*.

The significance of the event at first failed to impress the public. The news was received with mild interest, some amusement, and considerable incredulity: "The thing seemed absurd on the face of it; the 'common sense' of most refused to be hoodwinked by sensation–mongering journalists and for a few days the public remained tranquil on the subject. For a few days only."[43] Then, the news being absorbed by the public veins in repeated doses, the intoxication occurred. Tradesmen in London displayed X-ray apparatus and pictures in their shop windows. Cartoons satirizing the X-ray appeared in newspapers, popular lectures on the subject abounded, and a lively market developed for X-ray photographs of ordinary objects such as keys and chains concealed in purses. Cathode–ray tubes and theories of electricity became subjects of breakfast conversation. An experiment undertaken from February to March, 1896, by Thomas Edison received special publicity: an attempt to photograph a living human brain. Edison humbly described his scientific role: "[Roentgen] needs men like myself, whose chief aim is to turn the great discoveries of science to practical use and adapt them, so that the world will receive the benefit of them."[44] His effort failed; the skull bones were too thick for the weak rays generated by cathode–ray tubes of the day to penetrate.

But the public still believed that the X-ray was a "materialized eye" which could see to any depth of the human body and photograph any part of it desired by the operator. In fact, however, it could reproduce only very dense structures, lying close to the body's surface, such as bones or bullets. The statement of the charlatan to his gaping patient, "I've been looking at your kidneys, sir, for the last ten minutes, and they are badly shrivelled, sir, badly shrivelled!" seemed credible to many of the public and was typical of the excesses.[45] Some people feared for privacy in the home, for anyone armed with an X-ray tube might see through its walls. Writers quickly responded to the public's fascination with X-rays. C. H. T. Crosthwaite wrote a short story entitled "Röntgen's Curse,"[46] which described the experiences of a man whose eyes had X-ray powers. *Punch*[47] took note of the discovery also:

> O, Röntgen, then the news is true,
>   And not a trick of idle rumor,
> That bids us each beware of you,
>   And of your grim and graveyard humor.
>
> We do not want, like Dr. Swift,
>   To take our flesh off and to pose in
> Our bones, or show each little rift
>   And joint for you to poke your nose in.
>
> We only crave to contemplate
>   Each other's usual full–dress photo;
> Your worse than 'altogether' state
>   Of portraiture we bar *in toto!*
>
> The fondest swain would scarcely prize
>   A picture of his lady's framework;
> To gaze on this with yearning eyes
>   Would probably be rated tame work!
>
> No, keep them for your epitaph,
>   These tombstone–souvenirs unpleasant;
> Or go away and photograph
>   Mahatmas, spooks, and Mrs. B–s–nt!

Despite such barbs X-ray photographs became objects of great sentimental value. New York women of fashion had X-rays taken of their hands covered with jewelry, to illustrate that "beauty is of the bone and not altogether of the flesh."[48] "Women Not Afraid,"[49] read one headline, as single women clasped hands with their beaux for sentimental X-ray photographs, and married women gave bony portraits of their hands to relatives as family souvenirs. One woman exclaimed upon seeing a view of her vertebrae, "This is really the dearest picture, altogether and in every way, that I ever had taken."[50] Another woman, who discovered that she had dropped a ring into dough from which cakes had just been baked, located her ring by getting the cakes X-rayed. The family dessert was preserved.[51] And it was announced that the X-ray fulfilled for man Hamlet's aspiration, "Oh that this too, too solid flesh would melt."[52] However, the publicity given the X-ray also had a serious side. People with bullets, needles, and other assorted objects lodged in their bodies, causing no discomfort, insisted on having them located with the X-ray and removed by surgery. Death was sometimes the consequence for patients whose doctors acquiesced to the demand.[53] No previous diagnostic discovery had stirred quite so much public interest and involvement as the X-ray. It obliterated one distinction between the outer and inner spaces of the body – both were now susceptible to visual examination.

The X-ray's potential uses intoxicated physicians much as it did the public. The X-ray was rapidly accepted within the medical and scientific communities, for the general availability of the Crookes tube facilitated confirmation of Roentgen's findings. Within weeks of the discovery, articles filled the pages of medical journals in Great Britain and the United States describing possible clinical applications. The medical imagination was pleasurably lost "in devising endless applications of this wonderful process."[54] Shadow portraits of arm bones, leg bones, gall and kidney stones showed eager doctors the shapes of the new territory ahead of them (Figure 7). Rarely had the medical or scientific communities become so roused by an invention. The low cost of the machine (about $50 in 1896), and the simplicity of picture–taking, further motivated physicians and hospitals to purchase X-ray equipment.[55]

About one month after the X-ray's introduction, a machine called the fluoroscope appeared. It consisted of a screen coated with a fluorescing chemical, and an X-ray generating apparatus. The fluoroscope did not take pictures but cast transient images of objects placed in front of the X-rays onto the fluorescent screen. By eliminating the tedious wait necessary to develop the X-ray plate, the device allowed an instant view into the body. Even more important, unlike the X-ray picture, which revealed the state of the body at a given instant, the fluoroscope could show organs and tissues in motion. However, the fluoroscopic image had a key disadvantage: it was a transient image, which could not yet be reproduced or displayed. This prevented objective comparison with an established standard or with any evidence from other medical cases,

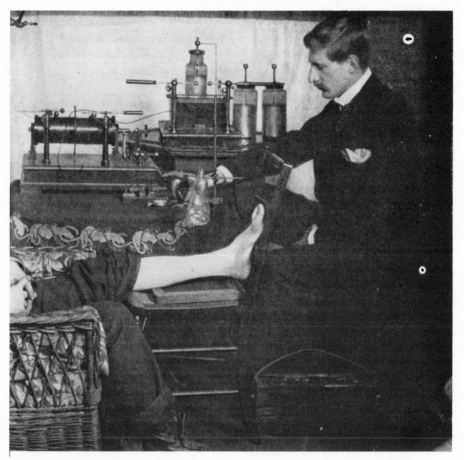

Figure 7. A patient being X-rayed in 1896. Reprinted from Sydney Rowland, "Report on the Application of the New Photography to Medicine and Surgery," *British Medical Journal*, vol. 1 (1896), p. 557

as was possible with the permanent, fixed image on the X-ray plate that froze movement, that represented " 'accumulated vision;' a record and something that can be studied at will by several."[56] At this period, correlation of fluoroscopic images was possible only in the mind of the physician; it was thus no more than a personal observation. As such, its critics asserted that it commanded no more credence than any other subjective opinion.

X-rays directly challenged the use of touch in diagnosis. Before their discovery, doctors had evaluated fractures by manually prob-

63

ing the injury to determine the position of the bone fragments. Often the swelling of the surrounding flesh made such evidence difficult to obtain and imprecise. With X-rays, the surgeon could locate the positions of the bones easily, and reassess their alignment after putting on the cast. Similarly, foreign objects lodged in the tissues, which previously had to be found with metal probes and fingers, could now be located precisely. Physicians cited many cases in which an unproductive tactile search for an object was followed by its detection through the X-ray. For example:

On February 29th [1896] a woman aged twenty-six years ran a portion of a needle into her right hand; it entered the web of the hand on the palmar surface at the base of the ring finger. The patient came to the Middlesex Hospital on the evening of that day and was seen by Mr. A. E. Griffin, the house surgeon on duty. He could not detect the presence of the needle, and as the patient was suffering a considerable amount of pain he applied a hot boracic fomentation. I saw the patient afterwards daily and made several careful examinations of the hand, but could feel nothing, so the treatment of fomentations was continued on account of the pain, which was constant. There was no swelling, but the patient could not flex her finger. On March 10th she had her right hand photographed by Mr. Friese–Green, of King's–road, Chelsea, and the following day she brought the photograph to me and begged me to explore her hand. This photograph showed a distinct shadow across the proximal end of the first phalanx of the ring finger. I again examined the hand very carefully, but could detect nothing, but as she was still suffering considerable pain and was unable to flex the finger I determined to make an exploratory incision and at the same time told the patient not to be disappointed if I found nothing, as I was still unable to feel any unusual resistance in the palm of the hand. I rendered the limb bloodless by an Esmarch's bandage and applied a tourniquet. Dr. A. H. Lister kindly gave the patient nitrous oxide gas and I made an incision in the palm . . .The knife struck the needle, and with a pair of Spencer Wells' forceps I extracted a portion of a needle half an inch long. I am greatly indebted to Mr. Friese–Green for the photograph, which has thus enabled me to relieve my patient.[57]

Physicians were commenting on the advantages of the X-ray over diagnostic techniques which involved touch solely in the context of accuracy. The fact that the X-ray's proponents did not suggest its use as a means of diminishing physical contact per se between doctor and patient shows how acceptable diagnostic examinations which used physical contact had become by the turn of the century.

The X-ray also challenged the stethoscope and diagnoses based upon sound. Earlier physicians had been required to conjure up mental pictures of anatomical defects from sounds that came through the stethoscope; now, with the X-ray, they could produce an actual image of the lesion and thus greatly advance the frontier of diagnosis.[58] Further, recognition of a disease in the chest from the sounds it produced was thought more difficult than detecting its presence by the shadow it generated.[59] And by 1899, the preponderance of evidence demonstrated that the X-ray picture usually unveiled disorders in the lungs earlier and more extensively than did auscultation and percussion, and that the fluoroscope revealed more information about the size, position, and action of the heart than did acoustic techniques. "Sight is a much more satisfactory agent of information than hearing or touch," concluded one doctor who expressed the sentiments of many.[60] The X-ray, however, like the photograph, drew attention to weaknesses in the perceptive power of the naked eye. The sensitive X-ray plate, which brought new objects within the range of human sight, demonstrated that man could appreciate only a very limited proportion of the waves that filled space. Although admirers of Roentgen's discovery extolled the visual sense, they did so mainly in the context of its technological extension by the X-ray.[61] This was demonstrated by the degree to which the X-ray modified opinions about the internal body structures gained from direct visual inspection during autopsy.

In the fall of 1896, the physiologist Walter B. Cannon, while still a medical student at Harvard, began his extensive investigation of the use of an ingested bismuth compound in X-raying the digestive tract.[62] By 1910, physicians were using bismuth with increasing frequency to explore the human intestine from end to end. To their surprise, they found little resemblance between the position of the stomach of the living person and the position shown in textbook pictures, drawn from post-mortem appearances. Generally vertical in the living, the stomach often became a horizontal, elegantly curved organ in the dead. Observations of the intestinal tract in the cadaver had led to the belief that its several parts occupied relatively fixed positions; this belief, which had been used as a basis of diagnosis in the living, was found to be equally mistaken. The X-ray now proved that various segments of the intestine could be discovered at almost any place in the abdomen during life.[63]

In 1896, the minimum length of time required to take an X-ray picture was 20 minutes, and for thick bones at least an hour. By 1898, only a few minutes were needed to produce an X-ray picture that could depict the deepest structures of the body. This shortened exposure time reduced the discomfort of patients attempting to remain motionless while the X-ray was being taken, and improved the quality of the image obtained. With fluoroscopy physicians spoke of leisurely watching the minutest movement of a patient's heart and lungs.[64]

By 1900, the X-ray had also acquired unique significance in the courts, as an arbiter of fault in malpractice suits. In a ruling made less than a year after Roentgen's discovery, an American judge allowed the introduction of X-ray evidence in testimony.[65] A short time later, the Supreme Court of Tennessee declared that if maps, diagrams, and photographs were admissible in juridical hearings, so were X-rays, provided the court believed in the skill and experience of the expert giving the testimony.[66]

This view evoked some concern in the medical profession. It now was possible for a patient to have some of his doctor's judgments evaluated by X-ray, and litigate if dissatisfied with the result.[67] As suits based on X-rays cropped up against physicians, the many ways for such evidence to be misrepresented were demonstrated. Some suits relied on X-rays that were technically poor, others on interpretations given by men unqualified to read them correctly; still others used X-rays willfully falsified by grasping patients and their attorneys. Just as the position of the subject, the lighting, and the focus of the lens were factors that could modify ordinary photographs of the same individual taken under circumstances supposedly identical, so could these conditions distort the evidence of X-rays. Apparent deformities within the body and misinterpretations of an item's location occurred when the angles between the X-rays and the object were changed.[68]

A 1900 report by the American Surgical Association confirmed the doctors' concern, that along with its considerable benefits to them, the X-ray increased their susceptibility to law suits: "It is surprising to see the number of damage suits now pending against corporations, individuals, and especially surgeons for supposed injuries sustained or for malpractice, depending entirely on the shadowgraph as evidence."[69]

Some physicians recognized the problems of X-ray reading. They sought to convince their colleagues of the important distinction between noticing and evaluating lesions shown in the X-ray (a problem also faced for example by physicians who used the laryngoscope), and of the need for experience and knowledge by the would–be X–ray reader. These critics doubted the propriety of

66

using X-ray evidence in court until further advances in technology had made it more accurate.[70] Nevertheless, pressure from the threat of malpractice suits and excitement with the revelations of the technique led many doctors to ignore such warnings, and they routinely X-rayed patients. Some physicians even believed they were open to litigation unless they took an X-ray before and after each operation; many took X-rays merely to satisfy the whims of patients, who thought the procedure a solution for all diagnostic doubts.[71] The misuse of the X-ray was fundamentally influenced, too, by the belief that an X-ray was the same as a photograph. Yet the X-ray did not show the object itself but a silhouette that often reproduced details poorly.[72]

Although reports that X-rays could destroy organic life and produce damage to the skin began to appear with increasing frequency by 1900, the harmful effects of the X-ray were minimized by many physicians. Ernest A. Codman, a Boston practitioner, pointed to the fact that among the approximately 8,000 patients X-rayed at the Massachusetts General Hospital by 1901, not a single case of dermatitis had been detected.[73] He and other physicians confidently asserted that the small number of cases of damage induced by the X-ray should not cause alarm; X-ray injury was unusual and was produced principally by unskilled use, and was not due to any dangerous properties of the rays.[74]

Stories of injuries from X-rays continued to be published. In 1905, ten men who had worked with the rays for three or more years were found incapable of producing sperm. Such human damage, in addition to laboratory experiments on plants and animals that demonstrated the X-ray's ability to destroy generative material, prompted investigators to warn that X-rays endangered the reproductive capacity of man.[75] News of radiation–induced injury to well-known scientists occasioned further concern. Much publicity was given to the damage sustained by Thomas Edison and his assistant as a consequence of their early X-ray work.[76] Still most physicians and patients thought of the X-ray as a remarkable invention with little capacity for harm, and thus tended to ignore the caution to use the X-ray prudently, and to view exposure as a dose of powerful medicine.[77] Even today the controversy continues over the relative benefits and hazards of X-rays in diagnosis.[78]

In the second half of the nineteenth century, technological advances such as the ophthalmoscope, laryngoscope, and X-ray permitted the physician to visually explore the body's interior without surgical penetration of its surface. While physicians continued to use and to refine their aural diagnostic techniques (auscultation and percussion), many found the visual evidence of internal disease more satisfactory. The aural techniques required the physician to form a mental image of the lesion represented by a sound – the visual techniques presented the image to him directly. Sounds also seemed less substantive, and more prone to personal distortion, than images perceived through the eye. Medicine was, as a physician concluded in 1899, "gradually relegating hearing to a lower intellectual plane than sight."[79] Of all the instruments of visual diagnosis, the X-ray produced the most significant changes in the methods physicians used to evaluate illness. Unlike the ophthalmoscope and laryngoscope, which could be used by only one person at a time, and whose evidence was thereby prone to the subjective distortions of the viewer, the X-ray enhanced the possibility of group evaluation of pathology by allowing many people simultaneously to view and discuss what they saw. Equally significant, while physicians using the stethoscope, laryngoscope, ophthalmoscope, or even fluoroscope, needed the patient before them, those who possessed an X-ray picture could ponder and debate the medical problems of the patient, and subject his anatomical flaws to searching review – without requiring his physical presence.

4 *The microscope and the revelation of a cellular universe*

Magnifiers have been referred to intermittently for a very long time, for example, as "crystalline spheres" by Pliny and "globules of glass" by Seneca in the first century A.D. Both the Arab scholar Alhazen in the eleventh century and the English experimentalist Roger Bacon in the thirteenth century wrote of the ability of a convex lens to form a magnified image. The use of spectacles to improve human vision began in the fourteenth century and encouraged the study of optics and lens making. But not until the late sixteenth and early seventeenth century did investigators using combinations of magnifying lenses study aspects of natural objects invisible to the naked eye. These lenses were incorporated into the design of what later became known as the telescope and the microscope.[1] The specific origins of both instruments are a subject of controversy, because of the vagueness and questionable accuracy of surviving documents and the dearth of instruments that can be clearly dated.[2]

Despite the obscurity surrounding the invention of the microscope, there is however, good evidence that Cornelius Drebbel, a Dutchman and mathematical tutor to King James I of England, displayed a compound microscope (in the modern use of the term, a microscope having at least two separated convex lenses) in London in the early 1620s, which was then sent to several European cities by emissary to demonstrate its magnifying capabilities.[3] In the second half of the seventeenth century appeared the most notable microscopists of this period; pre-eminent among them were the Italian physician Marcello Malpighi, the English experimentalist Robert Hooke, and the Dutch lens maker Antony van Leeuwenhoek.

Malpighi produced brilliant descriptions of the structure of the lungs, spleen, kidney, and other body parts, and successfully examined the minute development of embryos in animals. Perhaps

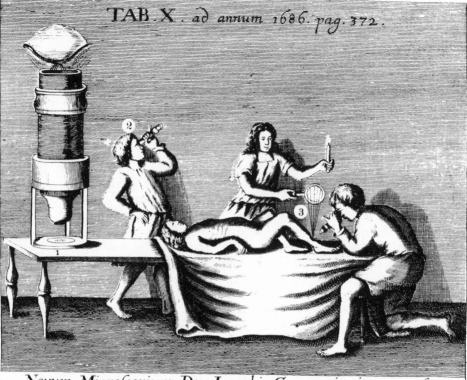

TAB. X. *ad annum 1686. pag. 372.*

Novum Microſcopium Dn: Ioſephi Campani, ejusque uſus.

Figure 8. A compound microscope constructed by the Italian instrument maker Joseph Campani in the mid–1680s. Fig. 1 is an oversized drawing of the microscope, whose maximum real length was 5 inches. Its removable base contained two pieces of glass between which liquid specimens were held for viewing. Fig. 2 portrays the use of the microscope to examine transparent objects. Fig. 3 depicts the instrument's value in medicine; here, the examination of a wound. Reprinted from *Acta Eruditorum* (Leipzig, 1686), facing p. 372.

most important, he observed and portrayed the minute capillaries connecting arteries and veins, whose existence was a crucial supposition in William Harvey's theory of the blood's circulation.[4] Robert Hooke's *Micrographia* (1665) was one of the earliest books wholly devoted to microscopic observations. It was based upon work conducted mainly with the compound instrument (Figure 8). Among other important observations, the treatise contains the first description of the biological structure the "cell," as Hooke called it, a term derived from the Latin word for "a small room." In one experiment, Hooke cut off a thin piece of cork and placed it under the microscope, using a black object plate for contrast. He then "could exceedingly plainly perceive it to be all perforated and porous. . .These pores, or cells [which] consisted of a great many little Boxes. . .were indeed the first *microscopical* pores I ever saw, and perhaps, that were ever seen, for I had not met with any Writer or Person, that had made any mention of them before this."[5] However, Hooke failed to recognize the cell's significance as a fundamental biological building block.

Antony van Leeuwenhoek holds a special place in the early history of the microscope because of the superb single–lens instruments he designed and the large number of careful observations he made. He attracted considerable attention with his accounts of biological structures, such as the facets of the bee's eye, red–blood cells, and spermatozoa. Simple microscopes had been developed in the early 1600s and consisted of single lenses mounted in tubes or between plates. Their power was gradually increased, reaching a peak in the instruments constructed by Leeuwenhoek. One of his best had a magnifying power of 270 diameters and could distinguish objects separated by as little as 1.4 microns.[6] At this juncture, they generally produced a better quality image than the compound type. Using and making a simple microscope for investigations that required high magnification sometimes posed greater problems than those encountered with the compound microscope. The very small space between the lens of the simple microscope and the specimen, and the closeness of the instrument to the observer decreased the illumination of the object and tired the eye of the observer. Robert Hooke described simple microscopes as "offensive to my eye, and to have much strained and weakened the sight, which was the reason why I omitted use of them."[7]

The only way to step up the power of a simple microscope was to increase the lens curvature until it was spherical. Further increase was then possible only by reducing the size of the sphere. Grinding the small lenses into perfectly shaped rounded surfaces posed a difficult problem, and few lens makers were successful at it: Leeuwenhoek was one of them. He could grind lenses smaller than the head of a pin. To overcome the difficulties of lens–grinding, methods were devised for melting glass into small beads, but the poor quality of the glass and the difficulty of melting usually made the ground lenses superior.

71

Among the fascinating phenomena revealed by the microscope were populations of tiny organisms, heretofore concealed from the human eye. In a letter written to the Royal Society of London in 1674, and in a more comprehensive and important one to the society in 1676, Leeuwenhoek described a variety of exceedingly minute creatures that he had observed floating in various types of water, such as rainwater and water infused with pepper. Modern commentators consider these organisms to have been protozoa and even smaller organisms, probably bacteria. Of the latter, Leeuwenhoek wrote that they were "so small, in my eye, that I judged, that if a hundred of them lay stretched out one by another, they would not equal the *length* of a coarse grain of salt."[8] These disclosures were received with great skepticism until Robert Hooke confirmed them and himself expressed wonder "that there should be such an infinite number of animals in so imperceptible quantity of matter. . . so perfectly shaped."[9] In 1681, Leeuwenhoek discovered that protozoa and bacteria inhabited the human body, but he did not associate them with disease.[10]

In 1687 the Italian physician Giovanni Bonomo established a causal relationship between a microorganism and an infectious disease by detecting the tiny mite responsible for a skin disorder, scabies, commonly known as "the itch." Bonomo had seen children having this affliction pull out, with the aid of a pin, little bladders of water from their skin and decided to investigate the composition of these bladders. His experimental design was simple and direct; "I quickly found an *Itchy* person, and asking him where he felt the greatest and most acute *Itching* . . . I took out a very small white *Globule* scarcely discernible: Observing this with a Microscope, I found it to be a very minute Living Creature, in shape, resembling a Tortoise, of whitish colour, a little dark upon the Back, with some thin and long Hairs, of nimble motion, with six Feet, a sharp Head, two little Horns at the end of the Snout." Bonomo now understood why the itch was so contagious. These small creatures passed by direct contact from one person to the next, "their motion being wonderfully swift."[11]

But the concept that microorganisms could generate disease was still not generally exploited by physicians of the seventeenth century. The idea bore no relation to the still-dominant humoral theories of disease, and became a casualty of the condemnation that opponents of the instrument heaped upon all microscopic disclosures. For example, using arguments that paralleled those employed to oppose anatomical dissection, Dr. Thomas Sydenham and his friend, the physician–philosopher John Locke, asserted that microscopic studies diverted physicians from interest in bedside observation by leading them to speculate about the cause of disease. They labeled as hopeless any efforts to investigate events inaccessible to the unaided senses, and believed that reasonable men would admit that Nature's inner structure was too esoteric to master. Locke further argued that even if physicians could describe the minute composition of matter, no logical relationship existed between the macroscopic and microscopic worlds, so that no predictions about the one could be made from knowledge of the other.[12]

Practice tended to confirm the skeptical views of Sydenham and Locke. The difference in the appearance of biological phenomena when magnified and when seen by the naked eye, the distortions in the visual field caused by the technical imperfections of early microscopes, and the tendency of many scientists of the period to develop elaborate theories from scant evidence, led to contradictory hypotheses about the composition of this microscopic universe. By the end of the seventeenth century microscopy remained essentially the province of a small circle of pioneers. Robert Hooke asserted in 1692 that microscopy was "now reduced to almost a single Votary which is Mr. Leeuwenhoek: besides whom, I hear of none that makes any other Use of that Instrument, but for Diversion and Pastime."[13]

With the advent of the eighteenth century, attention was given to increasing the magnification of the microscope, principally through the compound instrument, to which microscopists added lenses and intensified the illumination of the objects observed by inventing improved light–reflection systems. But the problem of image distortion with the compound microscope remained unsolved, causing many scientists to believe with the English scientist William Hewson that "the compound having a larger field, is more pleasant than the single microscope for many purposes; but the single should be always preferred by those who wish to ascertain the figures of minute bodies."[14] Professional scientists who used microscopes contented themselves with lower–power simple instruments. The compound microscopes were used mainly by amateurs curious about the microscopic world.[15]

Even when simple microscopes were used, eighteenth–century observers, like their predecessors, continued to mistake optical illusion for natural appearance and thus to build conclusions from false

73

data. A notable illusion was the supposedly globular shape of red–blood cells, a view held even by Leeuwenhoek who was expert in the use of the simple instrument. The globular shape of red cells was generally accepted by subsequent observers until 1774, when William Hewson produced experimental evidence showing otherwise. By diluting a sample of blood in additional blood serum, he caused the normally massed blood cells to separate so that they could be studied more easily, and found that the red particles appeared "as flat as a guinea."[16] Hewson lamented: "When we consider how many ingenious persons have been employed in examining the blood with the best microscopes, it will appear wonderful that the figure of those particles should have been mistaken; but our wonder will be lessened when we consider how many obvious things are overlooked, till our attention is very particularly directed to them."[17] Despite Hewson's work, for half a century more, many investigators clung to the belief that the red corpuscles were globular.

Other problems impeded the application of the microscope in the eighteenth century: investigators blamed inaccurate observations made with the microscope entirely on the instrument and not on themselves (a problem commonly met when inventions are introduced and which also occurred in connection with the stethoscope, ophthalmoscope, and laryngoscope); inadequate preparation and indelicate handling of specimens, which destroyed frail tissue; the belief that the instrument was exceedingly complicated to use; and the judgment that it was "a meer Play–thing, a Matter of Amusement and Fancy only, that raises our Wonder for a Moment, but is of no farther Service."[18] Although some of the criticism was unwarranted, it was true that unless placed in the hands of scientists skilled in optics and anatomy, able to thread their way through the illusions of observation, the microscope was not a reliable instrument and was still unsuited for general use.

These circumstances prompted many people to be suspicious of facts derived from microscopic observations, especially those made with the compound instrument. Typical was the attitude of a late eighteenth-century lecturer, who told his class in medical school that they could see anything they fancied in the objects examined through the microscope – that microscopic anatomy was essentially based on imagination.[19] Even eminent physicians and scientists, such as Albrecht von Haller and Xavier Bichat, foreswore use of the microscope in their work.[20] Great credit thus must be given to amateur microscopists, aided by skilled instrument makers, whose enthusiasm helped keep alive an interest in the instrument, particularly in the compound version. Such devotees from the leisured class filled eighteenth–century literature with their accounts of the minute structure of insects, animals, plants, and minerals.

The microscope's prospects seemed no better as the nineteenth century began. Noted medical figures criticized it. Laennec, for example, like Sydenham two centuries before him, feared that interest in the microscopic world would divert physicians from studying the macroscopic signs of disease in people. Laennec worried that "if the causes of severe diseases are sought for in mere microscopical alterations of structure, it is impossible to avoid running into consequences the most absurd; and, if once cultivated in this spirit, pathological anatomy, as well as that of the body in a sound state, will soon fall from the rank which it holds among the physical sciences, and become a mere tissue of hypotheses, founded in optical illusions and fanciful speculations, without any real benefit to medicine."[21]

Optical defects continued to impair observations. The distortions of microscope images which had bedeviled investigators since the seventeenth century, and were particularly augmented in compound microscopes, were of two kinds: spherical aberration and chromatic aberration. The first occurred because the rays of light passing through the outer portions of the spherical lens were bent more strongly, and thus converged at a different point than the rays which passed nearer to the center of the lens. The defect produced blurred microscopic images. It could be partially corrected by decreasing the size of an aperture adjacent to the objective lens to block peripheral rays. But as the size of the aperture was decreased, the quantity of light striking the specimen diminished too: this made observation difficult. Chromatic aberration occurred chiefly because the different wavelengths forming white light were bent unequally by the instrument's lenses. As a result, colored fringes encircled the visual field and greatly distorted its character and definition: the greater the number of lenses in the microscope, the greater the distortion. Scientists in the mid-eighteenth century had developed for telescopes a single unit which combatted chromatic aberration by combining several lenses of different refractive powers. Yet no one had succeeded in applying the invention to lenses as small as those in the microscope, until the end of that century. A Dutchman, François Beeldsnyder, in about 1791, made what ap-

75

pears to be one of the first achromatic lenses for a microscope. Then in the early nineteenth century, men such as William Tully, the English instrument maker, and Giovan Battista Amici, the Italian mathematician–botanist, reduced color aberration by improving the achromatic lens.[22] But single achromatic lenses provided low magnification. Efforts to increase their power by adding additional achromatic lenses often increased spherical aberration, whose damage to the visual field outweighed the benefit of correcting for color. The microscopist William Hyde Wollaston noted in 1828 that despite "the great improvements lately made in the construction of microscopes, by the introduction of achromatic object – glasses . . .whereby they are admirably adapted to make entertaining exhibition of known objects, hardly any one of the compound microscopes which I have yet seen, is capable of exhibiting minute bodies with that extreme distinctness which is to be obtained by more simple means, and which is absolutely necessary for an original examination of unknown objects."[23] It was not until 1829 that Joseph Jackson Lister, an English wine merchant and devotee of the microscope, solved the problem. Instead of attempting as other scientists and lens makers had, to remedy by trial and error the spherical errors of one achromatic microscope lens by opposing it with those of another, he developed through experiments a theoretical basis for combining lenses.[24] (A current evaluation of the optical performance of seven compound microscopes built between 1690 and 1790 reveals an average image distortion of 19 percent, while a microscope designed in 1838 which used Listerian lenses had a distortion of only 3 percent.)[25] Lister's work was crucial in transforming the construction of the microscope's lens system from an empirical art to a scientific discipline. His innovation, with others such as the introduction by C. R. Goring of standard test objects to measure the clarity of the microscopic image,[26] converted the compound microscope from an untrustworthy device to a powerful machine for investigation.

With these new instruments, a group of microscopically oriented anatomists began to fill major professorships at medical schools in Germany, France, and England. By the 1840s, the earlier skepticism regarding microscopic discoveries was lessening and a new interest in studying the minute elements of the body arose. As the physician John Hughes Bennett commented, "Observers, no longer confused by optical illusions, had no occasion to employ the imagination when the means of vigorous and exact research were laid open to them. The confusion and opposition which formerly existed amongst microscopists in consequence have diminished."[27]

The microscope was increasingly used to investigate products of disease, such as phlegm from the lung, and to examine blood, urine, and mother's milk for signs of pathology. Guy's Hospital in London established a microscopy department that issued periodic reports of their inquiries and findings beginning in 1843. Although gross anatomy still formed the basis of pathology, some physicians began to think of the tissue destruction produced by disease as an alteration of the tissue's elementary constituents, and criticized colleagues who ignored the microscope in their work. The German physician Carl Rokitanski was criticized when the new edition of his famous treatise on pathological anatomy appeared because, "while it abounds in much novel and useful information in relation simply to the *external character* of morbid structures, [it] presents us with few proofs of the author's having cultivated that more recondite division of the science of morbid anatomy, which seeks, by the assistance of the microscope, to resolve the solid products of disease to the simplicity of their elementary components."[28] Physicians in the 1840s and 1850s gradually embraced the viewpoint that naked–eye inspection of post–mortem tissues no longer furnished sufficient new facts to advance the science of pathology.[29] They believed that moving the station of observation closer to the more basic architectural features of the body proportionally increased their power to understand disease.

In no disease was the advantage of the microscope illustrated better than in cancer. The gross visual characteristics of the tumor in the living patient, and the grating sensations the pathologist felt when he scraped a tumor's surface after it was removed from the body – evidence that often failed to discriminate malignant from benign forms – became replaced by more reliable tumor classifications founded upon microscopic structure. The evidence of microscopy also improved the physician's understanding of the patterns by which disease became diffused throughout the tissues of the body. The instrument showed that ailments often produced widespread but moderate damage to tissues other than the one principally affected (which gave the illness its most characteristic features and name). It became recognized that these moderate changes accounted for complications in illness whose origins had previously been obscure.[30] Enthusiasts proclaimed that prospecting the microscopic world produced more surprises and intellectual gratification

77

than exploring the universe. As the 1850s wore on, more manuals began to appear on the use of the microscope, and good microscopes became less expensive, as well as lighter and more easily transportable from doctor's office to patient's bedside. Techniques of preparing material for observation improved too, such as the use of stains to delineate specific structures in tissues. There were also advances in the design of the microscope's optical system, such as those that led to the practical use of the immersion lens. With all these developments, inquiry into the microscopic world increased further.[31]

Although Robert Hooke had observed and named the cell in the mid–seventeenth century, a precise knowledge of the cell emerged finally only in the 1830s, and was stimulated in part by the increasing use of the microscope.[32] In 1831 Robert Brown, a botanist, drew attention to the importance of the cell nucleus, whose significance in the composition of plants was extensively analyzed by Matthias Schleiden in an 1838 paper that proved that the tissues of plants were composed of cells. In 1839, Theodor Schwann demonstrated that animal tissues were also composed of cells, and enunciated the principle of the identity of structural units in animals and plants. Schwann, elaborating on views put forth by Schleiden, proposed that cell development began from an undifferentiated fluid between the cells.[33]

Although a number of physicians agreed that cells were the starting point and immediate agent of all organic changes,[34] by the 1850s no physician had yet launched a systematic effort to bring together the facts that would establish their importance to health and disease. Then in 1858, the German pathologist Rudolf Virchow published *Cellular Pathology*.[35] In this epoch–making work, he brought together many old and new facts about cellular changes in disease. He demonstrated conclusively that a disruption of cellular function was the basis of disease, just as its orderly operation was the foundation of health, and showed that cells found in disease were modifications of normal types. He proved erroneous the notion that cells rose spontaneously from an undifferentiated matrix, and formulated the doctrine that a growth of new cells implied already existing cells – a doctrine summarized in the precept *Omnis cellula e cellula:* cell development is continuous. He insisted that no tissue could be called living if the constant presence of cells in it could not be demonstrated, and he made the cell the ultimate morphological unit within which life could exist.[36]

78

Virchow considered his cellular concept of disease an evolutionary development of Morgagni's anatomically rooted notion that each disease had a seat. "No physician can properly think out a process of disease unless he is able to fix for it a place in the body," Virchow declared.[37] To him, the fundamental question the practicing physician and medical scientist must ask was *"Ubi est morbus? Where is the disease?"*[38] Despite the anatomical basis of his cell theory, Virchow did not restrict his analysis of cellular function to a study of structural change; he insisted that chemical and physical investigations were also fundamental to comprehending cellular phenomena: "The cell is the locus to which the action of mechanical matter is bound, and only within its limits can that power of action justifying the name of life be maintained. *But within this locus it is mechanical matter that is active – active according to physical and chemical laws.*"[39] Virchow believed that even if future scientists isolated the molecules that composed the cell, and thereby advanced "to the last boundaries within which there remain elements with the character of totality or, if you will, of unity, we can go no farther than the cell. It is the final and constantly present link in the great chain of mutually subordinated structures composing the human body."[40] Virchow's *Cellular Pathology* provided a theoretical and factual foundation for microscopists, whose instrument became an essential means for studying this ultimate unit of biological activity.

Despite the growing esteem in medicine for the microscope during the 1840s and 1850s, even devotees cautioned that its findings must be subjected to rigorous scrutiny, because they were so easily distorted by the imagination. Discordant results from different microscopic investigations of the same subject still engendered distrust as to the microscope's accuracy and fidelity. It caused some pathologists to view microscopic evidence "as something like the spectres of an imaginative eye, or the refined delusions of a complex optical mechanism, or, at best, the obscure shadows of infinitely–divided particles of organic matter."[41] The problem led several physicians to investigate the sources of these deceptions. Henry Bence Jones, the English physician–scientist, hypothesized that all observers sometimes described what they thought should be there, rather than what they actually saw: "Each sense has its own fallacies, and our fears, our hopes, and our prejudices distort our perceptions."[42] This tendency was strengthened by a lack of definitiveness in the images presented to the eye, which allowed much of the image to be filled in by the mind. Accordingly, objects magnified 500 to 800 times, whose forms should have been dim and poorly outlined, might be represented in such a sharp and defined manner that they appeared "carved in wood, and drawn from observation by the naked eye."[43]

Errors also arose from a lack of attention to the influences impinging on the object being observed, such as the character and quantity of light that illuminated the microscopic field or the unique actions of the different liquids added to specimens to dilute and prepare them for microscopic inspection. The skill of the investigator likewise influenced his pronouncements, and here there was room for improvement. Lionel Beale, a pioneer microscopist, commented in 1857, "although there are many instruments, I fear it must be confessed that the observers are comparatively few."[44] For the belief prevailed among some doctors that it was necessary only to place an object in the microscope's field in order to determine its structure (a problem encountered too in introducing the ophthalmoscope and laryngoscope). To become a first–rate observer required a knowledge of optics, chemistry, and anatomy, accompanied by dexterity in manipulating the instrument, and time to educate the eye and to become acquainted with the illusions inherent in the best magnifying instruments. The microscope per se could not confer the power of observation upon the unlearned. Physicians were urged to distinguish between qualities of superior instruments designed to unveil medical facts, and the mental traits that enabled investigators to recognize the facts. Some physicians believed that bettering the human capacity for microscopic observations was even more crucial than improving the optical components of the instrument (a precept also advanced by some users of the stethoscope).

In the decades of the 1860s and 1870s, having profited from such discussions, growing numbers of physicians employed the microscope to settle diagnostic questions. One of the most important apprentices in this field was the American James Marion Sims. His conversion occurred when a friend, after holding up a glass slide to prove it contained nothing the naked eye could see, asked Sims to look at the slide under the microscope. "I am sure I was never more surprised in all my life, than I was then, to see, and read the Lord's Prayer," recalled Sims. "From that moment I was convinced that the instrument exhibited things just as they were."[45]

The microscope became a central device in Sims' edifying investigations on the causes of human sterility. Before this work, physicians had usually attributed barrenness in a marriage to sterility in the woman, and subjected her to numerous painful therapies, such as the surgical incision of the neck of the uterus. Sims used the microscope to examine the condition of the male semen, and to demonstrate that defects in it could also account for infertility. In pursuing this work, he had to overcome the criticism that his interventions were incompatible with decency and self–respect. In a rejoinder to his detractors written in 1868, Sims indicated how fundamental physical examination had become to medical practice by insisting that "there can be no indecency, and no sacrifice of self-respect in making any necessary physical examination whatever, if it be done with a proper sense of delicacy, and with a dignified, earnest, and conscientious determination to arrive at the truth."[46] Sims declared that physicians could not initiate therapy for sterility, in good conscience, without first ascertaining the viability of sperm; this required use of the microscope.

Despite much testimony to the microscope's value during the 1870s, many educators, students, and practitioners failed to put it to use. In the United States, only a few medical schools, most notably the Harvard Medical School and the University of Pennsylvania Medical School, had special laboratories devoted to microscopy and considered the subject an essential part of the curriculum. The medical student, although he heard of the microscope's utility, was oppressed by other requirements and gladly excused himself from attention to an instrument without knowledge of which he might still become a doctor. The view was also prevalent among physicians that acquaintance with an expert microscopist, to whom they could delegate work, made learning to use the instrument unnecessary. Nevertheless, in practice, they often neglected to consult the expert because they were embarrassed to ask for assistance in diagnosis, or lacked the time to do so. When they did consult the microscopist, doctors without microscopic skill often confounded him by giving him tissues carelessly selected, and hence not inclusive of the diseased elements requiring identification. Microscopists, in turn, themselves damaged the reputation of their instrument, by frequently changing a judgment that clashed with a previously announced diagnosis from a clinician. This circumstance sometimes prompted physicians to withhold bedside data from the microscopist until after he had rendered an opinion.[47]

The transformation in medical diagnosis engendered by the microscope's disclosure of the cellular world was rendered complete by the development of bacteriology, and particularly by the work of one of its pioneers – Robert Koch. It would be impossible in the scope of this work to give a full discussion of the development and acceptance of bacteriology. In brief summary, the study of microorganisms had regained some momentum in the 1830s when improved microscopes appeared, incorporating achromatic lenses. In research published in 1835 and 1836, the Italian physician Agostino Bassi demonstrated that a microorganism was responsible for the fatal disease of silk worms known as muscardine. In 1840, the German medical scientist Jacob Henle published an important essay, "On Miasmata and Contagia," in which he sought to establish that minute living creatures that parasitized the human body caused infectious diseases. He reasoned further that since physicians were "daily becoming more acquainted with the wide distribution, the rapid multiplication and the vital tenacity of the lower, microscopic plant world, it is even more natural to imagine the contagion having a vegetable body," a conjecture that he believed was given "powerful support" by Bassi's work on muscardine.[48] During the 1840s, other investigators also discovered bacteria and fungi in the wastes and body fluids of sick people, and would attribute illness to their presence.

But considerable opposition developed to the notion that microorganisms were the causal agents of infectious disease. Justus von Liebig, the chemist and physiologist, criticized investigators who too hastily interpreted "two things which occur frequently in conjunction, as standing in the mutual relation of cause and effect." He accordingly declared "nothing more deficient of a scientific basis, or more mischievous than the hypothesis which regards. . .contagions as animated beings. . .developing, propagating, and multiplying themselves in the body, thus creating diseases and causing death."[49] The English physician John Simon argued that the analogy drawn between the causal agents of infectious disease and parasites was false: diseases generated by parasites usually produced local, not general disturbances of body function.[50]

Bacteriological investigators also floundered in their inability to detect bacteria in a number of conspicuous and prevalent infectious diseases such as smallpox and measles – disorders later found to be caused by viruses, a group of organisms unknown to mid–nineteenth–century scientists. In addition, it seemed improbable to most investigators that a class of similar-looking minute organisms embraced a sufficiently wide range of species to account for the many infectious diseases then known.[51] Further, some scientists believed that the microorganisms found in the disordered tissues were the result of the spontaneous transformation of disease–damaged body cells into "low types of animal or vegetable existence."[52] And others attributed infectious disease to the actions of infectious "particles," rather than to organisms. The historian J. K. Crellin called the 1860s "the era of the particle," in which biads, bioplasts, globules, morbific ferments, and so forth were postulated as causes of infectious disease. Paradoxically, these theories aided the hypothesis that disease was caused by microorganisms – themselves particles – and did much "to demolish the widely-held idea that infectious diseases could arise spontaneously through miasmata such as emanated from filth."[53]

Significant new evidence to support the relation between microorganisms and illness appeared in the 1860s with the work of the chemist Louis Pasteur and of the surgeon Joseph Lister, whose father had refined the achromatic lens. Pasteur proved, through brilliant experiments, that putrefaction of organic matter did not occur in the absence of microorganisms, and that these creatures were not generated spontaneously in the course of putrefaction, but were visitors from the external environment. In 1865, a colleague of Lister called his attention to Pasteur's work. The enigma of why fractures healed rapidly when the bone did not break through the skin, and why a fracture in which a bone penetrated to the outer surface was specially liable to generate pus, engaged Lister's attention because of the frightful mortality from such wounds. With many others of his day, he believed that oxygen in the air stimulated pus formation; but it seemed hopeless to prevent air from acting on the wound. His reading of Pasteur furnished an alternative explanation for pus formation – bacteria suspended in the air fell into and contaminated the wound. Lister demonstrated that he could prevent putrefaction by applying chemical disinfectants to the wound and its dressings, mainly carbolic and phenic acid, which destroyed bacteria.[54] As a result of his antiseptic method, the rate of wound inflammation and surgical mortality in his patients declined dramatically. Yet, for lack of skillful application, many other surgeons who used his procedures failed to reproduce Lister's results and therefore remained unconverted to the premise that bacteria produced disease.

Investigators of microorganisms also were hampered by lack of trustworthy experimental techniques to demonstrate their association with disease. The development of such techniques, which eventually became crucial tools of diagnosis, was one of the important contributions of the German physician Robert Koch, whose pioneering bacteriological work began with his study of anthrax, a disease of men and animals. In 1850, a French physician Casimir Davaine had observed bacteria in the blood of a sheep killed by anthrax. During the next two decades, he wrote many papers in which he tried to establish a causal relation between a particular bacterial species and this disease.[55] Koch, a graduate of medical school in 1866, who pursued scientific interests while a general practitioner during the 1870s, was familiar with but skeptical of Davaine's work; he did not believe the bacteria alleged to cause anthrax could maintain themselves in a winter environment, as it appeared their life cycle required. Yet, reasoning that the bacteria might survive the winter if they formed spores, he initiated experiments in which this hypothesis was eventually confirmed.

Koch's work involved careful microscopic identification, cultivation, and transmission of the bacteria from animal to animal in order to establish a relationship between a bacterial species and anthrax. He demonstrated that a bacillus found in hay, morphologically similar to the anthrax bacillus, did not cause anthrax when inoculated into animals, and thus showed clearly that closely related bacteria differed in their ability to generate disease: "Only a species of bacillus," Koch asserted, "is able to cause this specific disease [anthrax], while other schizophytes have no effects or cause entirely different diseases when inoculated."[56]

Despite these experiments, critics contended that some factor in the blood used to transmit anthrax from animal to animal, rather than bacilli, was responsible for producing the disease. Yet Koch's work attracted the attention of the scientific community in Germany. In 1880, he received an appointment at the Imperial Health Department in Berlin, and just five years later, he went to the University of Berlin to fill a newly created chair of hygiene. Within this period, he helped to establish the foundations of modern bacteriology, and had begun training researchers who would become its leaders.

At the time of Koch's arrival in Berlin, tuberculosis was the predominant endemic disease in Europe, responsible for approximately one death in seven.[57] There had been convincing evidence that tuberculosis was infectious since Jean–Antoine Villemin had demonstrated in 1865 that it could be transmitted from animal to animal, and even from humans to animals through inoculation. Koch applied his ingenuity and techniques to search for a bacterial cause of tuberculosis. In 1882, he triumphantly announced success: "For the first time, the parasitic nature of a human infective disease, and, indeed, of the most important of all diseases, has been completely demonstrated."[58]

Koch proved that tuberculosis was produced by a rod-shaped organism he named the tubercle bacillus. This feat had required Koch to develop microscopical and chemical techniques far more complex than had ever been used before in bacteriology, and to proclaim what became known as Koch's postulates, a methodological creed by which a scientist could establish a cause and effect relation between a microorganism and a disease. The basic elements of the postulates had been suggested by Henle, a teacher of Koch's, in his 1840 essay "On Miasmata and Contagia." The postulates enumerated three conditions: first, the organism must be present constantly in the diseased parts; second, it must be cultivated outside of the body and separated from all other matter; third, the disease must be produced in an animal susceptible to it, which had been inoculated with the microorganism just cultivated.[59] To apply the postulates, Koch developed techniques for staining and culturing the organisms, and then inoculating them into animals.

The staining technique was a necessary component of Koch's research method, for unstained bacteria could be difficult to identify from their appearance under the microscope. Clinicians found staining a technique easier to use than bacterial cultures and animal inoculation, both of which required sophisticated laboratory equipment.[60] However, while easier to employ than these other bacteriological procedures, even staining bacteria was difficult. For example, one of the most common methods of staining the tubercle bacillus, developed by Paul Ehrlich shortly after Koch's announcement of his discovery, required clinicians to spread a thin layer of residue coughed from the lungs over a small piece of glass, dry it by carefully drawing it through a flame, soak the glass in aniline dye for 24 hours, then decolorize the specimen with hydrochloric acid, dry it, add canada–balsam, and finally place the specimen under the microscope. A medical journal editorialized: "However simple these directions may appear, they are only achieved by a nicety of manipulation, a good microscope with accessories, and an immoderate quantity of patience."[61]

Although the method could not be used in ordinary medical practice because of the experience and equipment required, Koch believed that the cultivation of bacterial colonies pure in strain was the crux of research into infectious disease. Before Koch's research, scientists had grown pure cultures of bacteria in liquids containing nutrients, but such cultures were easily contaminated with other bacteria. An observation Koch made (as several others had before him), that different strains of bacteria flourished, in separate colonies, on the surface of a boiled potato, prompted him to seek a solid material better suited to his experimental needs than liquid cultures. He found that the liquid nutrient he had been using to grow bacteria, solidified by the addition of gelatin, admirably suited his purposes. Koch implanted bacteria on it by drawing a sterilized platinum needle containing bacteria across the nutrient, which was layered on a glass slide. He controlled the purity of the culture by constantly examining bacteria under the microscope, sampled from the colonies that grew.[62] The solid culture allowed scientists not only to isolate pure bacterial strains, but also to distinguish different organisms by the topographic features of their colonies. These landmarks proved decisive in identifying the comma bacillus, the postulated cause of cholera. This bacillus belonged to a family of microorganisms resembling each other so closely that when examined individually under the microscope, scientists had no confidence in their ability to tell them apart. Only the diverse forms of their growth in colonies allowed them to be identified with certainty.[63]

Animal inoculation gave Koch another procedure to probe the causal relation between bacteria and disease. As used by his nineteenth–century predecessors, bacteria–laden fluids from an infected animal were injected into a healthy animal in the hope of transmitting the disease from the one to the other, and thus establishing the microorganism as the source of the illness. Critics, however, maintained that the possibility could not be ruled out that something in the fluids, other than bacteria, might be responsible for the transfer of the disease. The solid–culture technique that Koch developed permitted the extraction and certain isolation of the bacteria in question from the body fluid. The microorganisms, without the fluid, could now be injected into the healthy animal, thereby answering the principal criticism of the older inoculation technique.

If the same symptoms were produced in the healthy animal as those exhibited by the sick one, this provided further confirmation of the bacteria's role in causing illness. The time, however, required to apply this test (between two and four weeks), and the equipment and skill needed, also discouraged the average practitioner from using it.[64]

Crucial to Koch's work too was the technique of photomicrography. Hypotheses weighed down with subjective impressions and contradictory microscopic representations of the same object filled the pages of the bacteriological literature of the 1880s – an old dilemma in microscopy. Changes in the conditions of observation accounted for much of the disparity. With a single microscope, two observers could not simultaneously view the same object and form a joint opinion, but each had to look in turn. Even the slightest turn of its fine adjustment knob, or a change in the intensity of illumination, could cause bacteria to disappear from the field entirely, or seem to have different markings. Although agreement among scientists increased when observations were made with the same microscope, they commonly used instruments located in different places, produced by different manufacturers. Investigators compounded the problem by using a variety of mounting and staining procedures on the specimens. Their frequent inability to discuss what they saw with each other generated continued conflict.

For Koch, the only remedy to this was "photography, which comes both as a harmonizing mediator and as an instructress. Indeed, under certain circumstances, the photographic picture of a microscopical object is more valuable than the original preparation."[65] The photograph fixed the microscopic image, reproducing it in exactly the focus, magnification, and illumination desired. Several observers could evaluate the picture at the same time, each precisely concentrating on the object in question. The microscopist himself could exert control over his own observations through an accurate record of the objects he had viewed. Before the availability of the photograph, drawings of microscopic images had been the primary technique for preserving these data. Like others earlier in the century, Koch criticized drawings as almost never true to nature. The objects as drawn always seemed more elegant and invested with sharper lines and stronger shadows than the original; they portrayed the unconscious bias of the artist. The photograph helped free the investigator from subjective influences in presenting

87

his evidence. It placed the observations of the scientist directly before his audience, allowing them to share his perceptions. It represented a scientist's findings more accurately and thereby exposed them to more searching critical appraisal than was possible before. Photography led Koch and others to believe that such objective representation of the phenomena they witnessed would free bacteriology from the rancor of its past.[66] Koch was aware that circumstances such as the intensity of light, mode of film development, and the skill of the operator could influence the photographic record. He nevertheless believed that the photomicrograph, like the X-ray, provided a permanent record that transcended memory and subjective impression, and furnished a new, more secure path to medical truth.

Some physicians remained unconvinced by Koch's claim that a microorganism caused tuberculosis. A number of skeptics argued mainly that, along with the tubercle bacillus, some unknown factor was being introduced into the experimental animals, or that the mere presence of foreign matter in the body (such as bacteria), possessing no disease specificity whatsoever, could initiate tuberculosis. This criticism was effectively dealt with when clinical tests on patients verified Koch's laboratory experiments. In one of the earliest trials, physicians examined matter coughed up from the lungs of 120 patients who had symptoms of advanced tuberculosis, and found tubercle bacilli in all the samples. Analysis of similar matter produced by patients who showed symptoms of ordinary bronchitis did not reveal a single tubercle bacilli.[67] Other critics, however, called for additional investigations into the special conditions in the human body that allowed germs to breed. Although bacterial researchers might identify the organism responsible for a given disease, they had not explained why one patient became infected while another did not; why one patient who contracted the disease died, whereas another similarly affected lived. Now that proof had accumulated that bacteria played a crucial role in causing disease, it was urgent to uncover additional facts that could explain the varying resistance of people to infection.[68]

Despite some stubborn critics, the association between a bacterial agent and tuberculosis raised the hope that microorganisms were in fact the starting points of disease, for which medicine had hunted for so long. Medicine seemed "dominated by a new idea concerning the causative agency of disease, and one that seems to possess more rational grounds for acceptance than any that have gone before."[69] Many physicians began to elevate microorganisms to the pinnacle of diagnostic signs. Why bother seeking the secondary effects of disease when they could detect their true source?

Evidence about tuberculosis gathered through the main techniques of bedside examination, such as history–taking and auscultation, seemed inferior when compared with the more certain knowledge provided through bacteriology. In the 1880s the medical journals reported on numerous patients in whom bacilli were found before the other techniques had detected signs of tuberculosis. Typical was the case of

A. S., aged 31, a gentleman whom I have known for years, and treated for various ailments, but who, though [he had] a phthisical family history, had himself never suffered from cough, and was in the enjoyment of very good health, consulted me on December 27th for hemoptysis [coughing up blood], which had attacked him on the morning of that day. He could not in any way account for it, except for a very slight fall he had on December 25th, which, however, did not hurt him in any way. The physical examination showed absolutely normal relations; neither was there loss of flesh, loss of appetite, or pyrexia. Examination of the sputa on December 29th showed abundance of tubercle–bacilli.[70]

Physicians often concluded that the presence of the tubercle bacilli, in the absence of any symptoms of the disease, stamped the person as tubercular, while failure to discover the organism after frequent and careful study of the patient justified a conclusion that he either did not have tuberculosis, or that the disease had been arrested. Not only in tuberculosis, but in other diseases such as diphtheria and cholera, microorganisms seemed the earliest and safest guide to diagnoses, and superior to all other signs of these maladies.[71]

As the twentieth century began, the list of diseases in which various microorganisms were implicated was long. It included tuberculosis, pneumonia, plague, anthrax, typhoid fever, diphtheria, gonorrhea, cholera, influenza, leprosy, actinomycosis, malaria, amoebic dysentery, relapsing fever, and trypanosomiasis. For some of these diseases, physicians could make only presumptive diagnoses from microscopic disclosure of the offending organism in the fluids and wastes of the patient's body – additional methods such as cultivation of pure bacterial colonies and animal inoculation were required for substantiation. But for other diseases, such confirmatory procedures were set aside either because they were ineffective, or too complicated and time–consuming for ordinary diagnostic purposes. Here, expert microscopic observation alone reigned supreme.[72]

The microscope had thus become crucial in locating some major causes of physical suffering and death in man, and was considered by a number of physicians at the twentieth century's turn as the pre–eminent diagnostic instrument in medicine. Like the stethoscope, the microscope drew the physician into a universe of physical changes concealed from the natural senses. Unlike examinations made with the stethoscope, which required the patient's presence, examinations made with the microscope could take place in the absence of the patient, requiring only products taken from the body. The microscope – like the X-ray – encouraged a physical separation of the doctor from his patient in the diagnosis of illness. To some clinicians this separation did not appear to endanger accurate diagnosis, for they believed that the signs of disease elicited at the patient's bedside were secondary in importance – mere indications of more fundamental alterations in tissues that diagnostic technology such as the microscope could detect.[73] But this attitude troubled other doctors. The English clinician Sir Dyce Duckworth cautioned his colleagues in 1896 "that our eyes and our minds are rather apt in consequence to dwell too much on our detailed notes and manifold instrumental aids, and too little on the patient, his personal peculiarities and the ultimate nature of his ailments." He counseled: "We must, if we are to be great in medicine, sometimes lift our eyes from the microscope, and away from the engrossing researches of the laboratory. . .If we do so we shall certainly come to know more of the inwardness and due proportions of matters which relate to the life of man as he passes through his present environment."[74]

5 The translation of physiological actions into the languages of machines

Reappraisal of the viewpoint that unveiling defects in body architecture was the main task of medical diagnosis began when a number of nineteenth–century physicians recommended that the principal measures of illness should be changes in essential body functions, such as breathing, blood circulation, and temperature. Such changes, unless of long standing, generally were not associated with structural defects; consequently many physicians, who had developed confidence in disease indices they could verify by structural alterations, were suspicious of those not so associated. The diagnostic value of signs of change in body function also suffered as autopsies showed many such previously accepted signs as not reliable.

The situation changed when instruments appeared that could portray functional actions by inscribing them on graphs or measuring them in numbers. This transformed the functional actions from subjectively monitored phenomena (such as impressions gathered from pulse–feeling), to objective events several observers could jointly evaluate and discuss. The statement of the body's vivifying activities in numbers and graphs provided a factual transcription of pathology equivalent to the discovery of an anatomical lesion. Number, graph, and lesion – each connected subjective impressions that physicians personally gathered at the bedside to an objective form that permitted collegial debate and ready comparison with past, present, and future medical data.

The attachment of nineteenth–century physicians to the numerical measure of physiological operations began in earnest with John Hutchinson's 1846 monograph, "On the Capacity of the Lungs, and on the Respiratory Functions, with a View of Establishing a Precise and Easy Method of Detecting Disease by the Spirometer."[1] Hutchinson, an English physician, studied the mechanics of

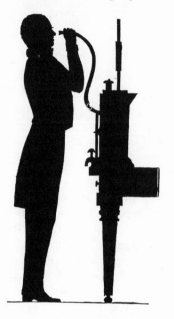

Figure 9. Measuring the vital capacity of the lungs (1846). The figure depicted has just inhaled and is ready to breathe into the spirometer. Reprinted from John Hutchinson, "On the Capacity of the Lungs" (1846), p. 236.

respiration through five variables, each relating the quantity of air breathed to the motions of the chest wall: residual air – the quantity of air remaining in the lungs after the deepest possible expiration; reserve air – the amount of air left behind in the lungs after gentle expiration; breathing air – the volume of air required to perform ordinary inspiration and expiration; complemental air – the volume of air that could be drawn into the lungs by violent exertion beyond the effort of ordinary inspiration; and vital capacity – the quantity of air expelled by the greatest voluntary expiration following the deepest inspiration.

Earlier investigators, such as the eighteenth–century cleric–scientist Stephen Hales and the physician–chemist Humphrey Davy, had studied the mechanics of breathing.[2] But since they had not taken account of differences in the body weight of their experimental subjects (often themselves), their findings were undependable and discordant. Hutchinson, who found a direct correlation between the weight of a patient and the volume of the lungs, produced more accurate data than his predecessors. Intent on demonstrating how the intake and expulsion of air from the lungs changed during normal growth and disease, he selected as the cardinal index the vital capacity, and constructed for its measure an instrument he called the spirometer. The device linked a tube, through which the patient breathed, to a delicately balanced receiver which was elevated by each increment of expired air. Hutchinson directed the patient undergoing the test to stand perfectly erect, head thrown back; to slowly fill his chest with air, and then to immediately empty his lungs (Figure 9). A graduated scale measured the amount of air expelled.[3]

After Hutchinson had tested his invention on more than 2,000 people, most of whom were healthy, he proclaimed that with a knowledge of vital capacity doctors could confidently judge the physical fitness of men for public duties, such as service in the armed forces, and could detect lung disease at an earlier stage than was possible with auscultation or percussion. He demonstrated this last point with Freeman, the nearly 7–foot "American Giant" upon whom Hutchinson obtained a vital–capacity reading while Freeman was in England for a prize fight. When a second measurement was taken two years later, although 20 percent diminished and thus a signature to Hutchinson of the lung's impairment, two skillful auscultators Hutchinson brought into the case failed to detect a trace of disease. Another year elapsed before Freeman developed unmistakable tuberculosis, the disease from which he died.[4] Such evidence moved some physicians to give greater value to the spirometer than to the stethoscope in diagnosis. They criticized the inability of Laennec's instrument to discover tuberculosis when it began its invasion of the lungs, and they praised Hutchinson's invention for the new and accurate data it produced.[5]

Hutchinson advocated an entirely quantitative examination of the lung: counting the number of respirations per minute, gauging the chest's circumference during inspiration and expiration, taking the patient's height and weight, and, most important, determining his vital capacity with the spirometer. These steps completed, a numerical portrait of the patient emerged. Hutchinson also arranged measurements of lung activity in tabular form so that observers could clearly perceive the difference between the patients represented by the figures. This all suggested a new precept to Hutchinson: observations susceptible to objective, numerical statement, and obtained with a minimal expenditure of mental energy, demanded the most weighty diagnostic consideration in medicine. "If a man breathe into the Spirometer 200 cubic inches [of air], it is neither 199 nor 201 cubic inches; it requires no delicate training of the judgment, nor sense of sight, to come to such a conclusion;

therefore, for the purpose of determining a *fact*, the Spirometer is ready and definite, without a long system of education."[6] Hutchinson explicitly proposed his machine as an equalizer of diagnostic skills. The spirometer obtained precise results, but no significant act of intellect, no exquisite sensory training was required to obtain or understand its data. The spirometer permitted doctors, whether able or inept, to make accurate judgments. When Hutchinson weighed numerical indices of disease derived from self–recording devices, against data derived by physicians directly through the senses (such as sounds heard through the stethoscope), he found the numerical indices the more easily comprehended and objective measure of illness.

A small amount of support for this viewpoint emerged during the 1850s, as some physicians concluded that evidence acquired through instruments which extended the sensory powers of the natural human faculties, such as the stethoscope and ophthalmoscope, could be unreliable because the person behind the instrument had to interpret the evidence, and thus crucially influenced its character.[7] The shortcomings of sensory data, even those acquired through instruments, made numerical, machine–produced information appear more trustworthy and objective to some doctors.

Nevertheless, as physicians tested the value of the vital-capacity index generated by Hutchinson's machine, they found that it was not an unerring signature of disease, only an early clue that required confirmation by auscultation and percussion. The yardstick by which the vital capacity was measured – its statistically deduced normal standard – came under attack when experience revealed that a deficiency of vital capacity could occur in healthy people. Critics doubted whether a numerical standard based upon a statistical average could be relied upon to distinguish normal from pathological states. Since all of the physiological activities of the body, such as respiration, changed from moment to moment, establishing a norm for any activity, even for a single person, was difficult. How then could physicians trust any physiological norm based on averages derived from groups of people? Opponents declared that physiological activities were too complicated for figures to represent adequately. The pulse could be counted, for example, but the numbers did not convey the character of its rhythm. Moreover, uniting a vague idea with figures, even if they were extended to the tenth decimal place, would not clarify it; the observer with a quick eye, sensitive touch, and experience did not require number–

dispensing machines such as the spirometer. Such machines were called "crutches to the feeble, which should be discarded as [the clinician] gains strength. . .To the vigorous and active, they are but as clogs and impediments to his free action and progress."[8] During the 1850s some physicians used and praised the spirometer, but doctors generally disregarded the device and the numerical measure of disease for which it stood. However, by this mid–century point, armed with new instruments, physicians had begun to study an old index of body function – the pulse – and to give new attention to the value of graphs as a way of depicting pathology.

During the second century A.D. Galen, the first significant commentator on the pulse, had developed doctrines about its qualitative alterations, ideas that dominated Western medicine well into the eighteenth century. He defined the pulse as a double movement of an artery involving an expansion and a contraction, with two periods of rest in between. The pulse depended upon and was synchronous with the heart, and was best appreciated at the wrists and the soles of the feet. One set of pulse characteristics originated with the artery's expansion. When pulsation occurred the artery became extended in all directions, giving the pulse beat properties of length (longitudinal dilatation), breadth (lateral dilatation), and depth (vertical dilatation). Other characteristics were the slowness or swiftness of the pulse, the length of time occupied by the expansion and contraction of a single pulse beat, and the interval of time between two expansions or contractions. Galen had applied the terms "strong" or "feeble" to indicate the force with which the artery struck the finger, "hard" or "soft" to define the character of the arterial wall. He used the terms "equal" and "unequal" to classify the pulse's rhythm and gave special names to some of the more distinctive beats: a succession of pulsations that regularly diminished in magnitude was called "decurate" or "sharp–tailed," from their resemblance to the tapering tail of the mouse; a pulse stroke with a weak, imperfect dilatation, a pause, and then a full, strong dilatation received the name "dorcadessans" or "goatlike," after the way this animal leaped – making first a short spring, pausing briefly, and then making a much larger bound. The terms "regular" and "irregular" he used to describe whether such peculiarities of the pulse were repeated or not: thus any unequal pulse of three weak followed by one strong beat, repeated consecutively, he called a regular pulse. Galen had also originated the idea of organic pulses –

unique characteristics given to the pulse by each one of the body's organs, which allowed deductions about the state of each organ. He defined, in addition, the critical pulses – those that allowed physicians to gauge when crucial periods in an illness would occur. All of his interest was however limited to a qualitative account of the pulse; he did not investigate the value of counting its rate of beating.[9]

Herophilus, an Alexandrian physician born in the last third of the fourth century B.C., was apparently the first person to count the pulse using a water clock, but physicians of that period seemed to believe that sensorial judgments could not be improved by their quantification, and so ignored such measurements.[10] In the Middle Ages doctors, following Galen's example, were almost totally absorbed with the qualitative features of the pulse. Consequently, when Nicholas of Cusa, in 1450, advocated the use of a water clock to time its rate, his suggestion represented a large departure from tradition, and was generally ignored. Cusa, a priest and mathematician, invited physicians to ponder: "Do you think if you would permit the water from the narrow opening of a clepsydra [water clock] to flow into a basin for as long as was necessary to count the pulse a hundred times in a healthy young man, and then do the same thing for an ailing young man, that there would be a noticeable difference between the weights of the water that would flow during the period? From the weight of water, therefore, one would arrive at a better knowledge of. . .various diseases. . .than from the touch of the vein."[11]

Over a century after Cusa, the quantification of the pulse attracted Galileo's attention. We are told by Vincenzio Vivani, Galileo's biographer, that while a medical student at the University of Pisa in 1582, Galileo had constructed a small pendulum suspended by a string, the upper part of which was attached to a scale. He obtained a numerical estimate of the pulse rate by pressing the string of the swinging pendulum with his finger at the point on the scale that caused its oscillations to coincide with the beat of the patient's pulse. Vivani declared that the idea for the invention came to Galileo when he noticed "the motion of a lamp when he was one day in the Duomo at Pisa, and thence, having made very exact experiments, he ascertained the equality of its vibrations, and thus it occurred to him to adapt it to use in medicine for the measurement of the frequency of the pulses."[12]

Yet Galileo never fully exploited the instrument's medical potential. This was subsequently done by Santorio Santorio, a physician at the University of Padua. In 1620 he described a device modeled after Galileo's, fashioned from a cord at the end of which was a lead bullet, which Santorio named the "pulsilogium." Santorio claimed that the pulsilogium allowed him to monitor the frequency of the pulse with a precision unattainable by the unaided senses: "On the same or on the following day, we can make trial with the same instrument whether the pulsation of the same artery be a very little quicker or slower; we say 'a very little,' because in the use of this instrument we do not seek those marked differences of rapidity or slowness of pulsation which can be carried in the memory of the physician, but rather these very slight ones of which the differences between one day and another are barely noticeable."[13] Although Santorio believed these distinctions would improve diagnosis, his efforts made little impression on his contemporaries. Nearly a century passed before pulse–counting attracted another dedicated advocate, Sir John Floyer, an English physician who seemed aware of Santorio's work. In his 1707 book, *The Physician's Pulse-Watch*, he praised the Galenists for their skill at detecting pulse characters, but described their pulse art as flawed because it lacked trustworthy standards by which to measure abnormality; the only pulse standards of the Galenists were subjective, tactile sensations, such as strength or weakness, which were difficult to remember. Floyer declared that counts of the pulse rate in different states of illness provided more trustworthy yardsticks to evaluate pathology with. To count he used common matches, pendulum clocks, and finally a pulse watch, made to order for him, which ran for sixty seconds.[14]

Floyer's reports on pulse-counting drew praise from a small number of physicians; but most of them, still attached to qualitative pulse doctrines, opposed Floyer. Many physicians were giving up using Galen's meticulous descriptions of different pulses. They substituted new pulse doctrines usually having a simpler vocabulary to describe the qualitative sensations of the pulse, which did not require the prodigious memory, great experience, or exquisite sense of touch necessary to apply Galen's theories. For example, Théophile de Bordeu, a Parisian doctor, proposed the equality and inequality of the pulsations, and the intervals between them, as the principal means of characterizing the pulse.[15] De Bordeu and others dismissed pulse–counting as largely uninformative, and magnified the virtues of qualitative descriptions. This attitude bred reports such as this: "The pulse during all this time is quick, weak, and unequal, sometimes fluttering, and sometimes for a few minutes slow, nay intermitting."[16] William Heberden, the well–known, mid–eighteenth–century English physician, denounced such minute qualitative distinctions as largely fabrications of the imagination and the cause of frequent disagreement among physicians. Heberden recommended numerical analysis of the pulse rate to his colleagues as "being most perfectly described and communicated to others."[17]

Heberden's efforts attracted followers such as the English physician William Falconer. He believed that physicians were beginning to appreciate the advantages of quantifying the motion of the pulse, even though he recognized the need for further study of why it beat at different rates in different diseases, and confessed in his 1796 monograph that the average rate per minute for the normal adult pulse was still unsettled.[18]

While some doctors in the early 1800s counted pulse beats, many complained that the excessive diagnostic refinements generated by pulse data, of any kind, complicated rather than clarified diagnosis and therapy.[19] Laennec called attention to the deficiencies of pulse as an index of the state of the heart and circulation, and cautioned physicians against relying on it.[20]

This was the climate in 1835 when a French physician, Julius Hérisson, introduced a machine he named the sphygmometer. It transmitted the impulses of the pulse beat to a column of mercury, thus rendering every pulse action apparent to the eye, such as the irregularity of the intervals between pulse beats, or the duration and force of contractions. Hérisson constructed the instrument from a thin glass tube marked with graduated figures, to which he attached a mercury–filled cup around whose rim was stretched a skin. Pressing the cup to an artery transmitted its impulse to the mercury, whose rise and fall in height provided a numerical portrait of all the pulse movements.

The idea of making the motions of the blood visible had occurred first to Stephen Hales. He had described, in his 1773 book *Statical Essays: Containing Hemastaticks*, an experiment in which he inserted a 9-foot glass tube into the artery of a horse, noted the height to which the blood rose in the tube (indicating its pressure), and the movements that occurred with each pulsation.[21] His main interest, however, had been in the blood's pressure rather than the characteristics of its motions. In 1828 the French physician Jean–Léonard-Marie Poiseuille, after examining Hales' work, conducted similar experiments; for Hales' long straight conduit he substituted a U–shaped tube partially filled with mercury which, like Hales' device, was directly inserted into an artery through a cannula.[22] Transmission of the blood's pulsations to the mercury permitted the force of the heartbeat to be calculated. The instrument, which he called a hemodynamometer, was an improvement over Hales' device because it was smaller and easier to work with. Poiseuille also used sodium carbonate to prevent the blood's coagulation and so to permit more lengthy experiments.

The inventions of Hales and Poiseuille were employed only on animals, however, for they all depended on the dangerous procedure of opening an artery. So Hérisson's sphygmometer, apparently developed without knowledge of Poiseuille's work, was the first device to visually portray and numerically measure the pulse beat without requiring puncture of an artery. Thus, clinical application became feasible.

Hérisson declared that the value of pulse – feeling had been debased by disputes about its characteristics: varying tactile sensations experienced by the physician when monitoring the pulse were too imprecise to allow an exact comparison to be made later. In contrast, the sphygmometer produced numerical results that gave the physician a description of the pulse he could easily compare with later observations. The instrument was eminently suited to the instructing of students, Hérisson believed, who now could judge pulse motions with their own eyes instead of having to rely, from lack of experience, on the word of their teachers. It permitted a group of physicians to observe the character of the pulse simultaneously, instead of one by one, each feeling the pulse and reporting his subjective sensations to the others. The sphygmometer also allowed for long-distance consultations by letter. Physicians in different cities distrusted the qualitative accounts of the pulses they had to accept when consulting each other through the mails, but "a far greater degree of accuracy may now be introduced into such a correspondence; the instrument being the same everywhere, the measure obtained at St. Petersburgh will be perfectly understood at Paris."[23]

The sphygmometer attracted several supporters. They claimed that the instrument could detect incipient disease in the heart and blood vessels by disclosing the slightest inequality of the pulse, and it therefore came to rival the diagnostic accuracy of the stethoscope. They further asserted that the numerical reports provided physi-

99

cians with results that could be more readily compared than the subjective sensations of touch. Yet to apply the sphygmograph to the patient required considerable skill. It was difficult to maintain the steady, unvarying maximum of pressure on the instrument necessary to make the column of mercury responsive to the pulse beat. This circumstance seemed to account for the discrepancy in findings of two observers, who were requested by the French Academy of Sciences to test the machine by taking pulse records on the same person. Another critic proclaimed the device a travesty: "One of the most silly and ridiculous baubles that was ever attempted to be foisted on the attention of the profession," and painted an amusing picture of using "a complicated piece of machinery for *seeing* the pulse, when it can be *felt* by the finger – the touch in this case, as in many others, being a thousand times less deceptive than the sight."[24] Although some physicians questioned the advantages of converting tactile into visual information, they also doubted whether the finer kinematics of the pulse could be appreciated through touch. The finger placed on an artery, they complained, detected only the grosser peculiarities of blood movement, such as force, frequency, and regularity.

In 1847, the German physiologist Carl Ludwig produced a variation of the U–shaped, mercury–filled tube that Poiseuille had designed to visualize arterial pulsations. On top of the mercury column Ludwig placed a float attached to a pen, which traced the motions communicated to it by the mercury onto a strip of paper stretched around a revolving drum. Ludwig called his instrument a kymographion.[25] The English physician–scientist Thomas Young was probably the first to conceive of recording the continuous motions of events taking place in extremely short intervals on a rotating cylinder. He had produced such a device in 1807 but did not exploit its potential in biology.[26] By modulating transient biological events into durable curves recorded on a graph, Ludwig's machine made these events more accessible to inquiry and transformed the study of circulatory and general physiology. The significance of this invention can be appreciated by recalling the problem William Harvey had encountered two centuries earlier, when he attempted to describe the beating heart as viewed by the naked eye, in his study of the blood's circulation. At first, he found the effort so arduous that he was tempted to think "that the motion of the heart was to be understood by God alone. I could not really tell when systole or diastole took place, or when and where dilatation or constriction occurred, because of the quickness of the movement. In many animals this takes place in the twinkling of an eye, like a flash of lightning. Systole seemed at one time here, diastole there, then all reversed, varied and confused. So I could reach no decision, neither about what I might conclude myself nor believe from others."[27]

Ludwig's kymographion was not used on human beings because, like the invention of Poiseuille, its application required that an artery be entered. The solution to this problem appeared in 1854 when Karl Vierordt introduced a machine called the sphygmograph, which connected Ludwig's pen and revolving drum device to an artery indirectly, by means of a spring pressed on the artery. The principle upon which Vierordt constructed the device – the application of pressure to detect motion – was the same one Hérisson had used in his invention; Vierordt, in essence, had substituted a graph–making component for the column of mercury employed by Hérisson. Yet Vierordt's machine was clumsy, tedious to operate, and produced tracings difficult to interpret. For these reasons, the device received only limited application but the principles of its construction survived – they needed only a more skillful mechanical interpretation.[28]

A turning point occurred in 1860. To help in research on the normal and pathological characteristics of the circulatory system, the French physician Etienne-Jules Marey developed an instrument he too called the sphygmograph.[29] His invention, the same in principle as Vierordt's but greatly simplified in design, had a lever, one end resting on a pulsating artery and the other connected to a pen. A clockwork mechanism moved a strip of smoked paper under the pen at uniform speed, converting the pulsations into a pictorial form (Figure 10). Since Marey lucidly explained the phenomena his instrument uncovered, and had carefully designed and constructed his machine, it met with a better reception than its predecessors. Its pulse tracing seemed to uncover some defects of the heart and blood vessels in their earliest stages, and so anticipated the sounds produced by these defects that the auscultator subsequently would hear. This sphygmograph's accurate monitoring of body functions enabled physicians to evaluate precisely the effects of certain drugs they administered to patients, and also restrained them from starting harmful therapy.[30]

Yet Marey and subsequent investigators warned that the character of normal circulation and the variations in the normal pulse trac-

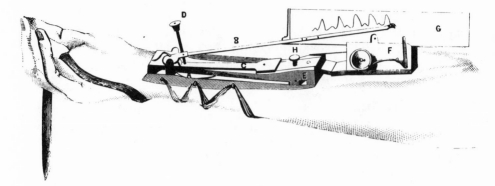

A, the pulse spring; B, the tracer, or writing lever; C, the lever for transmitting motion from the former to the latter (A to B); D, the pressure screw; E, the body of the instrument; F, the box containing clock-work; G, the traveller; H, the screw for adjusting pulse spring at a proper obliquity.

Figure 10. Marey's sphygmograph (1874). Reprinted from Edgar Holden, *The Sphygmograph: Its Physiological and Pathological Indications* (Philadelphia: Lindsay and Blakiston, 1874), frontispiece.

ing required further study, before definitive statements about sphygmographic evidence of disease could be relied upon. Physicians needed to understand the influence on the patient, and thus on the tracing, of work, effort, eating, heat, and emotion. The physician was cautioned against precipitate introduction of the sphygmograph into the consulting room, given the imperfect knowledge of the relation between the trace markings and the physiological disorders that they were supposed to indicate. If he disregarded this caveat, the clinician would "inevitably obtain fallacious indications, which will disgust him with the instrument, and induce him to throw undeserved discredit on a mode of investigation which he has really never properly understood."[31]

Despite such cautions, some physicians accepted too readily and exclusively Marey's views on the form of the pulse curve. As a result, they overlooked some unexplained undulations in the most significant portion of the curve, whose discovery cast doubt upon the reliability of the sphygmograph and pulse record. Eventually it was demonstrated that the undulations in question were normal features of pulse movement.[32] Trouble for users of the machine did not end with this episode. As the number and types of sphygmographs grew, different sphygmographs, varying in construction, bred different curves in response to the same pulse stimulus. The result was that for the old signs of disease, discovered by feeling the pulse, were substituted numerous sphygmograms, empirically linked to different disorders, which seemed to reflect idiosyncrasies of the instrument rather than peculiarities of the pulse.[33]

Physicians prescribed a two–pronged remedy to secure uniform and comparable sphygmographic tracings. One approach dealt with the machine's construction – either make a single form of the instrument, or standardize the building of different brands. The second related to the doctor's procedure – he should take sphygmographic readings from the same artery and should monitor his patient's activities, such as eating or exercise, to ensure that the readings were made under approximately equivalent physiological conditions. But even with such precautions, experience with the sphygmograph disclosed that no matter how the physician applied the instrument, he invariably introduced a bias into his work. Where and how much pressure to apply to an artery to obtain the best tracing; which of the many tracings produced most accurately revealed the pathology sought after – all required the investigator to make human judgments. Thus, while some physicians expected the sphygmograph to produce accurate records of physiological functions independent of the operator, and to generate the same record whether handled by a novice or an expert, other physicians were aware the instrument did not speak for itself. Its answers varied with the construction of the machine, the anatomical and physiological peculiarities of the patient, and the partiality and dexterity of the operator.[34]

Nevertheless, advocates of the sphygmograph continued to believe that the machine was a more accurate recorder of data than man, and that "the finer features of arterial pulsation which escaped recognition by our mere sense of touch have been elucidated by its aid. What appeared to our fingers as a single or occasionally a double beat has been broken up into its component parts."[35] The sphygmograph also reinforced the notion that when sensory phenomena were metamorphosed into visual form, they assumed a more objective character.

One of the problems lay in the fact that the physician still found it hard to transpose into words the information received by touch, and then to adequately communicate the message to others: he might acquire "the habit of discriminating pulses instinctively [and learn] valuable truths from it, which he can apply to practice. Yet how difficult – how impossible – is it for the skilled physician to impart his knowledge to his less experienced junior!"[36] Each new physician had to master the art of pulse feeling largely on his own. Under these circumstances, disagreement was inevitable, because physicians could not agree upon a yardstick by which to judge the meaning of a given pulse sign. Experienced doctors gathered together to examine the same pulse and to describe their impressions would give different accounts of what they felt.

But the sphygmograph transformed the subjective character of pulse feeling into an objective, visual, graphic representation that was a permanent record of the transient event, amenable to study and criticism alone or by groups of physicians. Some advocates were persuaded that the sphygmograph might reduce the diagnosis of heart and arterial disease to a process of self–registration. They raised the prospect of ending dependence on hereditary endowment or the first-rate education of outstanding physicians to produce trustworthy judgments, relying instead on the machine's certain and continuous superiority of performance.[37]

Paralleling this attention to the graphic depiction of the pulse, there were a few isolated efforts to transpose other fleeting motions of the body into lasting records. The English heart expert William Gairdner, in 1861, schematically represented in graphs the time intervals between normal heart sounds and abnormal murmurs heard through the stethoscope. While listening to the heart with his stethoscope, he converted evanescent murmurs into immutable visual portraits of hand–drawn rising and falling lines, and through this transformation of one set of signals into another increased the understanding of the heart's action.[38] Several years later, Hyde Salter described the spirograph, an invention which automatically produced tracings of chest movements during breathing. Salter compared his tracings to a photograph, and believed that the physician who used them would eliminate personal bias from medical judgments on the chest. The patient's breath would be, as it were, the hand that moved the stylus, uninfluenced by the subjective judgment of patient or doctor – a perfectly objective diagnostic system.[39] Yet during the 1860s, graphic depiction of body motions, mainly represented by the sphygmograph, still seemed unnecessary to most physicians, too complicated or untrustworthy to apply in general clinical practice.

During the 1870s, the English clinician F. A. Mahomed turned back to the generally neglected sphygmograph in a pioneering effort to establish that a persistently high blood pressure was a useful sign of cardiovascular disease. He believed that older methods to gauge the blood's pressure – feeling the pulse and analyzing the character of the heart's sounds – were unreliable, but he found that the sphygmograph provided an objective, more precise account of the phenomena.[40] The measurements taken with the sphygmograph proved, as before, excessively complicated for general medical use.

However, while Mahomed was at work with the sphygmograph, a notable advance in measuring blood pressure was occurring. In 1876 Samuel von Basch had introduced a machine called the sphygmomanometer, which eliminated the cumbersome mechanical problems of blood–pressure measurements using the sphygmograph. His invention had a rubber bulb filled with water, which the doctor pressed directly on an artery until the pulse disappeared anterior to the point on the limb at which the apparatus was applied. By connecting this bulb to a mercury–pressure gauge, the doctor obtained a reading of the pressure necessary to compress the artery, and hence the blood's force. Other physicians began to experiment with modifications of this design, among them Pierre–Carl–Edouard Potain, who substituted an air– for a water–filled bulb as the compressing force. Yet none of the instruments made before 1896 met all the requirements necessary for common use by physicians: reasonable accuracy, easy application, portability, and automatic results that left little room for human error. Then in 1896, the Italian physician Scipione Riva–Rocci overcame these technical difficulties by devising an instrument whose innovative character was constricting the flow of blood in an artery by circular compression of the arm. He fastened a rubber bag around the upper portion of the arm, raised the pressure in the bag by pumping air into it, and measured the pressure by connecting the bag to a mercury column. The level of mercury at the moment when the examiner felt the pulse disappear at the wrist represented the maximum blood pressure.[41] Riva–Rocci's invention became the prototype of contemporary blood-pressure instruments.

In 1905, the Russian physician Nikolai Korotkoff proposed that instead of feeling the pulse to determine endpoints in blood–pressure readings, the physician listen for a pulse beat from the artery in the pit of the elbow, while, by means of a Riva-Rocci device, the blood flow above the elbow was first stopped and then gradually allowed to return. The reading on the manometer when the first sound appeared corresponded to the maximum blood pressure. The time of disappearance or fading out of the sounds marked the minimum blood pressure in the artery. Although monitoring the pulse through touch had been accurate in determining the maximum, or systolic, blood pressure, it was not as reliable in detecting the point of minimum, or diastolic, blood pressure. The Korotkoff method proved superior to touch as a means of recognizing blood pressure. In little over a decade after its introduction, it had largely replaced the pulse–feeling method and continues to be used today.[42]

The new blood–pressure machines gained the support of Harvey Cushing, the American brain surgeon. During the twentieth century's first decade, Cushing was convinced that surgeons, even more than physicians, needed some practical instrument to record variations in blood pressure in precise, numerical terms. The surgeon's traditional reliance on the anesthetist's subjective, tactile–based impressions of the pulse's character as a measure of cardiac strength was one of the most trying aspects of operations. If the surgeon could know cardiac strength with the definiteness that numbers alone gave, the risks of operations would decrease.[43] Manufacturers of this period successfully reduced mechanical defects in the blood–pressure instruments, while doctors fixed a numerical standard of normal pressure by which to gauge abnormal readings, and defined those diseases (particularly of the heart and kidney) in which a change in blood pressure was a crucial sign. In 1912, doctors at the Massachusetts General Hospital in Boston began to measure the blood pressure of all entering patients.[44]

A machine that tracked the path of the heart's electrical current was also introduced at the dawn of the twentieth century. During the nineteenth century, research by Heinrich Müller, Rudolph von Kölliker, and Franciscus Donders had shown in animals that currents were generated during the heartbeat. A significant breakthrough occurred in 1887 when the English doctor Augustus D. Waller, using an electrometer invented in 1872 by Gabriel Lippmann which registered small and rapidly fluctuating electrical potentials, for the first time recorded the electrical currents generated in the human heart, and demonstrated the feasibility of transcribing these impulses from the surface of the body without penetrating the skin. He did this by strapping a pair of electrodes (zinc covered by chamois leather and moistened with brine) to the front and back of a man's chest. When he linked this to a Lippmann electrometer, the mercury in the electrometer moved slightly but sharply with the heartbeat: "If the movements of the column of mercury are photographed on a travelling plate simultaneously with those of an ordinary cardiographic lever a record is obtained."[45] Waller thus founded human electrocardiography. His disclosures led physicians to appreciate that alterations in the time sequence of the currents generated by the heartbeat could advance the diagnosis of its disorders. Nevertheless, the Lippmann electrometer was difficult to handle and liable to break down. Because its response was too slow to render an immediate and faithful record of electrical changes, the interpretation of the curves plotted from its readings required mathematical transformations. Except in the hands of a trained physicist willing to spend much time on it, the instrument was unsatisfactory.

Willem Einthoven, a Dutch physiologist, overcame these obstacles with his string galvanometer type of electrocardiograph, first described in 1901. Einthoven anchored the ends of a silver–coated conducting string midway between two magnetic poles. Each end of the string was connected, by wire, to a liquid–filled electrode jar, in which the patient immersed his limbs (Figure 11). As electrical changes occurred in the heart, the string oscillated from side to side between the two magnets. A projective microscope transmitted a magnified image of the motions of the oscillating string onto a moving photographic plate, thus creating a fixed record of the heart's electrical activity. The temporal sequence of these events was measured by a time marker placed between the photographic plate and the projecting microscope. Einthoven's lucid account of the principles of electrocardiography, together with the general interest in developing new uses for electricity, led physicians all over the world to experiment with the device.[46] Yet the high cost of the apparatus (between $400 and $1000),[47] and a number of other problems stood in the way of its immediate clinical use. Until a sufficient number of autopsies could be performed to correlate anatomical lesions with electrocardiographic tracings, a trustworthy standard by which to judge normal and abnormal actions of the heart could not be defined. In addition, the machine failed to register pathology in some patients who had a definite disease of the heart. These shortcomings, plus the machine's complexity and delicacy, and the need for considerable skill in operating it, rendered Einthoven's electrocardiograph unsuitable for gen-

107

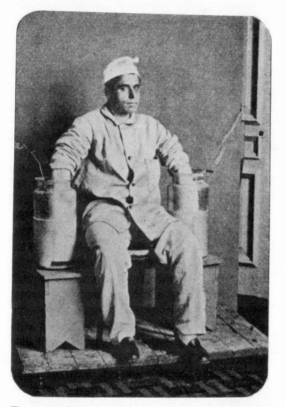

Figure 11. Patient attached to Einthoven's string galvanometer. Reprinted from W. Einthoven, "Le Télécardiogramme," *Archives Internationales de Physiologie*, vol. 4 (1906–07), p. 143.

eral practice, and confined its use chiefly to large hospitals and research laboratories.[48]

Nevertheless, an electrical record of the heart provided a totally new perspective on the normal and pathological behavior of the organ, by depicting the character of its contractions and rhythm better than any other existing procedure. The electrocardiograph could confirm diagnoses based on historical narrative and physical signs and, even better, could signal the beginning of disease before these signs appeared. It alone revealed the electrical impulses that produced the disturbances in rhythm detected by older machines, such as the sphygmograph, and helped to distinguish rhythmical abnormalities that did not adversely influence the health, from those that did. The electrocardiograph was not intended to supplant the trained hand, ear, or eye in diagnosing heart disease, but its reception clearly indicated the beginning of a movement toward that goal.[49]

By 1912, Thomas Lewis, an English physician whose work in electrocardiography won him international fame, declared that "the time is at hand, if it has not already come, when an examination of the heart is incomplete if this new method is neglected."[50] Physicians praised Einthoven's instrument as so accurate that any observer could duplicate the results upon the same patient, even if they did not use the same machine. Apart from certain unpredictable influences on the electrocardiogram, or EKG, as it became known, such as the unavoidable changes in resistance within the human body, Einthoven declared that "the form of the EKG. is independent of the instrument used, and every EKG., when and where it may have been recorded, is immediately comparable with every other EKG."[51] Belief in such standardization, which required minimal skill to procure good results and so equalized the abilities of different observers, was a crucial factor in the instrument's growing reputation.

While it was not yet possible to define a precise normal standard for the electrocardiogram, the curves produced by the hearts of different people being as diverse as their facial characteristics, the tracing from a given individual maintained a constancy in health, and did not radically depart from a recognizable form. This pattern encompassed three principal deflections – a small, rounded elevation, followed by a sharp peak, followed by another rounded elevation, usually larger than the first. During the decade 1910–19, physicians welcomed the electrocardiograph as a way of capturing transient clinical events through visual records; they referred to "the graphic age," and wrote reverently of the graphic record of the heart's electrical activities: "The little strips of paper, imprinted by the disease itself, form permanent and unquestionable testimony of events which have occurred."[52]

An important figure in making the electrocardiograph the widely used instrument that it is today was the American physician James B. Herrick. In a paper read before the Association of American Physicians in 1912, he had argued that an occlusion of the coronary arteries of the heart was not a rare pathologic curiosity, as then widely thought, but a common condition that physicians could diagnose from the patient's history and physical condition. His claim failed to stir interest at the meeting or when published shortly after. Herrick continued to press his view but drew little notice until in 1918 he presented a new paper on the subject to this same association. This time he bolstered his claim with evidence that coronary–artery occlusion produced specific and characteristic changes in a patient's electrocardiogram. He showed that an abnormal electrocardiogram, particularly if accompanied by clinical symptoms suggestive of coronary occlusion, enabled physicians to assert "with a reasonable degree of certainty that the patient has had obstruction in a particular portion of the coronary system."[53] This technical corroboration stirred the interest of physicians in his work. Subsequent studies established coronary–artery pathology as a major cause of illness, and gave a new and lasting measure of importance to the electrocardiograph in medicine.

Graphic and numerical methods in medicine received another important and widespread application in connection with the measure of body heat. Since earliest civilization, physicians had recognized elevation of temperature as an important sign of disease, and detected it either from the patient's own report or by placing a hand on the patient's body. The credit for inventing an instrument to measure changes in temperature should probably be assigned to Galileo. The device, which he invented between 1593 and 1597, is described in a letter by Father Benedetto Castelli, as he recalled an experiment he had seen Galileo conduct in 1603: "Galileo took a glass vessel about the size of a hen's egg, fitted to a tube the width of a straw and about two spans long; he heated the glass bulb in his hands and turned the glass upside down so that the tube dipped in water held in another vessel; as soon as the bulb cooled down the water rose in the tube to the height of a span above the level in the vessel; this instrument he used to investigate degrees of heat and cold."[54] Galileo apparently did not use the thermometer to explore temperature change in disease. In the seventeenth century, Santorio Santorio, who had also experimented with devices to count the pulse, became the first person to make extensive attempts to quantitatively estimate the temperature in the human body, and thus obviate the need for subjective evaluations by patient or doctor. He constructed for this purpose several thermometric devices (Figure 12) with which he could "closely measure the degree of the

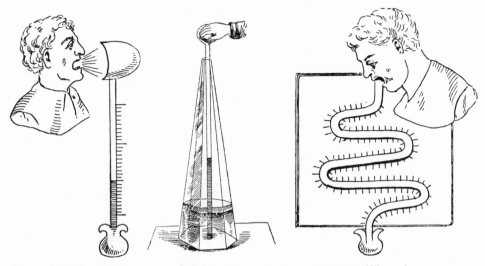

Figure 12. Thermometers constructed by Santorio Santorio (1625). When the upper parts were blown upon, or held in hand or mouth, the air in the instruments expanded, forced the water in the lower parts downwards, and so measured the person's temperature. Reprinted from S. Weir Mitchell, *The Early History of Instrumental Precision in Medicine* (1892), pp. 14–16.

recession of the heat of the external parts . . .so that we can thus tell, if the patient be better or worse."[55]

However, during the seventeenth and eighteenth centuries, controversy occurred as to the thermometer's value and accuracy, and limited its use. Robert Boyle, the English scientist reported in 1683 that the thermometer might seem to many "a work of needless Curiosity, or superfluous diligence." It appeared "impertinent to seek for any other judges of It [cold] than the Organs of that sense, whose proper object it is."[56]

Use of the thermometer was also hindered by a prolonged dispute concerning the instrument's accuracy. The disagreement centered principally on two aspects: the material used to indicate changes in heat, and the standards employed to graduate its scale of measurement. Early seventeenth–century thermometers which used the expansion and contraction of air acting on water to disclose heat changes, after the example of Galileo, were inaccurate because the air index was influenced by the weight of the atmosphere. The enclosure of a fluid within a hermetically sealed glass tube, an invention produced by Ferdinand II, Grand Duke of Tuscany, in the

111

mid–seventeenth century rescued thermometers from the influence of atmospheric pressure.[57] Yet debate continued about the question of what fluid would best register temperature change.

Highly rectified "spirit of wine," weakened spirit of wine, linseed oil, and mercury were among the indicators investigated. All of these fluids had defects in their temperature–measuring properties. The extremes of heat that spirit of wine could register were limited: it froze at very low temperatures, boiled at high ones. Moreover, different strengths of the wine responded differently to temperature. Linseed oil adhered too much to the sides of the thermometer, disturbing the regularity and uniformity with which the fluid moved in the instrument. Quicksilver seemed the most reliable fluid: it responded to heat and cold more rapidly than the others, never froze, boiled only at great temperatures, and did not stick to the sides of the thermometers, if well purified. But it did not expand as well as some of the other materials.[58]

More perplexing and controversial than the type of fluid to use was settling upon a standard by which to graduate the temperature scale. Various investigators and instrument makers fashioned thermometers according to different, often indeterminate standards. Thus, thermometers and the observations of different observers could not be compared. "We are very much to seek for a Standard or certain Measure of Cold," urged Robert Boyle, "as we have settled Standards for weight, and magnitude, and time, so that when a man mentions an Acre, or an Ounce, or an Hour; they that hear him, know what he means."[59] The boiling point of well–rectified wine was advocated as a standard by the astronomer Edmund Halley.[60] Boyle suggested the freezing point of oil of aniseed, or the temperature in a certain English cave, whose warmth did not vary in summer or winter. (This last suggestion drew criticism as a most inconvenient measure by which to construct thermometers: "Everybody cannot go to Mr. Boyle's grotto.")[61] But all of these standards based on a single index had a common flaw: the expansion and contraction of the thermometer's liquid indicator from one point subjected the graduation of thermometers to more errors than if two or more points were used at a convenient distance from each other.

To many observers, the boiling point and freezing point of water appeared most convenient as standards. Yet both of these yardsticks were criticized. The boiling point of water was objected to because it changed in response to alterations in atmospheric pressure. But supporters argued that the temperature at which water boiled was constant under ordinary circumstances of weather change, and that the standard could even be pegged to a specific atmospheric pressure – say boiling temperature at a barometric reading of 30 inches.[62] Distrust of the constancy of the temperature at which water froze was based on reports that it was influenced by climate and geography. But supporters of this standard thought these reported differences were artifacts – the result of careless observation or inadequate construction of the instruments used. From his own experiments, in the middle of the eighteenth century, the Scottish physician George Martine concluded "the *freezing point* to be a very constant and settled degree of heat, more fixed and determined than even that of *boiling water*, and consequently very fit to be one of the fixed limits in adjusting our Thermometers."[63] The diameter of the thermometer's base, the size of its bulb, and the character of its glass were other elements of its construction that could influence readings.

At least some of these problems were resolved at the beginning of the eighteenth century, when the Dutch instrument maker Gabriel Daniel Fahrenheit developed an improved technique of thermometer construction, and employed a group of points for the temperature scale that appreciably advanced the reliability of the thermometer. Using mercury as his registering fluid Fahrenheit pegged the temperature scale to three points: a zero mark – determined by the temperature of a mixture of ice, water, and sal–ammoniac or sea–salt; a 32–degree mark – the freezing point of water; and a 96–degree mark – the external temperature of the human body recorded by his instrument. It is a measure of his accomplishment that, when he gave two thermometers to the Chancellor of the University of Halle, Christian Wolf, which exactly agreed with each other in their register of temperature, the chancellor considered the event impressive enough to publicize in a scholarly paper.[64]

The improved thermometers available thereafter in the 1700s were used by Hermann Boerhaave, who persuaded Fahrenheit to construct for him a special thermometer to evaluate fevers.[65] However, Boerhave's applications of the instrument were limited in comparison with those of his pupil Anton de Haen. He used temperature changes as a guide to therapy, and regarded a return to normal temperature as a clear sign of recovery. De Haen was particularly impressed with the disparity in temperature readings when the feelings of the patient were compared with the numerical report of the instrument.[66] Noteworthy thermometric studies also were conducted in the eighteenth century by Martine, who investigated the heat of animate and inanimate bodies and variations in different thermometers,[67] and by James Currie, who tried to predict the course of certain diseases by following the alterations in temperature.[68]

None of these efforts encouraged the average physician to take up thermometry. Despite improvements, the thermometer seemed troublesome, untrustworthy, and inessential. The use of different scales to measure temperature, and the imperfection and inaccuracy of many instruments still in use, continued to prevent the ready comparison of observations made with different instruments.[69] Many physicians believed too, with one of Boerhaave's disciples Gerard van Swieten, that the pulse provided more important information about fever than the temperature.[70] Further, like their seventeenth–century predecessors, many physicians of the eighteenth century thought that a quantitative measure of body heat, made with an instrument, did not convey as much data as a qualitative evaluation, made with the hand. For example, at the end of the century a French physician criticized heat–measuring instruments as indicating "no more than the degrees of intensity of heat; and these differences are the least important in practice; . . . the doctor must apply himself, above all, to distinguishing in feverish heat qualities that may be perceived only by a highly practiced touch. . .There is, for example, that acrid, irritating quality of feverish heat."[71] But crucial for the acceptance of thermometry, and as yet unwritten, was a comprehensive treatise that would convince physicians that quantitative estimates of fever were valuable.

During the first third of the nineteenth century, diagnosis advanced by localizing disease through the techniques of physical diagnosis and the autopsy. Consequently, physicians tended to ignore signs of disease that represented general functional disturbances in the body, such as temperature alterations.[72] This became an added reason for the disregard of thermometry which, as a physician remarked in 1839, "has been more neglected than formerly, and indeed remains almost in *statu quo*."[73]

In the 1840s, however, interest revived in temperature movement during health and illness. Gabriel Andral, in his *Lectures on General Pathology* (1841), attempted to formulate rules about temperature variation in disease.[74] In 1844, Henri Roger published a monograph that examined the normal temperature of children at birth, and explored the course of the temperature in a great variety of illnesses,[75] a contribution whose significance was unfortunately reduced by the absence of repeated observations (he often measured the temperature only once during the course of an illness). Beginning in 1846, an army surgeon, George Zimmerman, began to publish essays which contained valuable observations on temperature, particularly its elevation in local inflammation, and which also reproached colleagues who neglected the thermometer.[76]

The evolution of medical thermometry entered a new phase when the German physicians F. W. F. von Bärensprung and Ludwig Traube, between 1850 and 1851, began to use temperature signs as basic data to diagnose diseases, predict their course, and determine therapy.[77] Von Bärensprung went beyond collecting fragmentary evidence about temperature, to construct a comprehensive statement of its expression in disease. Yet his work did not influence physicians in a manner commensurate with its merits, largely because of his excessive detail. He expressed temperature readings in numbers carried to two decimal places, attached significance to deviations of one–tenth of a degree or less, and recommended that the physician spend half an hour in taking a thermometric observation. These requirements made the instrument almost impossible to use during office practice, home visits, and even in hospitals. However, Traube took a more practical view about use, and was successful in persuading colleagues to employ the thermometer, one of whom was a young physician, Carl Wunderlich. He became a dominant figure in thermometry when, in 1857, he published his first paper on the subject.[78] an elaborate discourse stressing the importance of keeping daily temperature records. Wunderlich's paper stirred others to appreciate the importance of frequent temperature readings. By the end of the 1860s, physicians in England and the United States were beginning to applaud the value of temperature readings gained through the thermometer, and to criticize the accuracy of the subjective judgments of fever. Austin Flint, the American physician, advised his colleagues that "the information obtained by merely placing the hand on the body of the patient is inaccurate and unreliable. If it be desirable to count the pulse and not trust to the judgment to estimate the number of beats per minute, it is far more desirable to ascertain the animal heat by means of a heat measurer. The sensations of the patient with respect to temperature, as everyone knows, are extremely fallacious; he may suffer from a feeling of heat when, to the touch of another, the surface is cold, and *vice versa.*"[79]

Two factions of doctors still imperiled the thermometer's wide use during the 1860s: one group considered it an unnecessary medical detail, a scientific toy; another group, expecting too much from the instrument, claimed a use for it in almost every disease (often without adequate evidence), and evoked complaints of "practitioners brandishing the thermometer with such an air, and applying it to such strange purposes, as remind us . . . of the stethoscope in its early days."[80] A work that summarized thermometric theory and experience was obviously needed to analyze the vast store of facts being accumulated, and to forestall the growing danger that an altogether mistaken view of the function and value of the thermometer would prevail.

Into this climate Wunderlich, in 1868, introduced his treatise, *On the Temperature in Diseases;* it rapidly became a classic and was translated into English only three years after its publication in German. The book commented upon the information then known about thermometry and, like Morgagni's *The Seats and Causes of Diseases* and Laennec's *On Mediate Auscultation*, became the touchstone by which to evaluate all earlier and later work on the subject. Wunderlich had compiled thermometric observations on almost 25,000 patients, the number of single readings being in the millions. He amassed voluminous data to determine the actual facts, uninfluenced by theory, regarding the role of temperature in disease. He divided the volume into two parts. The first comprehensively outlined the fundamental components of thermometric observation, and the value of the thermometer in medical practice, the art of using it, and the genesis of temperature alterations in disease. The second discussed temperature variations in 32 common disorders, and served as a guide to everyday practice. Wunderlich declared thermometry superior to all other diagnostic techniques. Whereas other methods distinguished permanent or at best slowly changing damage produced by disease, ephemeral oscillations could be easily measured by the thermometer. The temperature also expressed the sum of physiological activity in the body; it opened up domains of diseased life inaccessible to other methods of exploration. Most important, the thermometric reading was expressed in numbers, which were more reliable than subjective impressions. Wisely, Wunderlich emphasized that complete accuracy was unattainable and was unnecessary for the clinical use of the thermometer. For the average case, errors of one–half a degree centigrade (or 0.9°F) were scarcely worth mentioning, and readings taken twice a day were sufficient. Although certain types of illness required greater precision and more readings, frequent repetition was more essential than absolute accuracy.[81]

Although he insisted that questions of purely scientific interest required the highest exactness, Wunderlich avoided the mistake of his predecessor von Bärensprung, by recognizing that adoption of the thermometer was unlikely if he imposed the standards of the laboratory on events at the bedside. He also considered it unnecessary for the physician himself to take the temperature readings. Any trustworthy, intelligent person with sharp eyes could quickly be taught the procedure, for the doctor's role was "not merely taking observations, but the superintendence, control, and right interpretation of them. The mere reading of thermometer degrees helps diagnosis no more than dispensing does therapeusis."[82] Other physicians agreed with this view point. If meteorologists and astronomers allowed technical observations to be made by people not involved in their interpretation, why could not doctors do the same? A dependable person with little or no medical knowledge might even make fewer errors than doctors in reading temperatures, because he would have no preconceived opinions to prejudice him and would see things as they really occurred. Hence, alert, well–instructed clinical assistants, nurses, or relatives could be more useful colleagues to the physician.[83]

A concept was thus elaborated that would help later physicians to justify their delegating diagnostic tasks to other health workers: that the skills needed to report objective information produced by self–registering instruments could be separated from those skills needed to interpret such information. The first could be acquired without extensive training, the second could be developed only by years of medical education and medical practice.[84]

Wunderlich had accomplished his transformation of medical thermometry by demonstrating that a constant temperature prevailed in a healthy human being, and that certain patterns of temperature variation were characteristic of certain diseases. He established the mobility of temperature as the cardinal hallmark of disease, and its normality as the principal sign of health. Wunderlich constructed for each patient a temperature curve that portrayed the rise and fall of body heat during the total course of the illness. By making a graph that represented the average swings of

117

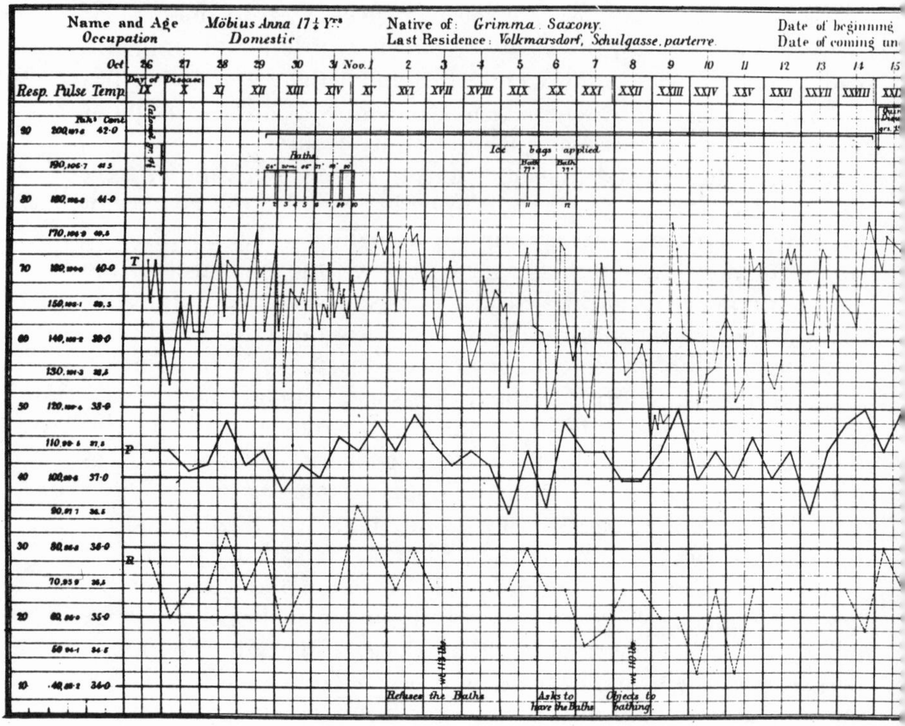

Figure 13. Graphic representation of the temperature, pulse, and respiration. Reprinted from C.A. Wunderlich, *On the Temperature in Diseases* (1871), Table I.

temperature from many patients with the same disorder, Wunderlich obtained the typical temperature portrait of a given disease. He believed that future doctors would extract from thermometric observations the principles that determined the natural course of disease and would thus establish, as Laennec and his followers also had hoped, "the domain of *law in disease*."[85]

Wunderlich's treatise elevated thermometry to a highly regarded diagnostic technique in the 1870s. Many physicians declared that thermometer readings were beyond control of the patient's will, or of extraneous circumstances, and thus were unerringly accurate. The instrument seemed to work by itself: "While the doctor is chatting with his patient, or interrogating the friends, the thermometer may be silently recording its truthful tale in the patient's axilla."[86] Patients, too, accepted the thermometer, while some even attributed therapeutic power to it. One young woman convalescing

118

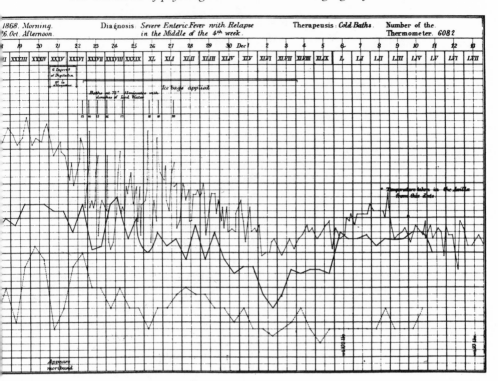

from an illness suffered a relapse and ascribed it to "having no glass under her arm for a week."[87] The thermometer also encouraged the growing belief that the physiological forces expressing health and disease could be measured precisely. It redirected the attention of the physician to numeration not only of the temperature, but to pulse and respiratory rates, thereby establishing this trio of signs, usually recorded in the form of a graph on the patient's chart, as the most important quantitative expressions of the body's healthy state (Figure 13).

Despite its triumphs, the thermometer continued to meet opposition during the 1870s and 1880s. Some practitioners distrusted the thermometric readings taken by nurses or others to whom the task was delegated, yet were unwilling to spend time in making the observations themselves. The large amount of data generated by the thermometer also caused dissatisfaction: "With its unavoidable escort of millions of facts, and with diagrams whose curves would compete with the waves of the ocean. . .clinical thermometry makes upon the mind of the practitioner first, an impression of awe, second, one of disappointment which too often is the last one."[88] Some fear existed that thermometry would become the special province of hospital clinicians, who could command the labor of a large staff; indeed, physicians paid greater attention to thermometry within than outside of the hospital.[89] Other doctors worried that by attaching so much importance to the thermometer's findings, colleagues would sometimes fail to adequately explore the other circumstances of illness, the object of therapy becoming only a reduction of the temperature: "The temperature chart, with all its graceful curves and geometric lines and angles, may please the vanity of the devotee of instruments of precision, while, undetected by the skilled touch, the depressed heart may suddenly 'cease at once to work and live.' "[90] This problem grew during the 1890s when drugs that could reduce fever became widely used: "The doctor, stimulated by the wish of patient and friends," pushed the antipyretics and noted "with satisfaction the temperature chart." But this sometimes led him to neglect other signs, and to misdiagnose or inadequately treat the patient's fever.[91]

Some patients objected to frequent temperature readings, or to the way the information was used. Although the patient and his friends often misunderstood the meaning of temperature variations, they would sometimes demand to know the exact figures, and become agitated at any increase. Some doctors tried to distract the patient's attention from the thermometer, by discreetly shaking the true reading down to a point that would please the patient. At other times, physicians were driven to use the thermometer to augment the credibility of their medical judgments:

Mrs. _____ with her daughter, after an opinion by myself that the daughter's trouble was purely 'bronchial.' 'Sure,' says the mother, 'doctor, you didn't try the little glass thing that goes in the mouth? Sure, Mrs. Mc_____ towld me that you would put a little glass thing in her mouth, and that would tell just where the disease was, entirely.' I used the 'little glass thing,' and thereby suited the interested mother at once; and I dare say, that while my opinion was taken as absolute after using the thermometer, it would not have been taken had I not used it; but a doctor would have been found who used the 'glass thing.' Again, where will it end? Shall we practice regular deceit, or shall we bulletin at each visit the exact condition to friends and patient?[92]

Doubt about the value of thermometric readings grew when flaws were found in thermometers that even reputable manufacturers produced. Leonard Waldo of the Yale College Observatory issued a report in 1880 showing that most of the several thousand thermometers, annually being made and purchased in the United States, were untrustworthy for want of a correct standard by which to set the instruments.[93] Experiments in the United States, Great Britain, and Germany, in which thermometric readings of different brands of instruments were compared with a standard, showed a disheartening variation: "One naturally asks himself, What use is thermometry at all?" wrote Moritz Immisch, himself an inventor of a widely used thermometer.[94] In the United States some physicians attributed the problem to competition in business, and the absence of a scientific institution to verify the accuracy of the instrument. The publicity had a salutary effect. Manufacturers and physicians in large numbers took advantage of an offer by Yale to certify thermometers at its astronomical observatory, following the example of the English who accepted a similar proposal from the Kew Observatory. Certification restored confidence in the device.

The conversion of physiological signals generated by respiration, circulation, and heat production, into graphs and numbers, allowed physicians to obtain clear and accurate records; to preserve these signals so that changes in pattern could be studied over time; to free these signals from the limitations of private analysis – necessary when they were individually monitored by the natural senses – and open them to group inquiry; to make them objective and to invest them with unambiguous meanings that were evident to all physicians. Hutchinson, Marey, Einthoven, and Wunderlich shared a belief that any physician who was industrious and moderately intelligent could successfully apply mechanical devices to monitor subtle bodily changes. Against the exquisite judgment and the extensive memory of talented physicians these advocates matched the impartiality and constancy of machines, believing that most of the time the physicians placed second–best.

6 *Chemical signposts of disease and the birth of the diagnostic laboratory*

The induction of chemistry into the service of diagnosis had its principal beginnings in the sixteenth century. This was an age when physicians widely resorted to uroscopy, an ancient art whose practitioners focused on the visible features of urine – a fluid then thought to reflect the state of many parts of the body – to gain knowledge of the patient's illness. Practitioners usually examined urine in a bladder–shaped glass called a matula (Figure 14), in which they generally distinguished four regions, each of which was supposed to represent a part of the patient's anatomy: the uppermost region stood for the the patient's head, the one below for the chest, the third down for the abdomen, and the lowest for the urogenital system. The seat of the illness and its nature were determined from the many shades of color that the urine could assume, and the movement of urinary sediments from one region to the next. This made a large number of variations possible, and suggested many different diagnoses.[1]

During the sixteenth century some physicians disapproved the diagnosis of disease from the visible character of the urine. One of the most prominent critics was the Swiss doctor Paracelsus. He recommended chemical analysis to expose signs of disease hidden from practitioners who merely inspected the fluid visually. His method was to distill the urine to separate its parts. From the quality and quantity of distillates and residue left he deduced the nature of the ailment.

Paracelsus' advocacy of chemical diagnosis was criticized, like the uroscopy based on the urine's visible characteristics, for drawing physicians' attention away from other indices of disease. Since Paracelsus had given instructions for "reading" the deposits produced by distillation, some followers constructed elaborate distillation stills, whose parts corresponded to the human body and were

122

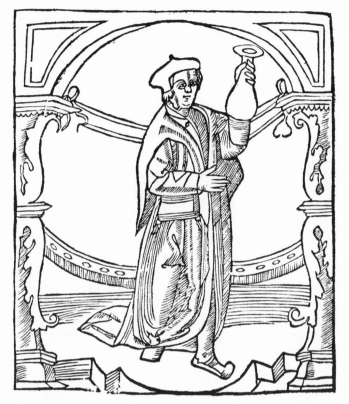

Figure 14. Inspection of the urine in the early sixteenth century. Reprinted from *The Judicial of Urines* (London: Peter Treveris, 1527), frontispiece.

used to determine the seat of disease from the sequence in which the distillates rose and location of the deposits. They have been therefore accused of merely maintaining "the old idea of 'uroscopy' – but with a chemical twist."[2] Nevertheless, the notion of Paracelsus and his followers that chemical analysis and quantitative evaluations of the weight and volume of urine should become features of medical practice was novel and far-reaching.

An advocate for chemical diagnosis in the following century, the English physician Thomas Willis, in his 1684 *Practice of Physick*, also criticized those who drew hasty conclusions from examining the urine's visible features, and commented that "the Medicasters and Quacks for the most part behold the urine sent in a Glass, shake it a little, and presently give Judgment."[3] To evaluate changes

123

in the body's elements caused by disease, Willis suggested evaporation, distillation, and precipitation of the urine; he illustrated his advice with a case.

Not so long since I evaporated the urine of a Gentleman, grievously subject to convulsive motions and painful stretchings out of the Muscles, in the bottom of which there remained a quantity of salt and tartarous matter, exceeding the weight of half the liquor. By this means it will be an easie thing to find the proportion of the saline Principle in the blood and humours: but whether this Salt be volatile, or becomes fixed beyond measure, the distillation of the urine will presently shew.[4]

In his 1684 *Memoirs for the Natural History of Humane Blood*, Robert Boyle made a plea for chemical analysis of the blood, similar to the one made by Willis for urine. Inspection of the appearance of the blood, like inspection of the urine, had been a long–practiced diagnostic procedure. Boyle criticized physicians who were content to remain mere observers and lacked the initiative to experimentally expose the blood's hidden properties, described his own experiments on human blood, and suggested research avenues for others who wished to explore the chemistry of the blood. His experiments included measuring the blood's temperature immediately after its withdrawal from the body; noting its reactions to flame and to various chemical reagents; and separating the blood's components through distillation, weighing, and examining their crystalline form. Boyle also analyzed the urine to evaluate its similarities with blood serum. Being a chemist, not a physician, he lacked opportunities to test the blood of people who were ill, but he stressed that knowledge of its normal state was "necessary to those that would discern, in what particulars and how far it deviates in the Sick. . .For having compared the Qualities and Accidents of this vitiated Blood, with those of the Blood of Sound Men. . .'twill not be difficult for a Physician to find, to what heads he is to refer those things that considerably recede from such as belong to Healthy Blood."[5]

This advice was acted upon in 1700 by the French doctor Raymond Vieussens who, in pursuing his work on the blood, believed that he was "treading in the Footsteps of the celebrated *Boyle*, and trying, if possible, to push it still farther than he had done."[6] Vieussens sought to determine the proportions of the blood's constituents represented in the population at large. He examined the blood "not of one or two Men only, but of a great many, and not only of healthy People, but of sick, neither of the same, but of different, and even contrary *Temperaments*, according to the exact Rules of *Analysis* [distilling and weighing the constituents], in such a Manner, as to separate the different Principles of it from one another, without any Loss of Substance."[7] His analysis showed that the blood contained "salts," "reddish spirit," "phlegm," and "fetid oil," and in his results, he gave the quantities of the component parts. The College of Physicians at Rome challenged his work; they not only disputed the existence of some of the elements in blood that Vieussens claimed, but denied that the proportions of the blood's constituents in the general population could be determined with existing knowledge and techniques. They argued, among other things, that some of the blood analyzed was inevitably lost through the distillation process then in use; that the individual composition of each person's blood, which varied according to differences in sex, climate, culture, diet, and exercise, made the idea of average composition meaningless. The College concluded that "to be able to find out one universal and certain Rule of that *Proportion*, which should agree with the *Blood* in all *Persons*, seems . . . to have more the Appearance of Truth, than of the Truth itself in it."[8]

Advocacy of chemical diagnosis was also taken up in the early eighteenth century by the English physician Browne Langrish. He urged the chemical analysis of urine during illness to detect changes in the proportions of its principal components. He reasoned that if knowledge about the urine could be gathered from mere inspection, then by "a more curious Search" into its contents, by "an exact *Analysis* we might see the different Contents of the Urine, and the various Proportions of its Principles."[9] Langrish also recommended analysis of the blood to determine the nature and causes of disease: "By proper Distillations, and the Force of Fire, we may compel Nature to an Account. . .It is satisfying and useful as well as curious, to reduce to Measure and Weight the constituent Parts of the Blood; and I am persuaded no inquisitive Person will judge it a vain Undertaking."[10]

During the second half of the eighteenth century, significant advances in the science of chemistry were taking place. Chemists now were generally convinced of the material nature of atoms, and were making progress in explaining their reactions and clarifying their individual properties. Several basic biochemical investigations were in progress on subjects such as photosynthesis in green plants, and animal respiration.[11]

Fresh efforts were made to apply chemistry to diagnosis. The

125

English medical scientist William Hewson, in 1772, chemically investigated the serum and solid components of the blood, and made diagnostic and therapeutic suggestions to practitioners based upon his work.[12] Interest also developed at this time in using chemistry to investigate diabetes. One of its chief symptoms, excessive urination, had prompted the physician Aretaeus in the second century A.D. to coin the term "diabetes" from the Greek word for siphon. Subsequently, sporadic reports appeared in the medical literature that diabetic urine had a sweet taste. This attribute is commented upon during the twelfth century in the medical aphorisms of Moses Maimonides, and again in the mid–seventeenth century by Thomas Willis who described the urine of a diabetic nobleman as "wonderful sweet water, that tasted as if it had been mixed with Honey."[13] Some doctors affirmed this attribute; others denied its existence, or would not accept it as a characteristic of the disease.

In 1776, the English physician Matthew Dobson sought the origin of this alleged sweetness by evaporating the urine of a diabetic patient. The residue smelled and tasted like sugar, and thus suggested that diabetes was caused by disturbances in the processing of sugar by the body. Dobson's work was a stimulus for experiments by the English physician John Rollo and his colleague, the surgeon and chemist William Cruikshank, that were published in 1797. The pair performed chemical analyses on residues obtained from the urine of several diabetic patients. They demonstrated that the chemical composition and weight of the residue changed during the course of the disease; it sometimes contained sugar and sometimes did not. Their work convinced them that chemical analysis not only provided important diagnostic evidence of the diabetic state, but that it also furnished accurate data on the patient's response to therapy and insight into the causes of the disease. Rollo recognized that the application of these findings to medical practice was difficult, since physicians were unlikely to be "sufficiently chemical, or have the advantages as we have had of the co-operation of an expert and intelligent chemist," but he believed that physicians might be induced to perform a "simple evaporation of the urine" of diabetic patients and thereby gain "a tolerably accurate state of the complaint, or convalescence from it."[14]

Cruikshank, like Rollo, was convinced of the importance of chemical analysis to medical practice. In addition to his joint work on diabetes, he demonstrated the diagnostic significance of chemical changes in the composition of body fluids in other disorders,

such as dropsy, rheumatism, gout, jaundice, and scurvy. Cruikshank hoped that his labors would induce doctors to apply chemical
analysis to illness, but he acknowledged that the subject was "much
neglected."[15] While a few European physicians used chemistry to
evaluate disease, particularly diabetes, most physicians disregarded
it. The sources of their indifference were examined in a three–
volume work on biological chemistry, written in 1803, by W. B.
Johnson. He noted that "the analysis of animal substances is the
most difficult and least advanced of any part of chemistry." He
enumerated as causes the unpleasantness of experiments with biological matter, the lack of good methods to separate or synthesize
biological products, and "lastly, the small degree of interest which
the chemist who was not a professed physician" took in analyzing
biological products.[16]

The use of chemical procedures in medical diagnosis was significantly furthered by the publication, in 1827, of Richard Bright's
Reports of Medical Cases.[17] Bright, an English doctor, demonstrated
that the widespread disease then known as "dropsy" (an accumulation of fluid in the tissues) was frequently accompanied by a characteristic shriveling of the kidney, and a large amount of a substance
called albumin that precipitated as a white opaque material when
the urine was heated. Bright's approach to diagnosis was exactly
analogous to Laennec's. Both selected alterations in the living patient – Bright's based on a chemical reaction, Laennec's dependent
on sound – that reflected and were connected with anatomical lesions revealed at autopsy. Bright forged the crucial link, therefore,
between the school of anatomy and the school of chemistry. Before
Bright, late eighteenth– and early nineteenth–century practitioners, notably the surgeon Cruikshank, and the physicians William Wells, and John Blackall,[18] had associated dropsy with precipitated albumin, and in some of their patients, at autopsy, Wells and
Blackall had even noted concurrent damage to the kidneys. But
they did not make the overall connection between dropsy, kidney
lesions, and the opaque precipitate. Although Bright could not
claim priority in relating dropsy and kidney disease, his colleagues
credited him with being the first to point out the frequent association of the two, to accurately describe the symptoms and autopsy
appearance in these cases, and, above all, to establish the fact that
this form of kidney disease, which became known as Bright's disease, could be detected during life by a simple chemical reaction.

The initial enthusiasm of physicians about Bright's discovery waned, however, because those who used the test often could not persuade their patients, who otherwise felt healthy, to remain in their beds solely because of the finding of albumin. Further, some physicians disagreed with Bright that a constant association existed between kidney disease and albumin,[19] and even Bright later qualified his statement. In his important 1827 monograph, Bright had declared that he had "never yet examined the body of a patient dying with dropsy attended with coagulable urine [albumin], in whom some obvious derangement was not discovered in the kidneys."[20] In 1836 he acknowledged the rare failure of the test when certain pathological products made their way into the urine, and either caused or prevented a white precipitate. John Bostock, the chemist with whom Bright worked closely, believed a variety of circumstances produced albuminous urine, "many of them of so trifling a nature, as to render it almost a constant occurrence."[21]

More confusion was introduced by Bostock's finding that the urine of some patients contained a form of albumin not precipitated solely by heat, but only when chemicals were added along with the heat. This raised the question of what the different albuminous matter in the urine indicated. Bright admitted that these findings diminished the value of the albumin test as an unerring diagnostic sign, if the observations were conducted over a short period of time, but he insisted that the continual presence of albumin was an accurate and dependable index of kidney disease. Bright's viewpoint was adopted by a number of physicians during the nineteenth century. However, as the century neared its end another view prevailed: while albumin's persistence in urine "most strongly" suggested organic kidney disease, it could "coexist with perfect health."[22] Bright had nevertheless discovered and publicized a significant chemical sign of a major disease. His work built an alliance between bedside observation, anatomical dissection, and chemistry. His strong advocacy of chemistry to serve clinical practice, rather than to clarify physiology (the task given chemistry by most of his predecessors), and the simplicity of the chemical test he developed, combined to make the albumin test the harbinger of further applications of chemistry to medical diagnosis.

Since Morgagni, the search for pathological change in the solid portions of the body had increasingly dominated medical thought; it had replaced interest in the body fluids, which at the time of humoral theories of disease had been the focus of pathology. But growing disenchantment with pursuing pathological change principally through the solids led physicians in the 1830s and 1840s to reassert an interest in studying the fluids,[23] particularly by means of chemical procedures. Many of them nevertheless retained the structural viewpoint of anatomists, and regarded chemical analysis as a refined type of dissection: it detected effects of disease that eluded the anatomist's scalpel.

It was in this atmosphere that, in 1841, Gabriel Andral, the French physician, called upon medicine to "commence and prosecute a series of researches similar to what have been done for the solids during the last 40 years. Pathological anatomy reveals to us the lesions which occur in the constitution of the organs of the body, and chemical analysis will do nearly the same for the fluids; it is in truth a sort of pathological anatomy."[24] In this new research effort, authorities in chemistry formed close collegial bonds with those in microscopy; both sought to study changes in parts of the body indiscernible to the naked eye. But the advocates of medical chemistry were not expecting a revival of the discredited humoral doctrines from the past. Rather, they anticipated the establishment of rational theories about the role of the body's liquid components in disease, firmly anchored by experimental evidence, theories that would not replace but would complement pathological doctrines based on the study of the body's solid parts. Just as there was no tissue which did not consist of solids and fluids, so advocates of medical chemistry argued that no organic change could occur without affecting both.[25]

The application of chemistry to evaluate disease increased during the 1840s. Early in the decade one observer commented that "the changes which take place in the fluids of the body, during the course of various diseases, seem to be daily acquiring increased importance in the eyes of medical men. Indeed, this disposition to return to the study of the fluids, forms a very prominent feature of the medical mind at the present time, as evinced by the number of interesting researches to which it has given rise."[26] Some physicians still worried, as had the College of Physicians of Rome in the previous century, that the data generated by chemical analyses were untrustworthy because exact knowledge of the normal composition of body fluids was lacking. Only when such studies were concluded would it become possible to confidently determine the alterations that they sustained in disease.[27]

Andral pursued this goal in his 1843 *Pathological Hematology*. He explored the blood's normal composition and charted the abnormal variations of some of the blood's constituents during disease. Andral investigated the blood from the triple view of its visible properties, microscopic features, and chemical composition. He considered the visible properties the least significant variables, realizing that the blood could look the same during different diseases, and that changes in appearance were but the effects of fundamental modifications. So chemical reactions and microscopic investigations dominated his work. Andral calculated the proportions in which the major elements of the blood – which he called globules, fibrin, solids, and water – existed in health and in illness, and described circumstances which changed the quantitative relationship of these elements to each other. He recognized that the absolute amounts of these elements, and the relative amounts in which they existed, could vary considerably within the healthy population. Accordingly, he set out to determine the average proportions of each element. In healthy people, he found that fibrin appeared in an average proportion of three parts in 1000 (without disturbance to health it could be as low as two or as high as four per 1000); globules – 127 parts in 1000; solids – 80 parts in 1000; and water – 790 parts in 1000. He linked different diseases with alterations in the amounts of these constituents, while he painstakingly distinguished normal from pathological variations of them. For example, an excess of red globules accounted for the disease then called "plethora." Its symptoms – dizziness, fever, ringing in the ears, and rapid heartbeat – denoted a surplus of vitality, the result of great numbers of red globules coursing through the body. In anemia, the cause and symptoms were reversed. Too few red globules produced a shortage of vitality and sluggish body function. Andral determined the proportions of the blood's elements to each other by separating them through heating, drying, and then weighing them.[28] From the proportional relations, he constructed a numerical portrait of the blood's appearance.

The anatomist and the microscopist used as a yardstick the visual configuration of the elements in a tissue. The chemist sought a fixed record of a similar kind through the proportional relations of the elements in a liquid, stated numerically.

Although Andral's work encouraged some physicians to believe that the normal composition of blood was no longer a mystery, many remained skeptical, as other distinguished chemists who analyzed the blood reached conclusions different from those of Andral about the normal proportions of its elements.[29] Nevertheless the study of the blood's chemistry accelerated, researchers being particularly interested in the relationship of sugar in the blood to diabetes, and of uric acid in the blood to gout.[30] This research was facilitated by the continuing popularity of bloodletting as a panacea for illness, so that investigators easily obtained the large quantities of blood they required. Andral, for example, carried out research on 360 bleedings from 200 patients.[31]

This work on the blood during the 1840s was paralleled by research into the normal composition and the pathological transformation of other body fluids. Notable was the publication, in 1841, of Alfred Becquerel's study of the urine, in which he estimated the quantity of such constituents as water, urea, uric acid, lactic acid, albumin, and inorganic salts. He determined the average amount of each constituent secreted by a healthy person in 24 hours, and compared these findings with similar observations on patients who had illnesses such as rheumatism, anemia, typhoid fever, heart disease, and liver disease. He emphasized the need to collect a 24–hour urine sample, since the long period decreased the errors caused by a changing food intake and the consequent variation in urinary products; only large departures from healthy standards were to be considered pathological. Becquerel hoped to prove that chemical changes in the urine constituents were valuable in establishing diagnoses and monitoring alterations in the course of illness; he wanted to demonstrate that diagnostic distinctions made by former generations of doctors, based on the appearance and color of the urine and its sediments, had "no real foundation, and should be entirely rejected, since they regarded as dissimilar and attached different significations to phenomena depending upon one and the same cause."[32]

Andral's effort to characterize the blood in numerical terms was continued in the 1850s by Karl Vierordt (who also pioneered in the graphic depiction of the blood flow with the sphygmograph). Vierordt developed a technique of counting red cells by making a dilution of a measured quantity of blood, and assessing the number of cells in a certain volume of that dilution with the aid of the microscope. His method was quite arduous to apply, sometimes imprecise, and little used. Subsequently, other physicians such as Louis Malassez, Georges Hayem, and John Burdon-Sanderson developed red–cell counting techniques but theirs had the same faults as Vierordt's and failed to attract the attention of either English or American physicians.[33]

A turning point came in 1877 when William Gowers, an English doctor, published a brief article "On the Numeration of the Blood–Corpuscles," in which he argued that a precise count of the red–blood cells provided doctors with the most accurate index of anemia.[34] The plea was accompanied by a description of a counting device that could be hooked onto any microscope (the counting instruments of Malassez and Hayem had required a special microscope eyepiece), and was more accurate than any of the preceding techniques. His invention, the "haemacytometer," had squares of one–tenth of a millimeter ruled at the bottom of a small indention of a glass slide within which cells were counted. Gowers actively publicized his invention. With it he demonstrated that iron therapy, a common remedy for anemia, worked by increasing the number of red cells. He established that skin color did not accurately reflect red-cell number, and therefore was an untrustworthy sign of anemia. Trials by other physicians confirmed Gowers' assertions. One physician described a visit to a young girl with a history of fainting spells, who had a rapid pulse, and a complexion "nearly as pale as the sheets which covered her."[35] Because her red–cell count was nearly normal, the physician avoided the conclusion, suggested by the patient's physical appearance, that she suffered from "anemia" and proposed what he considered the more likely diagnosis of "hysteria."

But the optimism generated by these early successes was tempered when flaws were found, first in Gowers' haemacytometer, and then in the counting technique itself. The trouble began in 1878 when two physicians, who bought several of Gowers' instruments in order to evaluate them, discovered that the instruments gave conflicting results because of slight variations in construction. The doctors then decided to compare Gowers' with other blood–counting devices on the market. They again obtained discordant red–cell counts, and concluded that one measurement of blood was untrustworthy, that at least two or more counts were necessary. Additional problems materialized when physicians experienced in blood counting complained about the many hours taken and the difficulties encountered in measuring, diluting, and mixing the blood sample and then correctly positioning the slide to examine the cells. "The eye strain, nervous excitement, and fatigue induced by three or four hours of the work were such as to make the most ardent clinical observer shrink from its too frequent repetition," lamented one commentator.[36] Even when all the steps were taken correctly, the errors inevitably involved in counting the cells hardly repaid the hard work attending preparation of the slide containing them. In a test of the procedure, two physicians independently enumerated the red cells in eight cases, and found that their totals varied as much as 25 percent. When a single observer counted the same specimen twice, his two totals shared a disparity of 15 percent. To the experimenters the evidence demonstrated "that in practical clinical work the results obtained in counting blood corpuscles are *extremely variable* – much *greater*, in fact, than one would infer from the literature upon the subject."[37]

Such criticisms led to the trial of an alternative to the counting technique: the use of centrifugal force to pack the red cells together and estimate their number by measuring the volume. The idea was first suggested by Magnus Blix in 1885, and then Sven Hedin developed a machine known as the "hematokrit," which he described initially in 1889. He connected a large wheel to a smaller one holding test tubes. One revolution of the large wheel caused the smaller one to turn 104 times. This whirling motion forced the cells to the bottoms of the tubes where, as a compact mass, their volume could be measured and the number of cells calculated. Some thought the accuracy of the centrifuge technique at least equaled, perhaps exceeded, that of the counting process. The hematokrit also required less skill, entailed no eyestrain, and took a much shorter time (about ten minutes). Physicians also used the centrifuge to separate the solid from liquid components of fluids such as the urine. As a technique the centrifuge soon gained many adherents for its varied uses and became important in many European hospitals and clinics.[38]

Gowers' interest in red cells, however, did not end with counting them. By 1878 he concluded that red–cell counts should be supplemented by determining the quantity of hemoglobin they contained. At that time several techniques existed to estimate hemoglobin: one determined the amount of iron (a key component of hemoglobin) found in red corpuscles; a second evaluated a solution of red cells by viewing it through a glass prism (spectroscopic analysis); and a third computed the amount of oxygen absorbed by a given quantity of red cells. All were difficult procedures not commonly used by

133

physicians. Gowers reasoned that since the hemoglobin content was related to the color of the blood, a simpler method of analysis would be to contrast a suspension of intact red cells with a color chart that corresponded to varying dilutions of red cells. His technique suited the exigencies of hospital work better than other hemoglobin–measuring techniques, and although not as accurate as some of them, seemed more likely to gain medical popularity.[39]

Drawbacks soon appeared in the use of color assessment to make numerical determinations. Physiologists and doctors spoke of a "personal equation" that influenced the accuracy of observations, and of differences in the ability to appreciate subtle distinctions in color. All the instruments devised to measure hemoglobin color were flawed in design: one by Georges Hayem, for example, did not take account of variations in color produced by different light sources. The standards used to estimate hemoglobin were arbitrary and often randomly set; the blood of one healthy person sometimes was the only yardstick used to construct a scale of tints. Circumstances such as age, diet, sex, or the region of the body from which physicians took the blood sample could influence the hemoglobin value, so that disparities of 10 to 20 percent could occur in the same person when blood samples were taken only a half hour apart. Hence, clinicians were advised to draw inferences about hemoglobin only when the result significantly differed from the standard, and was thus beyond the influence of deviations based upon normal physiological differences among people, possible instrumental defects, and observer error.[40]

The problems encountered with quantitative estimation of the red–cell and hemoglobin content of the blood (like the ones met during the introduction of the microscope), alerted some physicians – a small minority – to the fact that subjective and environmental factors beyond their control might affect the accuracy of instrumental observations. The attempt to characterize elements within body fluids quantitatively had originated, in part, from the belief that the infinitesimal alterations to which the fluids were subject represented important indices of health and illness, and that such small alterations were expressible only through numbers.[41] The recognition that the method itself involved small errors helped demonstrate that clinical significance could not be attached to minor deviations from normal standards and that, in any event, the demands of clinical practice and the available techniques of chemistry made absolute precision impossible.

Like physicians who numerically analyzed the blood, those who used chemistry to dissect the urine ran into difficulties. By the 1860s, quantitative tests for the urine had been developed that were divisible into two groups: those that did not require special knowledge or complicated apparatus, such as notation of volume, specific gravity, and weight of the solid residue; and those that needed a well–furnished chemical laboratory, experience in quantitative analysis, and more time than the practicing doctor usually could give. Both types of tests were subject to several kinds of error: the volume of urine produced by the patient could be misjudged when urine was lost by the patient himself or carelessly thrown away by a nurse; the quantities of its constituents, like the blood's, could be altered by material variations in the patient's physiology. And as in all chemical analysis, the skill and care of the analyst, the excellence of his instruments, and the purity of his reagents influenced the result. Since quantitative urine tests were so vulnerable to error, physicians were urged to repeat each test twice, and to distinguish cases that required great accuracy from those in which only an approximate quantitative estimate was satisfactory.[42]

Qualitative chemical tests for urine also produced difficulties. Doctors in the 1860s complained that the procedures demanded more time than they could spare, as well as a special knowledge of chemical theory and apparatus. The delicate apparatus and corrosive chemicals required for even the simplest urine test made it impractical to examine the fluid during a home visit. Further, so many tests for the same constituent of the urine were being developed that the ordinary physician was hard–pressed to distinguish good from bad tests. For example, of the eleven available tests for urinary sugar, which the physician could choose from, five were shown to be unreliable.[43] These dilemmas had been predicted several decades earlier by the clinician George Rees, who had concluded that "since chemists are not physicians, we shall scarcely benefit by their art, except by making the physician a chemist."[44]

Problems in the use of chemical tests of urine continued during the 1870s, when the invariability of the association between urinary sugar and diabetes was challenged. In the previous decade, sugar in the urine had meant diabetes to many physicians as surely as albumin meant kidney disease. The presence of sugar, like the presence of albumin, prompted insurance companies to refuse coverage to an applicant. Now it was asserted that unless other clinical evidence of diabetes was present, no amount of urinary sugar alone

135

justified a diagnosis of diabetes, and it was even demonstrated that constituents of the urine other than sugar would give the appearance of sugar when mixed with the most commonly used test reagent – Fehling's solution.[45] In spite of the imperfections of the chemical approach many physicians remained enthusiastic. One of them declared that "no urine–caster in his wildest dreams thought that the attempt would ever be made to do what is done now everyday by the least expert, when he finds sugar or albumen in the urine, and tells the accompanying symptoms or the consequences."[46]

During the 1880s and 1890s new chemical tests found growing application in diagnosis. In bacteriology, the chemical detection of typhoid fever was made possible by two events: Paul Ehrlich's diazo reaction,[47] described in 1882, in which chemicals added to urine produced a carmine–red color when the disease was present; and Fernand Widal's discovery, in 1896, that the blood serum of a patient with typhoid fever caused a culture of typhoid bacilli to lose their motility and to agglutinate – to clump together. Widal became the first person to diagnostically apply the agglutination phenomenon, which B. J. A. Charrin and G. E. H. Roger had originally described in 1889.[48] Investigators made great efforts to extend the "serodiagnostic" technique, as Widal termed this method, to other diseases. However, by the start of the twentieth century, the principal clinical application of the agglutination phenomenon remained the detection of typhoid fever.[49]

In hematology, the white cells became the object of intensive study. Their earlier neglect ended when physicians had become convinced that one of the blood's constituents – the leucocyte – played a significant role in the body's defense against bacterial invasion; and that white cells could be separated into several groups with sharply defined characteristics, through their distinctive chemical reactions with aniline dyes – another discovery of Paul Ehrlich's. Increase in the number of leucocytes now became an important sign that infection existed in the body.[50]

The development of blood chemistry has been hampered by a shortage of blood for experimental and diagnostic purposes, caused by the gradual abandonment of bloodletting as a therapy later in the nineteenth century. Thus, by the early 1900s, the 25cc of blood needed to evaluate the uric–acid content of the blood to diagnose a patient suspected to have gout,[51] was more than could be obtained except in special cases. But the situation improved as chemists such

136

as Ivar Christian Bang and Otto Folin developed techniques of chemical analysis that used only small quantities of blood – sometimes so small that enough for analysis of a single element could be got by only a prick of the finger. Such techniques were acclaimed in 1914 as "perhaps the greatest recent advance in diagnosis by chemical means."[52] They made possible, for instance, the estimate of blood sugar on a daily basis, and opened a new era in the study of diabetes. By 1919, from 10 cc of blood most of the commonly tested components of the blood serum could be quantitatively estimated – nonprotein nitrogen, urea, uric acid, creatinine, creatine, and sugar.[53]

Almost as far-reaching as the insights that chemistry provided for the blood, was the knowledge furnished about disorders of the stomach and the methods suggested to accomplish this. For centuries the stomach had been an organ enveloped in mystery. Before 1800 physicians studied dyspepsias through the characteristically vague and contradictory sensations of these disorders as reported by their patients. During most of the nineteenth century doctors poked, thumped, and listened to the stomach, using the major procedures of physical diagnosis – palpation, percussion, and auscultation; they even tried to see into it through a rigid pipe – the gastroscope – first developed by the German doctor Adolf Kussmaul in 1868. None of these techniques yielded good information, and the same therapy did not always relieve conditions that to all appearances were identical. This disheartening picture was transformed in 1871 when Wilhelm Leube suggested the diagnostic application of a flexible tube which, connected to a pump, had been used previously to empty the stomach for therapeutic purposes. In diagnosis, the tube was passed down the esophagus into a patient's stomach, and the digestive products, forced into the tube by movement of the abdominal muscles, were periodically removed and chemically analyzed. Such evidence was considered completely objective and scientific, in contrast to the obscure and uncertain information derived from the other diagnostic methods. This procedure attracted devoted followers.[54]

The most important question to be settled by chemical examination of the stomach was whether it contained hydrochloric acid. Some physicians insisted that its constant presence excluded the possibility of stomach cancer, and that its constant absence was a sure sign of cancer, regardless of any other symptoms. Other phy-

137

sicians believed stomach cancer could be present when the acid continued to be secreted. A heated debate, akin to the one over urinary albumin, ensued about the significance of hydrochloric acid. A moderate position finally prevailed: when the acid was not found in the stomach a presumption of cancer was justified; the secretion of hydrochloric acid allowed an obverse conclusion.[55]

A variation of this chemical examination, which constituted a new approach to medical diagnosis, involved use of the "test meal." Before inserting the stomach tube, the physician fed the patient definite quantitites of selected foods or chemicals. Allowing some time to elapse, he then evaluated the way in which the body dealt with the test meal by analyzing the contents of the patient's stomach or his waste products.[56] No subject was more discussed at the 1888 meeting of the American Medical Association than the new chemical techniques to diagnose stomach disorders. Some physicians called them as significant for the diagnosis of stomach disease as the stethoscope was for chest disease.[57] The patient's body could be made into a crucible within which a test reaction occurred, and became, as a doctor characterized it, "an analytical laboratory."[58]

The strategy of challenging the patient's body with substances that forced illness to reveal itself was next applied to the kidney. Doctors introduced foreign substances into patients by mouth and monitored the changes they underwent in the kidney by chemically analyzing the urine.[59] A 1910 study by the Boston physician Richard Cabot confirmed the value of using chemistry to test body function in the search for disease. Cabot discovered a disparity between anatomical lesions in the kidney disclosed at autopsies, and signs of kidney disease found by chemical analysis of urine. Structural defects could exist in the kidney without altering the chemistry of the urine; chemical pathology could exist in the urine without changing the anatomy of the kidney.[60] It seemed that anatomical and chemical change did not proceed *pari passu*. A deceptive appearance of health could be maintained by compensatory efforts of the damaged organs. Hence, new procedures and a different outlook on diagnostic testing were needed; challenge of the body's organs and chemical evaluation of the result seemed one answer.

Anatomical diagnosis, whether directed at lesions in the solid parts or at fluids of the body, sought a locus for disease. It asked, "Where is the lesion?" Functional diagnosis sought to evaluate performance. It asked, "What can the organ do?" Those physicians who emphasized function disavowed the maxim of practice: when

138

you find a lesion, treat it. The functionalist ministered only to defects that clearly threatened or interfered with the patient's activities.[61]

As physicians came to recognize that a chemical evaluation of disease, like a microscopical one, required skills, experience, and apparatus they generally lacked, they were increasingly inclined to forfeit their warrant to apply these techniques and interpret their findings, and to delegate this right to other physicians and lay experts. Many of these specialists organized their work in an institution that was to become prominent in and crucial to twentieth–century medical practice – the diagnostic laboratory. Laboratories, the organized workshops of science where investigators analyzed the objects of their interest firsthand, were largely a creation of the nineteenth century. Jan Purkyně, in 1824, had established in his own house in Breslau a laboratory for physiological research. Two years later Justus von Liebig founded a laboratory in Giessen devoted to the chemistry of life processes, whose organization became a model that later scientists emulated. It rested on three pillars: excellent facilities, competent direction of research, and openness to well–prepared students and mature investigators. In the latter half of the nineteenth century a number of important laboratories opened in Berlin. Among the most important were that of Rudolf Virchow for the study of structural and functional changes of disease in man, and the successive laboratories that Robert Koch organized during the 1880s and 1890s in which he developed new methods to investigate infectious disease. Such efforts stimulated the founding of other workshops for scientific research, which produced basic knowledge in anatomy, chemistry, physiology, and bacteriology.[62]

The clinical laboratory was an offspring of these efforts. Begun in the 1880s, its principal goal was to use knowledge gained about fundamental biological and disease processes to develop new methods to evaluate and treat illness and, secondarily, to provide diagnostic services to physicians. In 1885, Hugo von Ziemssen established in Munich one of the first clinical laboratories, followed in the United States by George Dock's laboratory at Ann Arbor, Michigan, in 1893, and the William Pepper Laboratory of Clinical Medicine in Philadelphia, opened in 1895.[63] The term "clinical pathology" was used at this time to designate the organized application to medical practice of the complicated chemical, microscopical, and bacteriological techniques often confined to research projects.

The clinical pathologist differed significantly from the morbid anatomist. The anatomist pursued the causes of symptoms and diseases, and helped to strengthen the clinician's skill by verifying or disproving his working diagnoses. However, the findings at autopsy could not help the patient. Clinical pathology on the other hand investigated the living. It used the scientific procedures of the laboratory to aid the clinician; it formed a bridge between medical research and medical practice.[64]

The clinical laboratory, in turn, generated another medical institution – the ward laboratory. Physicians in the 1890s increasingly urged that adjoining the main wards of the hospital should be laboratories that were small in size (a room 6 by 10 feet would do), simple in equipment (a sum of about $300 was required for the instruments), not devoted to research but solely to the ongoing problems of patient care. Laboratory development during the nineteenth century can be thought of as a chain of links that began with the laboratory devoted to basic research; was followed by the clinical laboratory, which split its efforts between research and patient care; and ended with the ward laboratory, the workshop next to the patient, where the knowledge and methods perfected in the other laboratories were most practically applied.

The ward laboratory encountered objections nonetheless: it was said to endanger ward cleanliness, house poisonous chemical reagents that patients might drink, consume too much space, consume too much money, produce facts unnecessary for diagnosis, and keep hospital doctors away too long from bedside observation and record keeping. Nevertheless, ward laboratories were established during the 1890s at well-known hospitals in the United States and Great Britain, such as The Johns Hopkins Hospital in Baltimore, the Bellevue Hospital in New York, the Royal Infirmary at Edinburgh, the St. George's Hospital in London, and in 1900 at the Massachusetts General Hopital in Boston.[65] During the first decade of the twentieth century, the ward laboratory acquired increasingly complicated scientific instruments, which intensified the pressure on the already overburdened house staff. Hospitals responded by hiring extra technicians, scientists, and physicians to run the hospital laboratories, and designated certain portions of the house physician's time for laboratory duty only. Now the clinical and ward laboratories had become indispensable to hospitals: "They are as essential to the proper equipment of the hospital as the internes. They are to the physician just as the knife and scalpel are to the surgeon."[66] proclaimed the American clinician William Osler. Hospitals thus became the home for the pursuit of a laboratory–based scientific medicine.

Public apprehension about bacterial–caused diseases, and physician frustration with the technical difficulties of bacterial identification, also generated the birth of government–supported diagnostic laboratories devoted to removing dangers to the public health. To prevent the outbreak of epidemics, and to administer curative remedies to afflicted patients at the earliest possible moment, rapid and certain identification of an infectious disease was acknowledged as crucial. Within a few years after Robert Koch announced in 1882 that he had isolated the organism causing tuberculosis, many doctors and laymen had accepted the finding of bacteria as the best sign of this disease. By the 1890s, this confidence had extended to other widespread diseases, such as cholera, typhoid fever, and diphtheria. Some physicians considered a possible bacterial cause in almost every departure from health. But the enthusiasm of physicians was curbed, in part, by the complexity of bacterial diagnoses. Their dilemma was exemplified by the problem of distinguishing the germ responsible for typhoid fever from a microorganism that resembled it. Six hundred and eighty–nine methods had been developed to separate them.[67] The knowledge and technical competence needed to judge these methods, to use the chemical staining procedures, magnifying instruments, and the culture media that were the everyday tools of bacteriology required specialized training and much time; the average doctor had an abundance of neither.

These circumstances led physicians to support the establishment of publicly financed laboratories to identify widespread contagious disease. The first laboratories opened were mainly devoted to detecting diphtheria, whose principal clinical manifestations – a throat that was sore and sometimes coated with a white membrane – were notably inadequate criteria to establish its diagnosis unequivocally. A serious contagious disease such as diphtheria also confronted the doctor with other dilemmas. If he failed to alert local health authorities, he could be socially censured and criminally prosecuted. If he reported the illness he might incur the wrath of the family, because of the consequences to them: forced isolation, household quarantine, and the disruption of business and social relations. Should he diagnose diphtheria, and be mistaken, the family could sue him. Accordingly, the doctor welcomed the aid of laboratory experts who would "formally relieve him of the risk and responsibility of making the positive diagnosis."[68] In 1893, New York City founded the first laboratory devoted to diphtheria diagnosis. The city furnished free to physicians tubes filled with nutrient that favored the growth of the bacteria that caused the disease. To apply the technique, the doctor drew the swab containing material from the patient's throat over the culture media, and could return the tubes to designated apothecary shops located all over the city. Each evening officials of the health department collected the tubes; by the next day the physician could learn the diagnosis in person or by telephone. In the first three months of its existence, the New York Board of Health examined 431 cultures and found 301 active cases of diphtheria.[69] Encouraged by these results, two years later the New York City laboratory began to examine sputum to locate the bacillus causing tuberculosis, and to widen the variety of diagnostic tests it could perform.

The idea of having a public bacteriological laboratory evoked favorable comment in Great Britain and in the United States during the 1890s,[70] and achieved considerable momentum in the first decade of the twentieth century when physicians discovered a laboratory test for the widespread and dreaded disease – syphilis. In 1901, Jules Bordet and Octave Gengou described the phenomenon of complement fixation, a method which used the serum of blood to determine the presence of a microorganism. The announcement by Erich Hoffmann and Fritz Schaudinn in 1905 that they had found the causative agent of syphilis, the *Spirochaeta pallida*, led a number of investigators to experiment with complement fixation to locate the organism in patients; in May 1906, August von Wassermann, Albert Neisser, and Carl Bruck succeeded. By 1911, boards of health in cities all over the United States had added the syphilis test, or Wassermann test as it became known, to their repertoire of procedures. So great was the faith of doctors and patients in the test that when it was positive, some physicians diagnosed syphilis in the absence of any other symptoms of the disease. The test was also of great value in allaying the anxieties of people obsessed with the idea that they had syphilis. Confidence in the Wassermann test induced some American states to require it as a prerequisite for marriage. More than any other procedure, the Wassermann test elevated the prestige of laboratory diagnosis in the eyes of patients and doctors.[71]

People skilled in laboratory techniques found increasing opportunities in the 1880s to earn money by publicizing their talent to physicians. To cope with the inconvenience and difficulties of using the growing number of chemical tests, the physician practicing outside of the hospital had three principal alternatives: to have a clientele limited in number so he could personally conduct these tests; to hire a scientific assistant to perform laboratory investigation; or to delegate the task to chemists or physicians skilled in chemistry. He generally chose the last option and thereby created a demand for private laboratory services. As early as 1883 a Philadelphia physician, Judson Daland, advertised his willingness "to make such examinations in the most careful manner, and to furnish promptly a written report of the results. A moderate fee will be charged."[72]

At the start of the twentieth century, commercial laboratories were organized in most large cities in the United States to meet the demand of physicians for chemical and microscopical examinations. World War I contributed greatly to the physician's respect for diagnostic laboratories, and created more demand. By 1918, nearly three hundred laboratories were established to supply analyses to physicians in the American Expeditionary Forces.[73] The war provided many doctors with their first experience in the regular use of the diagnostic laboratory. Upon returning to private practice, they encouraged the establishment of commercial laboratories, which have thrived vigorously up to the present. The introduction of chemistry into medicine established the laboratory as an important element of diagnosis. Delegating medical decisions to laboratory specialists as well as to specialists in other branches of medicine added certainty to the diagnosis of many diseases. This dependence however has created other problems that still trouble both doctors and patients.

7 Medical specialism and the centralization of medical care

During the first half of the nineteenth century most physicians were generalists. They tended to disapprove of those who narrowed their practice to a single aspect of medicine, because in their minds specialism was associated with quacks and itinerant healers who performed a single medical procedure, such as setting bones or extracting cataracts, and because of the specialist's limited perspective on illness. "I can remember," wrote the American clinician S. Weir Mitchell in 1891, "when older physicians refused to recognize socially a man who devoted himself to the eye alone. To-day we can only look back with wonder at such narrowness."[1] In such circumstances, few physicians limited their practices to specific diseases or parts of the body. Yet the anatomical concept, that disease attacked and resided in specific places within the body, provided an ideological basis, and an armory of technological devices now offered a material foundation, for the specialization of medical practice that began in the second half of the nineteenth century.

By the 1880s the number of specialist publications in medicine was growing at a faster rate than those of generalists.[2] One physician classified the specialties then existing into those based upon age and sex – the treatment of men, women, or children; those devoted to special diseases – notably mental disorders, gout, or consumption; those dividing the body along anatomical and physiological lines – such as the nervous, respiratory, or digestive systems; and legal medicine.[3] While the International Medical Congress needed eight sections to accommodate the interests of physicians in 1875, the one held in 1900 required seventeen. And in 1915 there were 34 medical specialties by one estimate.[4] In 1929, almost one out of four private practitioners in the United States was a full–time specialist; by 1969 the proportion had grown to more than three of four.[5]

The fragmentation of medical practice caused by specialization has engendered efforts to unite the elements of practice through organizations and some centralized direction. The changes as they occurred in the United States, during the late nineteenth and twentieth centuries are discussed in this chapter.

The generalists regretted the growth of specialism; one in 1897 wrote nostalgically of a past having "those old 'family doctors,' learned, sagacious, observant, friendly advisers and confidants, with an academic dignity which has been almost lost in the hurry and bustle and matter-of-fact directness of the last half–century. To follow one of these men through his daily rounds would be a curious experience to a modern specialist."[6] The generalists also looked with anxiety toward a future when medicine might be dominated by specialist practitioners, each focusing his expert attention on one disease or one part of the body but neglecting other pathology. They also feared that a specialist–dominated medicine would become so burdened by technology that the patient who called a doctor to the home would be confronted by a delegation. A patient of the future was pictured, satirically,

. . . in her boudoir, reclining on the sofa, in expectation of her medical attendants. A drag drives up, from which alight two servants with heavy bags, who assist four doctors to descend. The fraternity is announced, and, followed by the servants, enters the room. The bags are deposited; the servitors withdraw, and after the exchange of a few remarks the examination begins. Dr. Ready, the junior practitioner, conducts the first inquiries, makes the ordinary investigations of the different organs, and before finishing pulls out of his pocket a tablet containing the volumetric examination of every fluid in the body, completed since the last visit. This is looked at by all. Dr. Reckoner then takes traces of the movements of the heart, of the pulse, of the action of the muscles, records the velocity of their contraction, and estimates the amount of nerve–supply, showing the diagrams and figures to the patient, who inspects them with the look of a connoisseur. Dr. Eyeman now supplies the improved ophthalmoscope, which photographs as well as is used to see by. Again Madam shows active interest, and declares that the picture is very pretty. A mysterious nodding and whispering take place. There has been indigestion with pain at the pit of the stomach, – can there be anything wrong with the blood–vessels there? Dr. Magnet, who is a very accomplished physicist, steps forward: "If you will permit me, I will make you transparent." And by means of a modified, portable Ruhmkorff coil, and an instrument with lenses dexterously passed into the stomach, the fair patient is really rendered transparent. The examination is completed; fortunately no serious lesions exist, and a consultation held in the next room results in the advice to take a few glasses of soda–water, and a daily ride on horseback.[7]

Even the vision of such a future could not stop the growth of specialism in the United States, which increased during the early years of the twentieth century. It continued to be stimulated by the multiplication of scientific instruments whose skillful use required long education, the dominance of the anatomic concept of disease which facilitated the partitioning of the body among specialties, and the absolute increase in medical knowledge. But then other factors joined to accelerate the growth of specialism, such as the concentration of people in urban centers that could support specialized doctors, the desire of physicians to escape from the irregular hours and what some physicians thought of as the slavery of general practice, the hope of greater pay for less toil,[8] and the absence of professional or administrative barriers which prevented specialists from competing with generalists for patients.[9]

Events seemed to conspire against the American generalist at this time. He encountered keen economic competition from hospital clinics and dispensaries, who treated poor patients free of charge and sometimes unwittingly gave care to patients who feigned poverty. Practitioners of Christian Science, mental science, osteopathy, chiropractic, and spiritualism absorbed many of the generalist's clients, as did the patent–medicine hucksters who encouraged the public to treat themselves. The *Boston Medical and Surgical Journal* reported that an unparalleled number of respected citizens allowed public exhibition of their photographs, below which was appended a skillfully phrased declaration of their faith in the virtues of some nostrum: "Not a day passes but the lay press contains a villainous reproduction of the face of some well-known divine, accompanied by a testimonial overflowing with exuberant gratitude for the remarkable manner in which Dr. Charcoals Tablets have enabled him to overcome the ravages of a deadly disease."[10] As the reputation of specialists grew, the patient would often visit them directly instead of relying on the generalists to decide whether a consultant was necessary. Even when the specialist treated a patient professionally referred, he would sometimes criticize the generalist for his lack of knowledge, disparage his skill, or assume charge of the patient even though the generalist had asked him only for an opinion.

The generalist's confidence in himself tended to erode under

146

such attacks. One generalist in 1918 told the audience at a medical society that he often returned from their annual meeting wondering if he were competent to practice medicine:

I heard this morning one of our best men say that there was not one doctor out of fifty who is competent to tell whether a patient has tuberculosis or not. I heard another man say this afternoon, Mr. President, that the general practitioner was not competent to advise the public as to whether or not they were in the precancerous stage or whether they would have cancer. . .I wish to commend the idea of one of the speakers who said that the local practitioner was justified in making use of the ordinary measures to find out whether he could make a diagnosis or not before he applied the x-ray or called in a specialist. . .I want to say that we [general physicians] do not wish to go back home discouraged and feeling that all the years we have been practicing (twenty years in my case) that we know nothing and that the other man knows it all. [Loud applause].[11]

Many medical students declined to enter general practice because it was not scientifically appealing. They pictured the generalist as an overworked doctor who saw such a variety of medical problems that he could approach none of them as an expert, and who could carry his small stock of scientific paraphernalia around in his bag – usually a stethoscope, a device to measure blood pressure, a thermometer, a bottle to collect urine for analysis, and a pipette to draw blood for a white–cell count. The student, imbued with the belief that laboratory aids and complex instruments were indispensable to diagnosis, felt safer amid technology that he could use himself, or among specialists to whom he could delegate diagnostic questions. General practice, divorced from most technological and specialist assistance, seemed threatening to many students.

This picture of general practice applied principally to the rural doctor. While the generalist who worked in a city might more easily consult colleagues and keep abreast with new medical developments, the country doctor practiced without these resources – he usually met medical problems alone. He needed to find in himself the inspiration to do good work, for his county and district medical-society meetings usually were dull and poorly attended: "We feel that the old, old story of typhoid fever and appendicitis has been gone over again and again until the subject is threadbare. We feel that we have said all that we know how to say upon pneumonias, pleurisies and obstetrics, and all of these common–place topics."[12] Thus the students who believed technological and collegial supports indispensable avoided going into practice in the rural districts and small towns of the United States.

The economics of rural practice also contributed to its decline. In 1929, the gross mean income of generalists in American communities with a population under 5,000, was about $5,000, while in the remainder of the country it ranged from about $6,500 to almost $9,000.[13] A similar income disparity existed between rural and urban specialists: their gross mean income in communities of under 25,000 population was $12,000, while in larger communities, it ranged from about $14,500 to $19,000.[14] As a result, physicians settled in larger cities in growing numbers, increasingly turning to specialism, and left the rural countryside depleted of medical resources. In 1929, in communities with under 5,000 population (where almost half the American population resided), fewer than one–third of the doctors practiced, of whom only 1.5 percent were full-time specialists. But in cities over 100,000 (where almost a third of the people lived), nearly half the doctors could be found, of whom 35 percent were full-time specialists.[15] A survey taken in New York State about 1920 showed that rural areas were not attracting new doctors: 97 percent of the practicing doctors in the twenty communities studied had been there 25 years or more, and the remaining 3 percent, five years or less.[16]

Two other surveys that covered some thirty states revealed that more than 90 percent of older rural doctors were not being replaced by young ones.[17] Further evidence of the steady depletion of physicians from rural areas, and their growing concentration in urban areas, was a 1926 study of medical conditions in the largely rural state of Tennessee. It enumerated five principal problems: an unequal distribution of physicians but not necessarily a shortage; epidemics and other emergencies overtaxing the capacity of the country physician; the heaviest financial burden of medical care falling mostly on people in rural sections who were least able to meet it; the advanced age of physicians in small towns and rural districts which interfered with their ability to cope with the hardships of country practice; and a gravitation of population, wealth, and physicians cityward.[18]

This outflow of medical talent was encouraged not only by monetary considerations but also by the low prestige generally accorded rural practice by medical educators. Discussions of rural medicine focused mainly on its hardships. Most students believed that only those having a missionary disposition would seclude themselves in what was labeled the "backwoods." Hence, by the 1930s, American medicine faced a dual crisis: most graduates refused to go to rural districts where they were needed, and those who did go were not prepared to meet the conditions of practice they found.

Physicians in rural areas tried to neutralize this unattractive image of country practice, by turning its difficulties into circumstances that challenged an individual's ingenuity and strength:

If you can set a fractured femur with a piece of string and a flat-iron and get as good results as the mechanical engineering staff of a city hospital at 10 per cent of their fee;

If you can drive through ten miles of mud to ease the child of a dead beat;

If you can do a podalic version [childbirth] on the kitchen table of a farm house with husband holding the legs and grandma giving chloroform;

If you can diagnose tonsillitis from diphtheria with a laboratory forty-eight miles away;

If you can pull the three-pronged fishhook molar of the 250 pound hired man;

If you can maintain your equilibrium when the lordly specialist sneeringly refers to the general practitioner;

If you can change tires at 4 below at 4 A.M.;

If you can hold the chap with lumbago from taking back rubs for kidney trouble from the chiroprac;

Then, my boy, you are a Country Doctor.[19]

Many patients in the United States were distressed by the declining numbers of general practitioners, especially in rural communities, and complained of having to travel from specialist to specialist. The specialist, they felt, did not really understand them, and could not fill the role of counselor and confidante hitherto assumed by the general practitioner.[20] Another source of discontent was the financial and physical strain that making the rounds of specialists located in different places imposed on a sick person, a problem common in England as well. Wrote one doctor:

A relation of mine was lately the subject of a fatal and very painful illness, for the diagnosis of which an x-ray examination was needed. He suffered great torture in the transit from the nursing home to the house of the x-ray specialist and back again. He was a man of great physical courage, and the effect upon him was the more noticeable. It cannot be denied that our present system or want of system wastes the patient's money, and puts him to the utmost inconvenience, and sometimes to great distress. It also wastes everyone's time. Every special test that has to be made, every special examination, every special opinion that has to be asked, means that if the patient is up and about he has to trot round to a different door, and sit about in a different waiting–room, or else send various emanations from his person to another laboratory. Or if the patient is in bed each of these various authorities has to come to him and carry out the necessary details under the worst possible conditions.[21]

149

While a number of early twentieth–century physicians opposed specialism, many recognized it as an inevitable response to advances in medicine; the day of the individual practitioner, who could be competent in all aspects of medicine, had ended. There persisted "the beautiful thought of the family physician carrying cheer to his clientele, solving unaided his manifold problems, and delivering 100 percent efficiency to those dependent on his decisions, but the bold facts are that it cannot be done."[22] A medical diagnosis in a puzzling case was becoming increasingly difficult to make alone; instead it was assembled like the parts of a machine, each turned out by a person skilled in performing a particular procedure. Diagnosis without consultants, laboratories, or machines seemed more and more difficult as well as unwise. Yet, it was generally recognized that the specialist's perhaps narrow interpretation of symptoms must be avoided by integrating their viewpoints. At the beginning of the twentieth century there still existed a breed of supergeneralists who knew enough about each discipline to integrate their facts soundly. They prevented laboratory experts from overlooking the bedside features of illness; they kept clinical experts properly aware of the minimal knowledge of laboratory techniques. William Osler and William Welch performed this task at The Johns Hopkins Hospital, but they represented a type of physician destined to extinction by the technically expanding medical environment. In 1910, the American surgeon William Mayo warned the graduates of Rush Medical College that interdependence was an inevitable consequence of medical growth: "The sum total of medical knowledge is now so great and widespreading that it would be futile for any one man . . . to assume that he has even a working knowledge of any large part of the whole."[23]

A decade later, the belief prevailed that no person could be a universal diagnostician, except at the risk of harming his patients and damaging his reputation. As an alternative to the unifying knowledge provided by a brilliant clinician, proposals were made to link specialists through formally organized, cooperative medical associations. Advocates of this plan envisioned a cooperative practice as the only way to combine fields of knowledge, to give physicians access to the medical machines too expensive for an individual to purchase, and to achieve efficiency by locating patients, doctors, their assistants, and machines in one physical place. Cooperative practice was to involve a systematic division of labor among physicians possessed of different skills to diagnose and treat the patient's illness. This organization of specialists became a surrogate for the general practitioner. It performed tasks that the generalist would have performed, if he had had the knowledge of the group or time and energy to apply their knowledge.

The growth of cooperative specialism was aided by the support of physicians who had served in World War I, and of their patients; both had become accustomed to the organized delivery of medical care in the armed services and in general were impressed with its virtues. Cooperative specialism also reflected the tendency in medicine toward group effort that characterized industry and various social enterprises in early twentieth–century society. As one writer put it, "the bigger a man is, nowadays, the less he attempts a splendid isolation, the more he merges his personality in the membership of a group for he knows that, through the subtle interpenetration of the minds of its several members, feats become possible that are beyond the achievement of any isolated magnate."[24] The medical group, in this view, provided better service to the public and gave the physician a greater sense of self–realization than was possible when he practiced as an individual.

Several medical institutions began to emphasize a cooperative approach to medical practice. One was the hospital. The notion of ministering to anyone who was sick or suffering, homeless or hungry, through houses of hospitality or hospices, was principally a creation of the Christian era. These institutions grew in number and scope with the help and influence of Church authorities. By the eighth century, many hospices were specialized, some looking after orphans, some the poor, others only housing the sick. In addition, religious orders were founded devoted solely to caring for the sick and they embarked on a widespread program of hospital building. But in the thirteenth century the nursing and sanitary conditions of hospitals declined as ecclesiastical responsibility for them began to yield to civil control. The secular authorities did not maintain the standards of care set by the Church. This was particularly apparent in the deterioration of nursing services, as religious sisters were replaced by secular attendants. In England, the eighteenth-century secular nurse was described as "illiterate, heavy-handed, venal, and overworked. She divided her time between housework, laundry, scrubbing, and a pretense at nursing of the most rough and ready kind. She seldom refused a fee, and often demanded it. Strong drink was her weakness, and often her refuge from the drudgery of her life."[25]

151

The eighteenth–century hospital not only failed to provide diagnostic or therapeutic skills or facilities that were much better than those available at home, but exposed patients to the added danger of infections generated within its walls: "Every hospital, I fear, without exception, may in some measure be considered as a Lazaretto, having its own peculiar disease within it," wrote the English physician John Aikin in 1771.[26] At this period, with infectious diseases rampant and hospital epidemics unchecked, going into the hospital seemed (and in fact often was) to many people the equivalent of a death sentence.

Rehabilitation of the hospital occurred in the nineteenth century's second half. Florence Nightingale was a major influence in bringing about the reform of nursing, through the example of her own conduct in the Crimean War as well as the hard work and high intellectual and moral standards of the nurses whom she trained. She also helped, with others, to change the abysmal sanitary conditions of hospitals by advocating large space, much light, and fresh air as necessary elements in the building of hospital wards.[27] These advances in nursing care and hospital architecture, the introduction of antiseptic techniques in surgical operation by Joseph Lister in 1867, and the proof that bacteria caused disease in people, publicized by Robert Koch in 1882, were among the important factors that led to the growth in the numbers and prestige of hospitals both in Europe and the United States and made them attractive to doctor and patient for medical care. In the 1890s the success achieved by surgeons was attributed to the almost entire transfer of patient care from home and office to the hospital; an example that physicians were urged to follow. Patients began to use the hospital without the oppressive fear of earlier times: "Our great public hospitals have ceased to be grievous and infected places, and people are rapidly losing their dread of them," wrote the American surgeon Harvey Cushing in 1914.[28] By then, not only had hospitals shed their reputation as death houses, but they also stirred the pride of the citizenry who saw them as community assets. People now considered the hospital as the safest, most comfortable, and most economical place to go when seriously ill, or when they needed complicated diagnostic or therapeutic care. This new attitude toward the hospital is reflected in the statistics of hospital growth. Estimates of the number of hospitals in the United States in about 1875 range from 178 to 661. A Bureau of the Census survey in 1909 showed more than 4,000 with a bed capacity of over 400,000; by 1928 nearly

7,000 existed, having slightly under 900,000 beds. By 1973 there were almost 7,500 hospitals, with a total bed capacity of almost 1.5 million.[29]

Although the cooperative approach to medical care was integral to the functioning of the hospital, by the second decade of the twentieth century it was doing more to foster than lessen unrestrained specialism among hospital physicians. Richard Cabot, as the chief of medicine at the Massachusetts General Hospital, attempted to improve the situation by making ward visits with a team – a clinician, a pathologist, a surgeon, a chemist, and a physiologist – whom he encouraged to work together for the good of the patient. Group work was described as the mainstay of the modern hospital, which "moves and has its being in the idea and practice of cooperation between various medical and surgical specialists."[30] In many hospitals, however, the association among specialists was not binding. Although specialists issued reports on a given patient, there often was no substantive dialogue among them about the patient.

In spite of these problems, by the 1930s, a number of leaders in medicine looked to hospitals, and the cooperative model of practice, as the key to reorganizing the delivery of medical services in the United States. The final report of the Committee on the Costs of Medical Care, a panel of experts in medicine and the social sciences who wrote some of the most comprehensive studies on the organization of American medical practice ever to appear, proposed turning hospitals into comprehensive centers that would be the focus of all medical activities. The hospital would become formally linked to medical stations in outlying communities too small to support so large an institution, and also would house the private offices of doctors and patients. The typical hospital had already become a partnership, in the sense that its doctors were organized as a staff to conduct a practice, and that the functions of other agents of healing – nurses, laboratory technicians, and pharmacists – were integrated toward patient care. Accordingly, hospitals seemed to furnish the most appropriate foundation for an integrated medical service.[31]

A second form of cooperative clinical organization whose importance increased during the twentieth century was private group practice. Its chief model, the Mayo Clinic,[32] evolved from a joint arrangement made in the 1880s by the brothers William and Charles Mayo to practice medicine and surgery in Rochester, Minnesota. Gradually adding partners and laboratory facilities, they completed in 1914 a new building that housed the clinical facilities and laboratories under one roof. With this building the Mayo Clinic became a distinct institution.

After World War I the impetus toward private group practice grew in the United States. The physicians who banded together hoped to reduce overhead costs by using common facilities. They pooled income and considered a patient, though he was frequently under the charge of one physician, as the responsibility of the whole group. Some of these groups conducted general diagnostic surveys and instituted comprehensive therapies; others who were organized only for diagnosis, believed that if therapy were left to the referring physician, he would be encouraged to consult the group without fear of losing his association with the case, and could actively share in restoring the patient to health. At the one extreme, some groups worked under a single roof, its members legally related and incorporated. At the other extreme were groups of specialists who regularly sent patients to each other but had no spatial or legal relationship, except that of one consultant to another. Intermediate forms included independent physicians who leased offices in a "medical building," jointly shared a laboratory, and referred patients among themselves. Indeed by the beginning of the 1930s growing numbers of city physicians were leaving their offices at home for space in a building in the center of retail trade: almost half of the some 500 doctors in Dallas, Texas, for instance, practiced in a single building. Even in small towns physicians increasingly established their offices on "Main Street."[33] Advocates of cooperative out–of–hospital practice believed that it solved two major dilemmas confronting the generalist – his inability to know enough about all branches of medicine to work alone, and the confusing web of relationships he might encounter with independent consultants and with hospitals. The generalist could extend his own knowledge and skills by integrating with an organization of specialists, which might also enhance his prestige within medicine.[34]

During the 1920s and 1930s, many physicians, particularly the generalists, expressed misgivings about cooperative practice, in particular that it would lead to cliquism. Few things provoked more dispute within medicine than the possibility of coteries of physicians set up as superior and exclusive organizations that could attempt to monopolize practice. Some physicians charged that group clinics offered unfair competition to private practitioners. One group clinic was condemned by an independent practitioner for "doing tonsils and adenoids for $25 in their own building, supposedly being done by a 'specialist' while we independents have always received at least $35 plus hospital."[35] One study indicated indeed that the existence of a group practice impinged adversely on and tended to diminish the clientele of nearby independent physicians more than would an equal number of individual physicians practicing alone.[36] Many physicians declined membership in group practices for fear of endangering cordial relations with colleagues. One group physician complained that, with few exceptions, members of the local medical society were antagonistic: "Some of them would rather see a patient die than refer him to the clinic."[37] General physicians continued to believe that the ills of most patients could be adequately handled without assistance, but when they did require help they could call in consultants, without being formally tied to them.

The cost of medical care by a group likewise concerned the critics, who believed that cooperative practice led to the ordering of superfluous tests – blanket blood chemistries, unnecessary X-rays, and electrocardiograms. Diagnostic surveys in 1920 could last up to five days and cost up to several hundred dollars in fees ($20 to $35 for the laboratory, $10 to $75 for X-rays, $100 for the consultant in charge, and $10 to $25 for each specialist opinion).[38] Critics focused on the patient's vulnerability to large bills when visiting a group clinic, an expense that posed a serious problem for the patient of moderate means. It was said that only two classes of people were able to obtain good cooperative care: the very poor, whose bills were paid by welfare agencies, and the very rich. In response to such problems, the Massachusetts General Hospital in 1915 had established a consultation clinic for middle–income patients; $5 was charged for a group examination and $2 for X-rays.[39] The New York Diagnostic Society, organized in 1919 by a group of 400 physicians, also conducted a diagnostic survey including a history, a general physical examination, fluoroscopy of the heart and lungs, chemical examinations of blood and urine at a cost of between $5 and $20.[40] However, such arrangements had the appearance of charity and generally stung middle-class pride.

The reputation of cooperative practice was somewhat tarnished by the attempts of mediocre doctors to form groups. In some small–town hospitals, men with no specialist training tried to remedy the lack by taking brief courses in the needed specialties; and they sometimes took into their group laboratory and X-ray assistants improperly qualified. Cooperative practice was also charged with turning medicine from a profession into a business. The bookkeepers and systematized financial arrangements imported a commercial spirit seldom known to individual practice. The organized processing of patients by doctors and machines seemed akin to mass production methods of industry. The division of the patient among the group's specialists – "department store" medicine – produced an impersonal atmosphere the patients disliked.[41] Critics protested that the close personal relations between doctor and patient, essential for effective medical care, were often lost in cooperative practice: "A group diagnosis may be perfect in all of its parts; statistically, physically, chemically, quantitatively it may be correct, but as a whole it is only assembled and machine–made and may be a misfit. There is lacking the important feature of personal contact between physician and patient, with proper integration and estimation of the value of details."[42]

Independent physicians also believed that cooperative practice weakened personal relations by diffusing the responsibility of caring for the patients, who often complained of being shifted from one doctor to the next. Defenders of the group concept pointed out that a single physician usually coordinated the care of a given patient, and at least one man stated that patients were less interested in personal relationships than had been true in the past.[43]

Even those who opposed group medicine inevitably came to accept it, in various modified forms, out of necessity. Almost all doctors had to rely on others to make X-ray and laboratory tests, and occasionally had to consult with a specialist. Many physicians were affiliated with a hospital, and thus implicitly accepted the group concept. Of the some 142,000 active practitioners in the United States in 1929, about eight out of ten were affiliated with a hospital, and about one in twenty-five even had private offices or held hours for private patients in hospitals. By 1975 virtually no physician would consider practicing without the resources and consultants that hospital affiliation brought, and about one in four of the some 330,000 active American physicians practiced full–time in a hospital.[44]

As for formally structured and legally incorporated private group practice, defined as having at least three full–time physicians, it has grown in the United States at an annual rate of over 8 percent since 1932. At this time there were 232 groups, in which fewer than 1 percent of all active physicians practiced. In 1959, 546 groups were established which contained over 5 percent of practitioners. By 1975, 7,773 groups existed, comprising over 18 percent of all active physicians, excluding those employed by government. A significant aspect of this expansion has been the trend of physicians in the same specialty to affiliate in groups. While only one of ten groups could be classified as single specialty arrangements in 1946, they represented one of four in 1959, and about one of two in 1975.[45]

Considerable pressure was exerted toward accelerating group practice arrangements during the 1970s. It was becoming "an article of faith that larger units are 'more efficient' in providing medical care, and it is usual for sociologic or economic analyses of medicine to include a plea for 'group practice'."[46] The United States government now endorsed the group–practice concept by subsidizing the delivery of medical services through cooperative agencies called "Health Maintenance Organizations" (HMOs). The HMO brought together physicians, other medical personnel, equipment, and facilities in any organized way its members might choose. Its clients, for a prepaid yearly fee, had access to all services offered to the group.[47]

Physicians in the twentieth century have gradually accepted the idea that the interrelationship among doctor, patient, and technology requires some mechanism to integrate the provision of medical services. This notion has led American medicine to shed its essentially decentralized structure in which independent practitioners are scattered among the population, and become increasingly organized around hospitals and other types of cooperative–practice arrangements. This centralization has in many ways improved the quality of medical care available to the average patient. At the same time, it has created many pockets in which few or no local medical services are available to patients.

8 The shortcomings of technology in medical decision making

The modern technology of diagnosis unquestionably provides significant insights into the processes of disease. However, physicians who benefit from its help continually express their concern in the medical literature of the twentieth century over the possible harm done to medicine by overdependence on technology.

American medicine was often a focus of such concern. A Parisian physician touring American hospitals in 1912 reported his surprise at the number of laboratory tests routinely requested for the patients. To him the tests seemed "like the Lord's rain, to descend from Heaven on the just and on the unjust in the most impartial fashion," and he concluded "that the diagnosis and treatment of a given patient depended more on the result of these various tests than on the symptoms present in the case."[1]

Twenty years later a questionnaire surveyed a large number of American doctors – diagnosticians of local and international repute, professors of medicine, general practitioners – to learn how they used medical resources. Those who responded cited as the most common problem the large number of laboratory tests ordered in hospitals as a matter of course, without apparent relevance to the condition for which the patient was admitted, and without apparent understanding of the tests' meaning or limitations; next most common were redundant requests for X-rays and electrocardiograms. One heart specialist judged that 90 percent of the electrocardiograms made benefited neither patient nor doctor.[2]

Physicians continued to use large numbers of tests in the 1940s. Tinsley Harrison, a well-known American clinician and author of textbooks, noted "the present–day tendency towards a five–minute history followed by a five–day barrage of special tests in the hope that the diagnostic rabbit may suddenly emerge from the laboratory hat."[3] A study of laboratory use in five Michigan hospitals

158

from 1938 to 1958 showed a 100 percent increase in the number of tests given to patients in six diagnostic categories, when measured per day of hospital stay.[4]

From the mid–1950s through the 1960s, some hospitals reported that the number of laboratory tests ordered per patient doubled every five years. Typical was the Yale–New Haven Hospital, which in 1954 performed 48,000 laboratory procedures; in 1959, 98,000; and in 1964, 200,000 procedures. The patient census increased only slightly during this interval.[5] "The ever expanding role of the laboratory in clinical diagnosis and patient care is evident on the wards, in the records, in the building plans and, not least of all, in the finance office of every hospital," reported the *New England Journal of Medicine* in 1963. "Such terms as 'liver profile' – or perhaps one should now call these tests the 'liver image' or 'posture' – are a manifestation of this marvelous faith in laboratory tests. The use of 'routine' or 'baseline' tests is almost universal, and the category is ever expanding."[6] This trend continued despite studies which showed that physicians who received large numbers of reports containing normal laboratory findings were apt to overlook abnormal results when they appeared.[7]

In the 1970s, the rate of laboratory testing in the United States expanded at a slightly faster rate than in the 1960s. From an approximate 2 billion (American billion) tests performed in 1971, the number climbed to about 3 billion in 1974, and to roughly 4.5 billion in 1976.[8] Hospitals in Canada and Great Britain also reported substantial increases, prompting more than one doctor to speculate that the biochemical laboratory might soon appropriate the hospital's wards to meet its expanding needs, and force clinicians to occupy the narrow confines of the old laboratory.[9]

The increasing automation of laboratory analysis made possible and encouraged this expansion of testing. Automation had been advanced in 1956 when L. T. Skeggs Jr. invented the automatic analyzer, a machine which executed ten separate laboratory procedures on one biological substance, and could test 5,000 single substances daily.[10] By the early 1970s, an estimated four out of five of some 15,000 hospital and commercial clinical laboratories in the United States used some automated equipment. With this, they performed about 25 percent of all tests involving the blood, and up to 80 percent of selected laboratory tests. Paradoxically, the capacity of automated devices to carry out more tests at a lower cost has given rise to a routine of packaging so that today one orders a

"Chem 6" (a group of six tests), "Chem 12," or "Chem 18" instead of specific single tests. This in turn has increased the number of laboratory tests done. Indeed, some doctors have complained that their hospital laboratory was no longer able to perform single determinations.[11]

The use of X-rays, too, has increased greatly. In mid-century, much concern was expressed in Great Britain that the growing number and complexity of X-ray examinations, whose volume had doubled every five years between 1920 and 1950, might financially undermine the hospital system.[12] In the United States, a study showed that the number of X-rays given patients in six diagnostic categories, per day of hospital stay, rose sixfold from 1938 to 1958.[13] Some physicians doubted that the increased use of the X-ray in diagnosis was wholly the result of contemplative decision making. The ordering of an X-ray seemed to have become "routine"; consequently, the total number of X-rays made of a patient sometimes got out of hand. One radiologist disclosed that in records he reviewed he found cases in which 50 to 100 X-rays had been taken of a single patient when about five would have sufficed.[14] In some hospitals the practice of X-raying patients in the hope of finding an ailment in its early, often unsymptomatic stages continued, despite a low yield of benefits. One hospital routinely X-rayed the intestines of all patients with hernias, hoping to detect hidden cancer. A survey found that in the more than 300 patients who were subjected to the procedure, cancer had been detected in only one, a patient whose history gave ample, independent evidence of the disease.[15] Another study, in 1971, of 1,500 X-rays ordered to evaluate trauma to the skull, revealed only one fracture found for every sixteen films taken. The authors of this study concluded that in almost one-third of the patients, the X-ray could have been omitted or deferred on the basis of the clinical data available.[16]

Concern too has been expressed about the rapid growth in the use of computed X-ray tomography, a technique developed in 1972 in which a computer reconstructs data from an X-ray scan of the patient's body conducted from all angles in a single plane. The series of cross–sectional X-rays produced by this process enables physicians to locate disease in the soft tissues of the body that is difficult to find through other diagnostic techniques, and which may be painful or harmful. But the enthusiasm generated by its benefits prompted physicians to purchase the invention without thoroughly evaluating the engineering quality of the units on the market, to apply it in medical conditions for which its value is doubtful, and to cut short their customary diagnostic examination when using it. These problems, in addition to the high purchase price of computed X-ray tomography ($300,000 to $700,000), as well as the high cost per examination (up to $500 a patient), led the Institute of Medicine of the National Academy of Sciences in the United States to convene a panel of experts to study the innovation. They recommended, in a 1977 report, that although physicians should continue to explore the technique, some limits be placed on its acquisition and its clinical use.[17]

The growing volume of laboratory tests and X-rays ordered in general is costly. For example, in the United States roughly $8 billion (American billion) was spent on laboratory tests in 1974, and about $12 billion in 1976.[18] When the rising cost of such procedures was balanced against their utility and aftereffects, the outcome was not always favorable. Several studies and accounts by individual physicians in the 1970s furnished evidence that many laboratory tests and X-rays ordered by doctors yielded little information that was new or useful for diagnosis. Routine requests were frequent, and the information received often duplicated data already in the patient's record.[19] Concern was also expressed about possible harm to patients from excessive testing. Dr. David E. Rogers told the Association of American Physicians in his 1975 presidential address: "As our interventions have become more searching, they have also become more costly and more hazardous. Thus, today it is not unusual to find a fragile elder who walked into the hospital, [and became] slightly confused, dehydrated, and somewhat the worse for wear on the third hospital day because his first 48 hours in the hospital were spent undergoing a staggering series of exhausting diagnostic studies in various laboratories or in the radiology suite."[20]

Labeled "excessive diagnostic inquisitiveness" in the 1920s,[21] and "shot–gun testing" in the 1950s,[22] the routine ordering of technological procedures without a clear orienting thought was called by some physicians in the 1960s "decerebrate medical practice."[23]

The attachment to machine–produced evidence during the twentieth century originated in part from the contemporary faith in science and technology, and a belief that a scientific spirit entered clinical practice through technology. The doctor who depended chiefly on technology in diagnosing and following the course of illness could think of himself as using the same rigorous methods as did the scientist who pursued truth in his laboratory. To many doctors, the laboratory "seemed pervaded by a purer light" than the hospital ward, and the laboratory analyst was pictured as superior to the clinician – "the incarnation of all that is scientific in medicine and whose word cannot be questioned."[24]

Data supplied by technology also seemed to satisfy the medical appetite for precisely expressed clinical evidence. Medical facts recorded in numbers or graphs gave an appearance of exactness and finality. Some physicians measured progress in medicine by the degree to which quantitative measures of illness replaced qualitative ones; they felt uncomfortable in using terms such as "a little" or "a good deal" in clinical situations, but gained confidence when they could express themselves in degrees centigrade, grams, and seconds. Some physicians also used laboratory investigations as a way of reducing the anxiety generated by the uncertainty under which they often had to act. As one observer commented, the physician's belief in the existence of "strictly objective methods" created by laboratory technology was a comfort to him.[25]

Medical education, too, sometimes seemed to encourage an overdependence on the laboratory. One doctor recalled a teacher who always had his students take the route into the wards via the laboratory, to signify to them the true path to diagnostic knowledge.[26] Other physicians, and legislators concerned about laboratory use, cited the small amount of systematic teaching of medical students and hospital residents in the application, interpretation, and costs of laboratory tests as a cause of overuse. They characterized instruction in this subject as generally informal, and usually only an aspect of discussions about hospitalized patients.[27]

Some patients in their attitudes also encouraged excessive appeals to technology for clinical decisions. Many patients are themselves fascinated by the technological resources of medicine, a fact noted by psychiatrists and clinicians early in the twentieth century, who pointed out that often beneath the surface of the modern patient existed traces of primitive attitudes, a feeling that he was surrounded by unknown powers, which could be mobilized for him by the complex medical techniques, and the physician who controlled them.[28]

The early electrocardiograph exemplified the science and mystery of the new technology. A patient, arriving at the doctor's office, was "told to thrust his hands or one hand and one foot into mysterious receptacles connected by electric wires with the dark monster at the other end of the room! It is an 'electric picture' of the heart, of his own living, beating heart, which is being taken; every throb, every subtle movement is being written by that beam of light which quivers so mysteriously in the distance! Imagine, too, the thrill of scientific ardour which the manipulation of such a wonder must afford to any physician."[29]

The X-ray also fascinated the patient. Since Roentgen's discovery of the rays in 1895, and Walter Cannon's work, started a year later, showing that the tubes and organs within the body could be X-rayed if filled with an opaque substance, doctors had introduced dyes and air into the lungs, kidneys, spinal column, and even the heart, to outline the body's organs.[30] Physicians in the 1930s reported that patients often demanded "an X-ray all over" to evaluate their diseases, and were encouraged by a popular press that surrounded the activities of medical science with an atmosphere of omniscience and omnipotence. Sensational news stories could prompt a patient to demand his doctor use the "most scientific" instruments possible, whether or not diagnostically necessary or economically prudent.[31] Many patients believed that when physicians applied elaborate diagnostic procedures, an answer to their problems was almost certain. "When they go to see a physician they hardly think it necessary to give a history or to have a physical examination," commented the American medical consultant Walter Alvarez in 1943. "Thus, one day the vice president of a big company came in and said, 'Send me for an electrocardiogram; I want to check up on my heart.' Did he care to have me ask him any questions, or even to listen to his heart sounds? No; his idea was that the records made by a machine would tell everything he wanted to know, and that they would do this with an accuracy and infallibility far beyond any attainments of mine."[32] Accordingly, the doctor who, wishing to conserve the patient's finances, refused to order needless tests and consultations, might find that the money he saved the patient was used to see another physician, who did not object to ordering every conceivable test: "All the average patient in a consultant's office wants today is tests and plenty of them; he wants to 'be given the works.' "[33]

The growth of malpractice suits against physicians for alleged failure to use all available technology in a particular case also contributed to excessive testing. Early twentieth–century physicians learned to protect themselves by ordering X-rays routinely in cases of fracture, whether or not clinically necessary, to avoid possible liability claims against them in the future. As the century progressed, the growing battery of procedures that could be used to locate disease proportionately enlarged the risk of suit for the doctor. In the 1930s, some physicians felt that they were "forced by public opinion – the patient, his family, his friends – to utilize every laboratory test. In fact, we are compelled in the process of law (accident cases, etc.) to send to the laboratory even those cases in which physical examination gives the unquestionable diagnosis."[34] During the 1950s physicians often justified routine ordering of laboratory procedures as "for the record," or "for protection."[35]

In the 1970s, "defensive medicine" was the label applied to the use of diagnostic procedures to avoid litigation. A survey of the almost 16,000 members of the American College of Surgeons in 1972 revealed that over half requested more X-rays, laboratory tests, and consultants' opinions than they believed they needed to reach medical judgments, in order to ward off malpractice claims.[36] Some three–quarters of 111 randomly selected American physicians responding to a 1977 survey indicated that they ordered extra tests as a protection against legal suits.[37]

A further stimulus to excessive testing, despite its growing expense, appears to be the increasing proportion of medical costs paid for by private and government insurance plans and the growing number of people who receive such benefits. For example, between 1962 and 1974 in the United States the number of people covered for laboratory and X-ray examinations by private insurance plans more than doubled, from 35 to 73 percent of the population.[38] It seems likely that when less constrained by cost, physicians and patients have been more willing to call upon technology for help in evaluating illness.

How many tests physicians should give to their patients has become a part of a general but unresolved scientific and moral problem in contemporary medicine: where to draw the line in seeking facts about a patient's complaints, and whether and how far the line should be extended to include examining patients for latent disease.[39] This problem has grown more perplexing with the development of effective therapies that cannot be chosen and used until after a diagnosis is established.[40] The American internist David Barr has said that "discriminating selection of measures may be more important than unreflective completeness."[41] It is improbable that a formula can be devised that will tell a doctor how many or which tests to administer. Many physicians are concerned that the art of selecting appropriate actions from a wide spectrum of possibilities – one of the greatest skills in the practice of medicine – is declining as doctors become less willing to make independent clinical judgments based upon their own observations, and depend more on the judgments of specialists and machines. Too often the physician has been willing, as one doctor put it, "to let the instrument do it. The Wassermann test will decide as to syphilis. The roentgen ray will tell us whether there is an aneurysm or pulmonary tuberculosis. We can test the metabolic rate or get the blood chemistry, and disregard the time honored symptoms of exophthalmic goiter or nephritis."[42]

It has been suggested that a too ready acceptance of voluminous laboratory reports as evidence of clinical study could lead physicians to distrust their own observations, and those of colleagues. "There is one kind of clinician who has become submissive in the presence of laboratory reports. He resigns his art in the face of instrumental devices."[43] Such critics argue that as the physician's ability to conduct and trust his own examinations diminishes, his personal diagnostic powers are endangered; if he believes he will receive the answer in a report from the laboratory, he tends to stop his own search for clinical evidence of disease. A distinguished foreign physician visiting American hospitals remarked: "It seems to me that in your enthusiasm for the pursuit of laboratory evidence you have forgotten the patient."[44] Radiologists also report having to urge physicians to conduct clinical examinations on patients before sending them for diagnosis: "They apparently feel that if an x-ray examination is made, nothing more is necessary."[45]

Some physicians seem to have become apprehensive about the possibility of committing errors, distrustful of their own capacities, and confident that others who used techniques they respected, but could not fully understand, could make better judgments about illness. Such misgivings have encouraged them to group close to each other and to machines, in medical–care centers such as hospitals. One hospital resident expressed this attitude when, in 1950, he assumed temporary responsibility for the private medical practices of several vacationing doctors:

Of the patients I saw, I could seldom pick out a disease which I could recognize; for the most part, I found that patients came in complaining of a multitude of symptoms that did not fit any of the disease pictures I had seen or read about in textbooks. Often, there was not even a physical sign to point the way to a physical diagnosis. I welcomed the day when I could take up my next resident appointment back in the sheltered atmosphere of the hospital. The pathology laboratory and x-ray department would exclude 'organic disease,' my chiefs could confirm there was 'no abnormality detected,' and the patients could be sent back to their own doctors.[46]

Physicians have also worried that the central role of the laboratory in the evaluation of illness engendered an attitude in which the patient was less a person and more an object of study, and the doctor more a biologist than a physician. The laboratory worker was pictured by one observer "on his throne, the high stool, garbed in his royal robe, the long white coat. All undisturbed by the smell of garlic on the patient's clothes, the worker tests the body fluids, or examines pieces of his body under the microscope with that tranquil and detached and almost non–human air which so well marks the mien of the advanced laboratory man. Laboratory methods tend to make one forget the patient altogether in the nicety of the scientific."[47]

Another observer remarked that an impersonal clinicial attitude and a wall of technology were ways of shielding medical personnel from anxiety–producing thoughts prompted by the critically ill or dying person, about their limitations and failures as healers, and their own mortality. Thus a critically ill patient might "get a dozen people around the clock, all busily preoccupied with his heart rate, pulse, electrocardiogram or pulmonary functions, his secretions or excretions but not with him as a human being."[48]

By the 1970s, for a number of doctors the main feature of diagnosis seemed no longer to be the intellectual act of using facts to deduce conclusions, but the managerial act of choosing what tests to order, which specialists to consult. This practice involved the danger that patients might one day conclude that the doctor's personal skills were less important than the tests and consultations he ordered.[49]

Reliance on technologically produced evidence at the expense of physical examination and history–taking has long been a matter of concern in medicine. When the British physician Sir Humphrey Rolleston visited the United States on a tour of medical facilities in 1908, he pointed out what he considered the American physician's serious inattention to bedside observation and examination of the patient.[50] Confidence that the senses provided fundamental and trustworthy evidence for clinical judgments had encouraged many nineteenth–century doctors to work hard at developing their perceptual faculties, while confidence in technologically generated evidence appeared to discourage efforts of this kind among twentieth–century doctors.[51] "For years, physicians and many of our well known teachers have leaned so much toward laboratory methods that physical diagnosis has almost become a lost art,"[52] wrote one. Another, beginning practice in 1902, called his patients "peculiar people here; they all expect you to look at their tongues and feel their pulses, and most of them expect you to sound [auscultate] them."[53]

By the 1930s the new generation of professors of clinical medicine in the United States seemed interested principally in the biochemistry of disease; growing numbers of doctors stepped directly from the laboratory into a professorial clinical chair at a hospital.[54] Physical examination was often relegated to second place and in some hospitals was assigned to the younger, least experienced members of the staff. Attention to physical examination also declined in medical–school curriculums. A number of doctors expressed impatience with the physical examination as imprecise and time–consuming.[55] The laboratory's dramatic discoveries increasingly appeared to diminish the doctor's inclination to use his senses. The American physician James Herrick reported in 1931 that there was good reason to ask questions such as, "Should we no longer feel for an enlarged spleen, a presystolic thrill? Are we to give up the attempt to locate by percussion an infiltrated area in the lung or fluid in the pleural cavity? Are we to discard the stethoscope and cardiac murmurs and bronchial breathing and rely on the X-ray and electrocardiograph?" Medical teachers, Herrick complained, perhaps unconsciously were leading undergraduates "to place the emphasis on the instrument of precision rather than on the eye, ear, hand of the physical examiner."[56]

Typical of the decline of the physical examination were physicians' attitudes toward auscultation. By the 1930s the stethoscope was being characterized by some physicians as an almost archaic survivor of the past – like the blood–letting lancet. It was criticized in medical journals, at medical societies, and in conversations among physicians. The X-ray delivered the most serious blow to the prestige of the stethoscopist. The story is told of two well–known doctors who met at the Saranac Lake tuberculosis sanatorium: "What have you there under the arm?" asked one. "X-ray

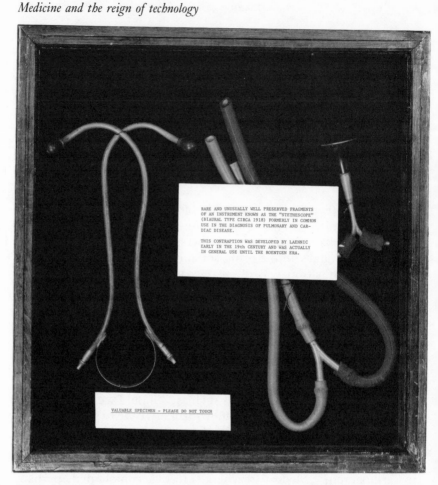

Figure 15. Stethoscope encased in glass presented to Dr. Merrill Sosman by several surgical residents of the Peter Bent Brigham Hospital, Boston, circa 1935. Reproduced by kind permission of the Francis A. Countway Library of Medicine, Boston.

films!" replied the other, "I now carry them instead of the stethoscope!"[57]

A humorous recognition of this situation occurred in the mid-1930s. In the X-ray viewing room of the Peter Bent Brigham Hospital in Boston, the chief of radiology, Dr. Merrill Sosman, conspicuously displayed a stethoscope encased in glass (Figure 15). A label within the case read: "Rare and unusually well preserved fragments of an instrument known as the 'stethescope' [sic] (biaural type circa. 1918) formerly in common use in the diagnosis of pulmonary and cardiac disease. This contraption was developed by Laennec early in the 19th century and was actually in general use until the Roentgen era."[58]

A formal debate held in 1945 at the Royal Society of Medicine in London, entitled "Stethoscope Versus X-Rays," concluded with general agreement that the stethoscope had descended from its diagnostic throne, that its clinical uses had to be redefined. Why really bother with "vague mysterious sounds, when something quite definite could be seen on the *x*-ray film?"[59] Auscultation was declared of little help in the early diagnosis of lung disease, important only when a poorly taken X-ray failed to reveal disease, when the lesion could not produce a radiological opacity, or when the stethoscope had a good psychological effect on the patient. Indeed, many clinicians used the stethoscope only because patients expected it, and were not satisfied with an examination unless it was applied.

Some physicians protested this characterization of the stethoscope by other doctors as primarily an object of display and reassurance to the patient. Such doctors seemed to the instrument's defenders like clerks with a medical background "busily signing the requisition for life–saving help from radiological and pathological colleagues."[60]

Despite these protests the effectiveness of teaching and using auscultation and other means to discover the physical signs of illness continued to decline. The decline was epitomized during the 1950s by such disparate events as the essay, "A Plea for the Stethoscope" by the Harvard professor of medicine Samuel Levine,[61] and by a brief dialogue on television between an intern and the comedian Groucho Marx:

Groucho: If I were found unconscious on the sidewalk, what would you do?
Intern: I would work up the patient.
Groucho: How would you start?
Intern: Well, I would do the laboratory work first. I would do a red count and hemoglobin and then a total white and differential count.[62]

In the 1970s the teaching of clinical skills was frequently encumbered by assigning too many pupils to instructors who, following a trend established earlier in the century, were usually the less experienced members of the staff. These conditions increased the chance that students would learn incorrect techniques of examina-

169

tion, which they often carried over into practice.[63] The American physician George Engel made informal polls of students in over 50 North American medical schools visited between 1960 and 1976. Only a few reported that in making physical examinations or interviewing patients, were they monitored by an instructor more than once or twice. Engel attributes the decline in clinical abilities, of which this was one cause, to the prevailing reliance on technology.[64]

The importance of history–taking had diminished when techniques such as auscultation and percussion became available, which enabled the doctor to use his own senses to gather data. By the second half of the nineteenth century, the long narratives of patients and their relatives had come to seem tedious and unprofitable, compared with data elicited through physical examination. Two minutes spent in such examination, many practitioners believed, could be more valuable than 30 minutes passed in listening to statements that were often exaggerated and inaccurate. "You ask when you visit a patient whether he slept. The wife answers – 'not a wink,' and yet you know from the patient's expression that he has rested during the night . . . You ask if he has passed urine – 'Oh, yes, sufficient,' yet you see by the pinched, anxious countenance, and position of abdomen and pelvis, that he is suffering from retention or suppression of urine."[65]

Neglect of the patient's comments increased with the development of the complex technology used in twentieth–century diagnosis. History–taking frustrated twentieth–century as it had nineteenth–century doctors. Young physicians increasingly tended to neglect history–taking, in some cases because their teachers had not emphasized the diagnostic importance of sitting down with the patient and questioning him about his illness.[66] A few doctors frankly stated that since patients' preconceptions and vague language often made the information gathered from them undependable, they tended to disregard the patient's own impressions of his illness. Instead they emulated clinicians such as one who remarked: "Let me test the patient, I don't need any history."[67]

Throughout the twentieth century physicians have written that no information is more neglected than the subjective symptoms of illness experienced by patients. Some assert that a correct diagnosis can be made on a majority of patients from the history alone. Critics contend that patients are frequently subjected to a long series of technological examinations before their doctors inquire very particularly into their history; that "too often the history of the patient is relegated to a relatively untrained person when it would be safer to turn over any other part of the examination," as the American cardiologist Paul Dudley White put it.[68] Advocates of history-taking argue, basically, that while instruments and the senses may reveal crucial facts about the causes of disease, only the patient can reveal how the illness affects him. Concern has been expressed for the patient, whose illness cannot be adequately evaluated through technology. What happens when he comes under the care of a physician whose education emphasized technological skills rather than person-centered, fact-finding skills such as history-taking?

Many modern physicians thus seem to order the value of medical evidence in a hierarchy: facts obtained through complex scientific procedures they regard as more accurate and germane to diagnosis than facts they detect with their own senses, which, in turn, they value more than facts disclosed by the patient's statement.

The delegation to technical experts of responsibility for diagnosis raised basic moral problems for twentieth–century medicine. Notable among those concerned was the English bacteriologist and physician Sir Almoth Wright, who in 1910 cited an example from his own relatively young field of work. He pointed out that the average physician, lacking a thorough education in bacteriology, often entrusted bacteriological work to a specialist, and the arrangement seemed to work well. The clinician obtained his diagnosis from one laboratory, and his remedy (a vaccine or antitoxin) from another, yet he thought he could keep a dignified role as a middleman between patient and bacteriologist. But new bacteriological discoveries made it essential to consider the question of when, and under what circumstances, the physician could delegate the skilled work necessary for diagnosis and therapy.

Wright distinguished three general situations in which delegation occurred. In the first situation, the consultant came face to face with the patient and hence with the problem to be resolved. The consultant conducted his examinations, discussed the case with the practitioner, and considered with him the errors that might have been made. The final decision, along with responsibility for it, was made jointly by the physician and the consultant. This was the usual outcome when a practitioner sent a case to a specialist.

In the second situation, the doctor sent a specimen to the bacteriological laboratory. In this instance, the bacteriologist was not

171

brought face to face with the patient. He could not obtain his specimen in the way he judged best, but was obliged to use the one submitted to him. When the written report reached the physician, who was not himself a laboratory worker, he was not qualified to expertly evaluate it. He lacked personal knowledge of the methods used to gain the results and had no opportunity to question the laboratory worker; therefore he could not weigh the human errors that might have entered the findings. Here was a situation in which a man arranged to delegate a medical task he was not competent to perform himself, but kept the responsibility for all medical procedures on the patient, along with the higher scale of rewards that went with it.

In the third situation, the physician, totally skilled in the work he undertook, entrusted part of it to an assistant. He could determine whether the work was conducted in the proper manner, and he accepted responsibility for it. This was the case when the physician delegated his duties to the resident staff of the hospital, the director of a laboratory to his staff, or the practitioner to his nurse.

Wright believed the morality of these three kinds of delegation differed. The third was proper and necessary in carrying out work on any large scale; the first was also appropriate. But the second situation was not clearly distinguishable from the case of a layman who undertook to treat a person, on condition that the layman be permitted to consult competent medical authorities. If doctors objected to treatment by laymen, must they not also criticize the diagnosis of grave bacterial infections by those unskilled in bacteriology? If twentieth–century doctors disapproved of consultation by letter, on the ground that no trustworthy opinion could be based on medical data furnished by an undependable patient, how could they tolerate a system in which a doctor with little bacteriological expertise used its findings to conduct his practice?[69]

Wright's concerns were expressed again by subsequent twentieth–century physicians, who realized that many doctors ordering laboratory tests had little working experience with the wide range of techniques used to analyze specimens in the laboratory, or with the criteria by which laboratory workers made judgments. They often did not know how the tests were performed, the assumptions used in calculating results, or the physiological and pathological circumstances that could influence the test result.[70] Without this knowledge, they could not adequately subject laboratory evidence to medical scrutiny. The clinician George Pickering, who became the Regius Professor of Medicine at Oxford, commented in 1955: "To rely on data, the nature of which one does not understand, is the first step in losing intellectual honesty. The doctor is peculiarly vulnerable to a loss of this kind. . .And the loss naturally leaves him and his patients poorer."[71]

The historical experience of medicine thus reveals diagnostic technology to be a double–edged sword. Its use can enlarge the doctor's knowledge of disease, but it also can erode his confidence in his ability to make independent judgments. The doctor can rely too much upon machines and technical experts but not enough on techniques of gathering data founded upon his own abilities and experiences. If the doctor develops a distrust for his nontechnical judgments, he risks becoming merely an intermediary between the patient and the medical judgments rendered by technical experts and machines.

9 Selection and evaluation of evidence in medicine

Two movements developed in the late nineteenth and twentieth centuries which raised important questions about medicine's uncritical reliance on technologically generated facts. The first attempted to reverse the growing neglect of the patient's views – his history and his description of symptoms. It emphasized that they constituted important evidence and should be carefully considered by the doctor evaluating an illness. The second emphasized that all techniques used to gather and evaluate medical evidence, including those based on technology, were liable to significant error.

An effort to persuade doctors to listen again more carefully to the patient's view of his illness was made by the British physician James Mackenzie. After several years of working at a general practice begun in 1879, Mackenzie discovered that his patients suffered mostly from subjective complaints that often gave him no clue about the nature of the illness. Equally discouraging, Mackenzie found that the physical signs of illness which he himself could observe, and which had been the chief focus of his training at medical school, often failed to clarify medical problems. In evaluating an illness, Mackenzie sought the meaning of his patients' sensations in textbooks of the period, but learned little; textbook writers appeared to believe that the data latent in the patient's report of his sensations were untrustworthy, exaggerated, vague, and distorted in a thousand ways.

Believing these assumptions to be wrong, Mackenzie set out to examine the significance of his patients' complaints by tracking individual symptoms over long periods. His goal, for each sensation or physical sign of disease reported, was to determine its physiological causes, its bearing on diagnosis, and on the future health of the patient. Mackenzie found that the patient's reported feelings usually produced the earliest clues to the presence of disease; they also furnished firsthand evidence of how an organ functioned and

174

so provided a continuing index of the status and likely outcome of the illness.[1]

At the time Mackenzie was practicing, prognosis – assessing the signs of illness to learn its most likely outcome – was an aspect of medicine generally unappreciated and poorly studied (and it remains poorly cultivated today). Nineteenth-century British and American literature contains few works solely devoted to a general exploration of prognosis. Some commentators on the uses of new information–gathering techniques occasionally discussed their prognostic value, most notably in connection with the sphygmograph and the thermometer. But prognosis was usually subsumed under diagnosis which, by naming the species to which an illness belonged and thus describing the typical and expected course of that illness, implied prognosis. As one physician told the International Congress of Medicine in 1913, "What physician, failing an accurate diagnosis, could venture on a prognosis or prescribe a treatment? . . .For us diagnosis signifies the recognition, as perfect and precise as our means of investigation will allow, of a morbid condition considered in regard to its origin, its present state, its future course. Thorough diagnosis is almost one with scientific prognosis."[2]

While Mackenzie was urging that illness could be better understood and detected earlier if doctors listened to what patients said, some of his contemporaries were also arguing that attentive listening could illuminate the emotional and social components of their patients' complaints, and thereby improve the effectiveness with which illness was managed. These practitioners took pains to distinguish the art from the science of medicine. Through medical science the physician investigated the mechanisms of pathology, through medical art he pursued the intricacies of personality; through medical science he studied parts of the patient to find the causes of biological breakdown, through medical art he kept the whole patient together, and observed him as he lived and worked. While medical science could be learned from books and in laboratories, medical art could be learned only from experience with patients. Essentially, the argument concluded, the art of medicine was a talent for understanding the human needs of the patient and using this knowledge to manage his illness better.

Enthusiastic young graduates of the early twentieth century who considered medicine mainly as a science were often bewildered when confronted with the human problems of practice. Schooled

175

chiefly in laboratories, wards, and morgues, and too briefly in out-patient departments or in the community, the newly qualified practitioner excelled in treating unusual, scientifically complicated cases, but often felt inadequate in handling ill-defined, every-day complaints and uneasy when dealing with human nature. Before the introduction of diagnostic technology during the nineteenth and early twentieth centuries, medical art was applied often; knowledge of human nature was considered more necessary for successful practice than was scientific knowledge. Ignorance of the causes of disease had frequently compelled pre–nineteenth–century physicians to treat patient rather than the disease. But the success they achieved, or the success that the most ignorant quacks achieved if they handled the human being with tact and sympathy; the failure of some of the best students at medical school to attract a large practice; or the success of others who had barely passed their examinations – these circumstances, which showed the power of the art, impressed only a few doctors in the medical climate of the early twentieth century, attracted more and more by technological methods.[3]

Into this picture came psychoanalysis and allied explorations of the human mind and emotions, whose data were not readily amenable to observation and measurement in the laboratory. As the twentieth century progressed, problems that could be dealt with only by the art of medicine were redefined in the new psychiatric and sociological terms and gradually brought within the framework of "scientific" medicine through theories about mental and emotional life and social behavior. The Viennese physician Sigmund Freud stimulated this reinterpretation through his work on emotional development, which by 1910 had spread from Europe to the United States. Freud was the principal exponent of a theory that attributed many emotional and physical disturbances to the continual reliving of unpleasant episodes of childhood, the memory of which the patient had erased from consciousness. By inducing the patient to relate in full detail his life history and the circumstances surrounding his present illness, physicians sought to retrieve this lost memory and to connect it with the symptoms displayed by the patient. The history became the cardinal focus of the new method, called psychoanalysis. Unlike the history–taking of the past, psychoanalysis was conducted under special conditions and according to a special methodology. The patient lay upon a couch in a quiet room, the analyst seated outside of the patient's field of vision. The patient was urged to say whatever came to his mind, however trivial or unrelated to his problem it seemed. The doctor listened to the patient, making no effort to direct the unfolding of the story by questions. The doctor neither took notes nor focused his mind on anything in particular said by the patient. Freud had urged doctors to maintain an "evenly–hovering attention" to everything heard, to avoid exerting a selective censorship that would bias their subsequent interpretation of events as the patient's story unfolded. The demand on the doctor for "evenly–hovering attention" was the corollary to the demand on the patient to disclose without selection anything that entered his mind. The physician who practiced analysis must himself have been analyzed, to uncover the hidden conflicts in his own unconscious mind that might introduce a damaging selection and bias into the therapy he chose. The crucial diagnostic instrument of psychoanalysis was the physician's own mind. As Freud advised, the physician "must bend his own unconscious like a receptive organ towards the emerging unconscious of the patient, be as the receiver of a telephone to the disc. As the receiver transmutes the electric vibrations induced by the sound-waves back again into sound-waves, so is the physician's unconscious mind able to reconstruct the patient's unconscious."[4]

Psychoanalysis focused attention on the importance of the patient's life history in relation not only to emotional but also to physical illness, which had two basic components: one perceptible in the physical destruction of tissue; the other in what the patient associated, feared, and apprehended from the destruction. Psychoanalysis elevated the importance of the patient's history: some doctors now interpreted it as a record of the mind's reaction to its environment, as a functional test of the mind. Those who practiced "the art of medicine" had attempted to learn about human nature by linking the patient's life with his illness, but they had usually done so in a haphazard way, and without penetrating deeply into his mental life. In providing a theory and a method for probing deeply into human nature, psychoanalysis demonstrated that for effective therapy, kindliness and humanity often were not enough

The difficulty of mastering the psychoanalytic method, and the length of time it often required, made it inapplicable to general medical practice. As an alternative means to evaluate and relieve emotional problems physicians developed a technique called "conscious psychotherapy," which used persuasion, explanation, and education in a rational appeal to the conscious mind. With this

177

technique they often successfully treated disorders such as hysteria, insomnia, and fatigue.[5] Although conscious psychotherapy totally differed in concept and application from psychoanalysis, it represented an effort by physicians to link man's inner life with his illness.

Medical social work complemented psychoanalytic emphasis on the patient's experiences and thought. In 1905 Richard Cabot established at the Massachusetts General Hospital the first social service department in American medicine. It trained social workers and doctors to examine how a patient's home and work environment influenced his illness. Cabot believed that the neglect of the social circumstances influencing illness produced ineffective treatment. He gave as an example the problem of the woman with diabetes, whom medicine could not help much but dietary change could. It was

useless to hand her out a diet-list without finding out whether she can get at her boarding-house any such diet as we recommend. It turns out that she cannot, that there is no boarding-house for diabetics, and that she had no money to spend on specially-selected diets. Shall we simply pass to the next case and let the woman's disease run on to its fatal termination unimpeded? The physician in charge has no time to investigate her case or to discover what resources, if any, the city of Boston contains for supplying her need. . .He needs the help of social workers to *make his treatment effective.*[6]

Like those who cultivated the art of medicine, proponents of psychoanalysis and medical social work reminded physicians that body organs were connected to patients, that patients were part of environments, and that physicians must understand these links or risk failure in therapy.

Despite Cabot, Freud, and others who followed in their footsteps, before World War II American physicians generally did not spend much time in exploring their patients' social or emotional experiences, and seldom appreciated how great an influence the doctor's personality could have on the diagnosis and the therapeutic outcome. To most physicians the social milieu of the patient seemed much too formidable to attempt to change, and its study was left mainly to the growing cadres of medical social workers. The doctor's exploration of the emotional components of illness was hampered in part by the attempted use of psychoanalysis by laymen who lacked proper training in its principles; the sometimes deplorable results tended to discredit Freud's entire method. The American public adopted psychoanalytic terms, with only a vague understanding of their technical meaning. Literary critics used its terminology in their writings, often incorrectly; novelists and biographers "psychoanalyzed" their characters in ways that often gave a false impression of the technique; laymen were even told (usually by other laymen) how to psychoanalyze themselves; and there appeared a flood of books, magazines, and newspaper articles that distorted both the methods and the consequences of the method. With the popularization of psychoanalysis came protests from religious groups. *Catholic World* in 1923 criticized Freudian doctrine for endangering morals, and objected to what it considered the psychoanalyst's displacement of the priest as doctor to the soul. In this climate, many physicians, who might otherwise have accepted Freud, could not distinguish between skilled and unskilled psychoanalysis, but judged it from the excesses they saw about them; thus they were deprived of insights into the relationship of emotions to illness to which psychoanalytic writings would have alerted them.[7]

Other reasons existed for the early neglect of the emotional components of illness. All physicians had to choose how to spend the limited time and energy available for practice: ordering laboratory tests, examining prominent physical signs, taking a brief history, and assessing the pathology they revealed took relatively little time; exploring the emotional life of twenty or thirty patients a day consumed time and energy that the average practitioner simply could not give. Another factor was that medical–school instruction in mental disease was usually based on demonstrations with grossly psychotic people who had little chance of recovering, and often were displayed like exhibits at a side show. The practicing physician was inclined to ignore what he regarded as the medicine of the madhouse. Psychoanalysis also roused opposition from patients; they resented being labeled as mentally ill, for to them, as to many doctors, the label seemed more a sentence than a diagnosis. And the average doctor, like other people, had built his own defensive mental walls against the fantasies and impulses of the mind and avoided confronting these forces in others for fear of stirring them up in himself.

Thus, while the taboo of physical examination had been broken in the nineteenth century, before World War II both doctor and patient strove to avoid inquiry into emotional life, despite the widely reported estimates that in the United States from 30 to 75 percent of patients' complaints had emotional origins.[8]

A change began during World War II, when medical evidence

179

from the armed forces focused attention on the men's emotional and social experience. Because over a third of Americans rejected for military service were rejected for neuropsychiatric disorders,[9] physicians began to question the wisdom of their preoccupation with physical illness. They began to listen more attentively to colleagues who thought of disease as a maladaption to biological, familial, or environmental circumstances – as disturbances of thoughts, feelings, and social relationships as well as disturbances of tissues and body fluids, whose cause could be a bacterium or a bayonet, a cancer cell or a seduction, a lack of calcium or of love. For some of these disorders, medical terms existed; for others, only the words of everyday speech.[10] While the view of man as primarily a physicochemical organism has remained the dominant view in postwar medicine, the reality of these disorders is accepted by growing numbers of physicians, and has influenced their practice.

The relationship of mental life to illness shown by psychoanalysis also prompted a number of doctors to reexamine their technique of history–taking. With the start of the twentieth century, it became increasingly routine for students and hospital physicians to take histories and do physical examinations by following an outline. This approach represented an effort to prevent distortion of the information from the patient by collecting answers to a standardized set of questions. It also helped deter the patient from attempting to reveal to the doctor irrelevant experiences. Such a medical history was patterned after the conduct of a physical examination on a passive patient; it was far from the two–person interchange of dialogue in which both participants probed deep into the nature of the issue at hand. In the outline method, the human relation between doctor and patient during history-taking, while perhaps more personal than when the doctor was listening to the heart or feeling the abdomen, was minimal. Not surprisingly, students who were taught to take histories with a standardized set of questions tended to believe that they could acquire a complete story of the illness if they asked the patient all questions in the outline, regardless of the fact that forcing rapid answers to the many questions often obscured the patient's main reasons for seeking medical care. And even after a student had given up rigid adherence to an outline, his earlier tactics in gaining information from patients tended to lessen his capacity for effective dialogue with them; as a practicing doctor he had learned to phrase questions in ways that allowed more or less yes–or–no answers, and so he might miss important leads provided by spontaneous remarks. Sometimes if a question revealed a problem that might take considerable time to investigate the doctor, having other questions to ask, might cut off the patient.[11] Audio and visual tape–recordings of doctor–patient interviews, used in medical education since the 1950s demonstrated that preoccupation with charting could result in the loss of valuable leads from the tone of voice, slips of the tongue, and facial expressions.[12] The recordings helped some students and physicians to recognize that the clinician who concentrated on the examination to the virtual exclusion of the patient was not listening with the "third ear," as the psychiatrist Theodore Reik put it.[13]

Psychoanalysis helped generate a change in history–taking methods, particularly after the 1940s. In this new type of history, or interview as it was often referred to, the physician sought not only to identify a disease, but also to discover what sort of person the patient was; to establish a relationship that fostered some understanding of the problems created by illness. Through such an inquiry into the sensations and life of the patient, the physician sought to uncover aspects of illness hidden from all other information–gathering techniques of medicine, and to keep the unique characteristics of the patient and his illness constantly before him. Through the interview, physicians attempted to uncover the implied meaning, as distinct from the logical content of words, to read the silences, and the rich communications made by expression, posture, and gesture. A casual parenthesis, a fleeting change in countenance, often provided a significant clue to the nature of the illness. The patient's problems were usually more extensive than his stated complaint. As the American psychoanalyst Erik Erikson's apocryphal patient told his physician, "Doctor, my bowels are sluggish, my feet hurt, my heart jumps – and you know, Doctor, I myself don't feel so well either."[14]

However, this change of attitude did not pervade all of medicine: many doctors continued to believe that the patient's story yielded less significant findings, obtained at a greater outlay of time, than those provided by other modes of diagnosis – notably ones organized around a technology.

Another effort to persuade twentieth–century physicians to listen more to their patients, and also to depend more on their own sensory judgments, was based upon reducing the doctor's reliance on technology in evaluating disease. James Mackenzie was a key figure in this field too. He advocated that no instrument should be accepted in medical practice until its inventor had shown that its revelations were pertinent to evaluating the health of the patient. Going still further, he urged that after a mechanical device had proven its value in clinical medicine, physicians should stop using it and try to obtain the same information from symptoms recognizable by the doctor himself. Mackenzie applied this logic even to his own ink polygraph, a variation of the sphygmograph: "For routine practice no instrument is necessary, and as soon as I had found out the knowledge it could convey, I set about discovering means by which the information could be obtained by the unaided senses."[15]

Mackenzie was not the first to argue that instruments could be used to sharpen the doctor's powers of observation. The sphygmograph, for example, diminished the importance of data gained through touch, by manifesting the pulse to the eye of the beginner and preserving a permanent record of it; but by improving the physician's understanding of the pulse, the machine also instructed the hand, which on occasion might be substituted for the machine. The thermometer, too, was supposed to improve the tactile evaluation of temperature, the blood-pressure machine to increase tactile sensitivity toward the pulse, and the electrocardiogram to improve the ability of the palpating fingers and listening ears to gain information about the condition of the heart. Of the doctors who praised such sensory education, only Mackenzie urged his colleagues to disregard the machine from which they learned.[16] He was convinced that laboratory methods and machines revealed but a fraction of the symptoms in any given patient, and that in every case, the doctor should search for other clues perceptible to the unaided but trained mind and senses. If the patient did not feel ill and showed no physical signs of illness, any facts revealed by technology were probably not important to his health. The mind and senses of the physician were to reign supreme; instrumental aids would serve as guides to new phenomena. Except for use in teaching (and chiefly for the purpose of training the senses) or research, diagnostic technology should be to the general practitioner what the bureaucratic apparatus of the state was to the Communist – programmed from its creation to ultimately wither away. This extreme point of view understandably never gained wide acceptance, but Mackenzie was perhaps the most influential twentieth–century supporter of the idea that the doctor was more important than the instrument.

Those who like Mackenzie seek to show the limitations of technologically generated evidence have pointed out that facts obtained from the laboratory are in one sense no more objective than those gathered at the bedside – both types of evidence must be interpreted by a human mind. Instruments are only powerful transmitters. Essentially all data are subjective: in all observations an opinion is registered at the same time that a fact is recorded.[17]

The influence of human subjectivity on all medical evidence is nowhere better demonstrated than in studies of observer error in medicine. During the nineteenth century, some physicians had been troubled by the faulty data that could be produced by mechanical flaws in their instruments – particularly in the microscope, thermometer, sphygmograph, and blood-cell counter – and by differences in the perceptions of observers who viewed the same data. These problems were not comprehensively investigated until the early twentieth century, when several empirical studies appeared.[18] These papers linked observer variation and error to flaws in the physician's personality (the fearful doctor who hesitated to make judgments or the rash doctor who reached decisions too quickly); to carelessness; to inexperience; to untactful behavior with patients; to faulty medical education; and to shortcomings in medical knowledge and techniques. These studies concluded that medical techniques and their human users were prone to similar degrees of variation and thus were jointly responsible for errors in medical judgment.

As concern grew about this problem, the laboratory received the most intensive scrutiny, because its results were assuming great importance to physicians.[19] Careful examination revealed that the physiological constitution of the patient himself repeatedly changed, and that its inconstancy could produce misleading results in laboratory tests – a conclusion that had been reached earlier by nineteenth-century chemists. Variables such as digestion, emotion, work, and weather caused unpredictable changes in body chemistry, and hence in the outcome of tests. Misinterpretation could also be traced to such factors as damage to specimens sent to distant laboratories for analysis, and random variables in the substances used to perform tests. For example, variations were detected in the guinea–pig serum used in the Wassermann test for syphilis, and in the media used to culture bacteria. Other sources of error in laboratory tests were foreign substances present in the material being examined, dirty equipment, or wrongly labeled specimens.

183

A far more important source of error than flaws in technical laboratory testing lay in human mistakes in performing the tests and judging their results. Laboratory workers not only exhibited widely diverse skills in executing technical procedures, but also had different understandings of what constituted an end reaction in a test.

By the 1920s, the increase in the kind and number of determinations that the laboratory could make, widespread confidence in the results, and the doctors' tendency to delegate even the simplest technical examinations to others had brought about a proliferation of laboratories, few of them under the direction of properly trained physicians. Some doctors did limit their work to laboratory pathology, but graduates fresh from medical school tended not to adopt this specialty; practice paid better and brought more prestige. Thus both hospital and private laboratories were often forced to place technicians, nurses, or inadequately trained doctors in charge of their complex bacteriological, chemical, immunological, and microscopy laboratories. Responsibility for the work drifted gradually into the hands of the lay technician, and the private laboratory, in particular, was often run for profit. Not all such laboratories were inadequate, but many owed much of their reputation to a display of glittering instruments and bombastic advertising reminiscent of the patent medicine man. "Behind the glass-topped tables and the polished armamentarium; ready and prepared with a 'prompt, reliable' and sure–fire test for whatever ails you," one found only "a technician capitalizing [on] the need of the patient and – must it be said – the carelessness of the physician for whom laboratories are laboratories."[20]

Some owners of laboratories hired untrained people willing to work cheaply, and gave them superficial instruction in performing a few routines. Yet, even the best laboratory worker was handicapped in that he had no contact with the patient. The blood, urine, and tissues of patients came to the technician, but usually not the patient himself, or even a report of the patient's history. Understandably, the technician often failed to recognize how heavy a responsibility he bore. A mistake in his report might result in prolonged or dangerous therapy for the patient, but the laboratory technician was too remote to feel a personal interest in the individual patient, as did the doctor. The technician's sense of responsibility was weakened further by the large number of tests ordered. A request for a specific test with a statement of why it was wanted, such as "hemoglobin and blood cell analysis for evidence of lead poisoning," focused his attention and skill but a general request for a "routine blood chemistry" tended to dull his interest in his job. Many laboratory workers repeating endless routine tests for faceless patients, viewed their daily work as a dreary procession of technical acts rather than as a contribution, made in partnership with the doctor, toward helping sick people get well.[21]

Physicians themselves unknowingly encouraged the generation of laboratory error in other ways. Their confidence in laboratory accuracy often blinded them to the errors caused by carelessness in collecting, preserving, and transporting the material to be examined. Typical of the problem was the preparation of slides smeared with blood, used to diagnose malaria. If the microscopist was to have an even chance to detect the presence of malaria, the blood had to be drawn at a definite point in the cycle of disease, be evenly spread on the slide, and this had to be done before the patient had been saturated with quinine, the normal treatment for the disease. The test was useless if, as sometimes happened, the physician fed large doses of quinine to his patient, and later collected a drop of blood on the slide. Often a doctor neglected to send the details of the case along with a specimen, to ensure an unbiased judgment, or restricted the type of procedures to be performed, thus tying the hands of laboratory experts who might have suggested other relevant tests.[22]

In 1919, Boston health department officials initiated a pioneering study of laboratory accuracy,[23] in their concern for false diagnoses of a communicable disease which could affect public health as well as the private individual. A false negative result opened the possibility that a carrier could unknowingly transmit his infection to others. A false positive test, particularly for venereal disease, could stigmatize the person involved, psychologically and socially. In the investigation, specimens of body fluids were submitted to fourteen laboratories run by the government, and large private hospitals. They were asked to evaluate the specimens for five diseases – diphtheria, tuberculosis, typhoid fever, gonorrhea, and syphilis. Their reports showed wide disparities in the analysis of identical specimens.

These results, and the poor reputation of some laboratories, in 1923 prompted a number of private organizations representing chemists, pathologists, and bacteriologists to ask the American Medical Association to consider with them a means of supervising clinical laboratories. Discussion among the groups in the following year led to the choice of the AMA's Council on Medical Education and Hospitals for the oversight job. The council, with the cooperation of the laboratory experts, established standards for laboratories and issued a yearly list of those that met the committee's criteria. Because of the committee's actions, physicians began to urge that laboratory technicians pass licensing examinations. An increasing number of laboratories formerly run by technicians came under the control of physicians, while some of the worst commercial laboratories went out of business. Although gradually a better knowledge of the requirements for a good laboratory spread through the medical profession, and the prestige and salaries increased for physicians who chose laboratory diagnosis as their specialty, problems persisted.[24]

In the late 1930s, the United States Public Health Service undertook several studies to gauge the accuracy with which municipal and state laboratories conducted blood tests for syphilis. Despite previous efforts to upgrade laboratories, these studies showed "conclusively that many laboratories have not met the minimum standard of efficiency of serologic test performance."[25]

Studies conducted in the following decade revealed the problem of laboratory error had not yet been solved. A 1949 evaluation of eighteen laboratories in Connecticut found the test results unacceptable in over one–third of the specimens analyzed. This outcome was ominous because among the institutions surveyed were large hospitals whose laboratories were overseen by full–time physician–pathologists. "One can only guess at the level of performance in most of the very small hospitals employing a part time director or in commercial laboratories with one or two unsupervised technicians," the researchers concluded.[26] An examination of laboratories in Pennsylvania at about the same time produced the equally disheartening conclusion that "the accuracy of the measurements is below any reasonable standard. . .The unsatisfactory results outnumbered the satisfactory and. . .no laboratory had a perfect score."[27] In the Pennsylvania study, both the poorly trained and the able but overworked technicians seemed the principal factors in the poor performance. Even at this time, technicians' salaries continued to be too low to attract people of the intellectual caliber required for the work. Many physicians and hospital administrators of the period still regarded laboratory pathology as the mere performance of simple mechanical techniques which demanded neither much training nor judgment.

In the 1960s, laboratory accuracy remained a widely debated subject in American medicine. A mid–decade study by Dr. Henry Bauer, director of medical laboratories for the Minnesota Department of Health, showed that 34 states lacked laws establishing scientific standards for the performance of tests, or educational standards for employment in laboratories. This study linked laboratory error to a shortage of staff – the result of continued low pay and status for laboratory technicians – and to their varying level of education: those with more education made fewer errors. From evidence he had gathered, and that of others, Dr. Bauer asserted that laboratory tests in the United States "were performed at levels of quality that can be described as far from adequate for today's clinical needs."[28] Others shared his opinion. In testimony before the United States Senate, Dr. David Sencer, director of the Center for Disease Control (CDC), a federal government health agency, stated that the results from over 25 percent of all laboratory tests in the country were unsatisfactory.[29] He based his statement on investigations of the accuracy in New York City laboratories and federal medical laboratories. Another examination conducted by the College of American Pathologists found a high rate of accuracy (85 to 95 percent) in the laboratories investigated.[30] The variation in accuracy reported for different laboratories disturbed a number of officials. They cooperated to gain passage in the United States Congress of the 1967 Clinical Laboratory Improvement Act, which placed the performance of some 700 laboratories doing business in more than one state under the regulatory eye of the CDC.[31]

During the 1970s the problem of error concerned not only physicians and laboratory specialists, but also a growing number of congressmen (now concerned about laboratory costs as well), who wanted to extend federal regulation of laboratories. By 1977 barely half of the states had enacted laws which set scientific standards for laboratories or required the licensing of technologists. Direct federal oversight was restricted to laboratories engaged in interstate commerce, and to some which participated in federal health insurance programs. But these numbered only about 4,000, a small portion of the total. There were about 15,000 hospital and independent commercial laboratories; and nobody was quite sure either how many physicians, with or without the aid of technicians, maintained laboratories for doing simple tests in their private offices (estimates ranged from 50,000 to 80,000), or how accurate were the tests done in them.[32]

A number of studies indicated that the accuracy of many hospital and independent laboratories needed further improvement. For example, one conducted by the state of New Jersey from 1967 to 1973, evaluated the performance of 257 laboratories in a basic test – the level of hemoglobin in the blood. Almost one in five failed to provide an acceptable result more than 70 percent of the time they were tested.[33] Data from the 1975 CDC laboratory evaluation program revealed about 20 percent of some 500 bacteriology laboratories incorrectly identified bacteria one out of four times, or less. The accuracy of chemical analyses of elements of the blood varied widely. While less than one laboratory in twenty failed within acceptable limits to gauge the amount of one substance (sodium) in the blood samples analyzed, more than one in four failed to gauge the level of another substance (creatinine). The director of the CDC laboratory licensing and testing division noted that the performance of participants in these evaluations "often reflects the best quality that a laboratory staff can provide rather than the quality of service provided an ordinary patient specimen."[34]

Several remedies for these problems were proposed. One was additional federal legislation to establish broader and stricter oversight of clinical laboratories. A second was an increased effort to automate laboratory procedures, which was known to improve the dependability of some tests. For example, the precision of estimating hemoglobin in the blood almost doubled when an automated instrument replaced manual techniques. Automated instruments also had the advantage over manual methods of requiring fewer technologists to run them. However, automation created new problems. There was concern that automated devices would foster a potentially dangerous propensity to diminish human supervision of laboratory procedures. Yet the technicians who maintained and supervised the equipment needed more than ordinary training and skill to ensure dependable results. An instrument might be precise (repeatedly giving the same analysis of a biological substance), but if flaws existed in quality control procedures, the answer it gave might not be accurate: "It is important to realize that in most cases precision is the result of instrumentation. Accuracy is the result of people."[35] There was worry too that the results of automated tests might be accepted by physicians even more uncritically than those

188

performed manually: "Very few [physicians] now feel comfortable in arguing with data generated by pumps, color–coded tubing, bubbling or mixed chambers, and automated print–outs."[36]

Beginning mainly in the 1920s, physicians also explored the problem of errors in reading X-rays. They found that misinterpretation could stem from faults in the materials – changes in the composition of plates, chemicals, or temperatures of the solutions used to develop X-rays could alter the outcome – as well as from an inadequate knowledge of the normal structural variance in the body. Errors resulted also from the pressures some radiologists felt to elevate the esteem in which their relatively young specialty was held. Toward this end, radiologists sometimes tried to hide from clinicians, and often from themselves, the existence of subjective factors that influenced judgments about X-rays, such as sensory acuity. Another source of error was what has been characterized as the "blind, unswerving, thoughtless belief in the infallibility of the roentgen ray by the medical profession as a whole,"[37] that had developed in medicine by the 1920s.

Because of their belief in the X-ray's dependability, many doctors did not think it necessary to provide a history of the patient being X-rayed so that the radiologist, like the laboratory worker, was often isolated from contact with patients. He was given little information about the patient's medical condition partly because many doctors considered the radiologist more a physicist than a physician. Furthermore, since the average doctor of the 1920s thought of radiology as an automatic procedure – take a picture "and presto! there is the diagnosis all but labelled for him on the film, like the pink ticket of the fortune-telling machine!"[38] – physicians without experience in radiology began to install X-ray and fluoroscopic machines (now made simple to operate by enterprising manufacturers) in their offices and to produce and interpret X-ray shadows. This led to dangerous illusions. The patient left the doctor's office thinking he had had an accurate X-ray study, and the physician believed that he had made one. Even laymen were permitted to operate X-ray laboratories, not only making but sometimes interpreting X-ray films.

The magnitude of observer variation in radiology was not fully apparent until publication of a 1947 study conducted by a group of radiologists, the American physician Carl Birkelo and his colleagues.[39] Their original objective was to determine whether film size altered diagnostic accuracy – a question raised by the introduction of small X-ray films to expedite the mass screening of military recruits for World War II. As an unexpected consequence of the study, the doctors found that they differed with the film interpretation of their colleagues about a third of the time, and upon a second review of films even with themselves about a fifth of the time.

These circumstances prompted the appointment of three radiologists of international repute to investigate the problem thoroughly. They read a prepared set of 100 films twice, and to their dismay produced results similar to those of the Birkelo study.[40] Unconvinced by these findings, the Danish government in the early 1950s conducted a study of the accuracy of X-ray reading before embarking upon a mass public health X-ray campaign.[41] It had each of three experienced radiologists read 2,500 films; they agreed on only about 12 percent of the films labeled by any one of them as pathological. For each confirmed pathological finding, they reported more than two false positive shadows. In spite of this bias toward labeling a shadow pathological when in doubt, the radiologists missed about one-third of the actual lesions revealed in the films. Even the assumption that the lesions missed in such investigations were of no clinical importance was disproven when Zwerling and his colleagues documented that active lesions were just as likely to be overlooked as inactive ones.[42] Subsequent studies have shown the continuing presence of such problems.[43]

Examination of the reliability of another widely used and respected technology, the electrocardiogram (EKG), produced equally disheartening results. In one study conducted in 1958, ten physicians, not experts in cardiology but representative of the general physicians who took and interpreted electrocardiograms, read the same 100 EKGs. They could agree unanimously on only about one–third of the tracings.[44] Yet the many textbooks written on the subject during the period gave little hint that such difficulties existed in agreeing on the meanings of EKGs. Inquiries conducted in the 1960s showed that an observer, on reexamination of EKGs, differed with himself in his interpretation about one–fifth of the time, and with colleagues about one–third of the time.[45]

When the unaided sense or simple instruments were used in diagnosis, disagreement among observers was no greater, but no less, than when complicated machines were used. A 1930 study on tonsillectomy had produced unexpected results. Of 1000 school children surveyed, almost two-thirds had had their tonsils removed. The remainder were examined by a group of twenty doctors who evaluated the tonsils visually in order to select those requiring tonsillectomy. They chose nearly one–half. The remaining half, presumably in good health, were reexamined by another group of doctors, who again recommended about half for tonsillectomy. The children declared to have healthy tonsils were examined by a third group of doctors, who also judged that about half needed the operation. Here the study stopped; of the original 1000 children, there were only 65 left whose tonsils had neither been removed nor been recommended for surgery. The physicians' possible desire to earn a fee played no role in these judgments – the children had access to a free clinic. The investigators concluded that the chance of being recommended for tonsillectomy depended more on the physician's preconceptions than on the child's health.[46]

In another study made during the 1950s on the perception of physical signs, eight experienced internists carried out a physical evaluation of twenty patients who had the lung disease emphysema. No more than two-thirds of the doctors could agree on the presence of any one sign of the disease, or on the diagnosis of emphysema. "Most of us assume that except in occasional borderline cases, the signs we observe are present and those which we do not observe are absent. However, experiment does not support this view and great disparities become apparent," concluded the investigators.[47] Equally disquieting was a test conducted in 1960 of the ability of over 900 physicians to identify heart lesions, by auscultation. It revealed that generalists who had practiced twenty or more years were correct only 41 percent of the time, and heart specialists correct about 79 percent of the time.[48]

Tests on the accuracy of history–taking also produced discouraging facts. In one study, six physicians interviewed almost 1000 coal miners to seek symptoms of four lung disorders. They asked the same questions of all, and each question could be answered by yes or no. Nevertheless, significant variation appeared in the responses different doctors obtained from the same patient.[49]

A crucial factor producing differences among observers was the lack of knowledge or agreement on the criteria for normalcy or pathology. For example, clinicians who were quick to see the potential value of the X-ray, after its discovery in 1895, began to use the method before systematic study of healthy subjects had provided the necessary baseline for judging pathology. The problem worsened as the twentieth century progressed. With the general decline in the frequency with which patients were brought to autopsy, X-ray signs were not well controlled by autopsy findings. Many radiologists rarely saw an autopsy, and few ever attended vivisections in an operating theater.

Laboratory tests also lacked clear standards to distinguish normal from abnormal findings,[50] the same problem that hampered the correct evaluation of heart murmurs, blood pressure, pulse rate, and electrocardiograms. Equivocal statements in textbooks that categorized as abnormal the innumerable variants that bordered on normal added to the confusion. Variation among observers also was encouraged by a standard of behavior that became particularly ingrained in twentieth–century medicine. Most doctors learned early in their training the informal medical canon that to misjudge and call a well person sick, was a far less grievous error than to misjudge and call a sick person well. If the person were in fact well, but diagnosed as sick, most physicians believed that the person suffered unjustified expense and anxiety – little more. But if a person were in fact sick, a diagnosis of health destroyed all chance of his being treated when the condition was in its earliest stages.

This double standard in viewing the seriousness of a wrong diagnosis was maintained by the differences in the consequences, legal and professional, to the physician who made the mistake. If he dismissed a patient as well, who in fact had a detectable disease, he might be sued for negligence, deprived of his license, or censured by his colleagues for incompetence. But committing the opposite offense – calling a well person ill – carried little penalty; indeed some physicians regarded the mistake as indicative of a good, conservative approach to illness. Interpreting a test so as to detect the greatest number of people who were sick, inevitably increased the number of well people who were classified as sick – false positives. Conversely, interpreting the test to exclude as many well people as possible, increased the number of sick people who went undetected by the test – false negatives. When faced with which interpretation to give the data, physicians usually chose to detect the greater number of people who were ill.[51]

Disagreement among observers in interpreting data is a problem not confined to medicine. Experiments in psychology, and the circumstances underlying discoveries in the physical sciences, make it clear that people often see what they expect to see. Similarly, doctors sometimes shut their eyes to observations incompatible with their ideas, close their ears "to bits of history which seem out of place," or to noises heard with the stethoscope not included in their "catalogue of official sounds."[52]

One response of physicians to varying interpretations among observers was to standardize ways of gathering facts: suggesting that instruments be tested by the United States Bureau of Standards to determine their average range of error; that a statement of the methods employed accompany each test result so that the error inherent in it could be estimated by the person who ordered the test.[53] A further suggestion was the multiple repetition of a procedure, the expedient that became most commonly applied. Although this strategy uncovered more cases of true disease, it also increased the number of people falsely diagnosed as having the disease in question.[54]

Other doctors believed that knowing the factors influencing one's own judgments would eliminate error.[55] Laboratory workers were urged to calibrate themselves to learn their own standard error in the technical procedures they performed. Radiologists were urged to do the same, but they had a more complex problem because their technique involved not only a technology but a large vocabulary. Some radiologists believed that differences in the interpretation of films resulted more from semantic misunderstanding than from differences in sensory perception. To deal with this problem, a group of radiologists carefully examined all the words commonly used in interpreting chest films to see whether they meant the same to each radiologist in the group.[56] Most conventional terms were found to be subject to variations in meaning. A shadow labeled "hard" by one doctor could be read as "soft" by another. Efforts to simplify the terms used, and to agree upon explicit meanings, had little effect on differences among individual radiologists.

The American physician Alvan Feinstein, during the 1960s, sought to standardize performance in the conduct of physical examinations by inviting each physician on his staff to specify all of the features that led him to judge physical characteristics observed in a patient as normal or abnormal. He refused to accept vague explanations such as "it sounded or looked that way." He found that the principal source of variability among observers was not sensory differences – all heard and saw essentially the same thing – but the different criteria each used for interpreting the events. For example, one physician might choose pitch and quality to weigh the character of a heart murmur, while another would add duration, site of maximal loudness, and variation with posture. Feinstein and his colleagues identified, for each other, the yardsticks they used to elicit a sign, and established specific criteria to be used in identifying the sign. When they did this their diagnostic disagreements became less frequent, or actually vanished. Feinstein hoped that bedside observations might not be displaced so readily by laboratory observations if physicians could improve the reliability of their own judgments.[57]

Yet some physicians did not believe the widespread evidence of observer disagreement justified such optimism. In 1975, a review reported on research conducted during the previous decade on observer variance. The physicians studied "almost always disagreed at least once in ten cases, and often disagreed more than once in five cases, whether they were eliciting physical signs, interpreting roentgenograms, electrocardiograms or electroencephalograms, [or] making a diagnosis." The review's author cautioned that "disagreements of this magnitude, if characteristic of clinical practice in general, cannot safely be regarded as inconsequential."[58]

Precision in medical diagnosis seems to depend on three characteristics: the intrinsic accuracy of the measurement or test, the constancy of the phenomena being measured, the ability of the observer to interpret and record the phenomena. In dealing with the problem of observer variation, doctors have usually given most weight to the measurement's accuracy, and assumed the constancy of the organ or function being evaluated, even though few biological functions are in fact unchanging – a heart murmur, for example, varies from day to day, even from hour to hour. Least attention was given to the third factor in observer variation, the physician's own possible mistakes in observation and judgment. The findings of the studies on observer disagreement were not widely accepted by physicians, for acceptance would have increased the already considerable doubt inherent in their daily confrontation with illness. It was even suggested in the 1950s that the research be discontinued because it disturbed morale too much,[59] and that the studies had little importance because decisions in medicine seldom were made on the basis of a single observation. In defense of the studies, it was pointed out that one error could reinforce another: an electrocardiogram erroneously judged abnormal might confirm an erroneously interpreted clinical symptom. Moreover, physicians often did act on the basis of a single positive sign in which they had faith.[60]

194

A number of physicians in the twentieth century have maintained that central to a comprehensive evaluation of illness is a penetrating insight into the patient's feelings and environment. To meet this they have suggested that the physician carefully listen to the patient and put searching questions to him. Other physicians have sought to alert colleagues about the significant risks they face in misperceiving and misinterpreting all types of medical evidence. In different ways both groups have raised doubts about the wisdom of overdependence on information gained through technology. In different ways they have also urged physicians to turn inward, to explore their own attitudes toward illness and ways of reaching medical judgments.

This cautionary advice generally had little effect on the diagnostic habits of most physicians or their reliance on technology. Rather, this reliance was intensified in the 1960s by the development of a new generation of machines to cope with the glut of medical data – created, largely, by the increased use of the mechanical devices for diagnosis that preceded them.

10 *Telecommunication, automation, and medical practice*

Concern with improving the standards of diagnosis and therapy, and with meeting the growing demand for medical care, prompted a number of physicians during the 1960s and 1970s to explore novel ways of organizing medical services through techniques that transmitted data over long distances, and of evaluating medical evidence through machines that processed data speedily and accurately. This chapter will focus particularly on the United States, where concentrated efforts were made to apply these techniques and machines.

During the seventeenth and eighteenth centuries medicine had been practiced in a decentralized framework. A physician performed many medical tasks by himself and did not require a host of nearby consultants. Since physicians relied heavily upon the patient's narrative as evidence, messengers or letters could be used to carry and return information; this meant that diagnosis and therapy could take place without a physical meeting between doctor and patient.

The advent of pathological anatomy, auscultation, and the other techniques of physical diagnosis changed this situation. Practitioners decreased their reliance on what the patient said or what his friends reported. The new medicine distrusted "second–hand" information – any report of illness that could not be verified. Instead, it demanded a methodical analysis of physical signs of illness, obtained firsthand from examination of the patient, and verified when possible by autopsy. The canons of physical diagnosis thus required doctor and patient to be in close proximity and diminished the possibility of diagnosis at a distance.

As the nineteenth century progressed, an increasing division of medical tasks among specialists occurred, stimulated by the anatomical and technological foundations of physical diagnosis. The

196

greater number of specialized skills now available for medical care required doctors to have more intense association with colleagues than in earlier centuries. Thus the transition from the narrative to the physical–diagnosis stage in the development of medicine encouraged physicians to abandon the decentralized form of medical care and to practice in an increasingly cooperative, and hence geographically centralized, manner.

The hospital provided physicians and patients with the cohesive structure now demanded not only by the practice but also by the learning of medicine. Laennec and other clinicians who practiced during the first half of the nineteenth century believed that the new techniques of examination could be studied properly only in a hospital. There, in a place controlled by physicians, students and physicians could carry out the time-consuming, often embarrassing physical intrusions of the new diagnostic methods upon patients far more easily than they could have in a patient's own house, or even in a doctor's private office. They could readily remove the clothes to explore the movements and sounds of the chest; they could always obtain the excretions and have the necessary chemical reagents and microscope at hand to examine them.[1] With its large number of patients, the hospital ward also offered medical students and physicians a diversity of pathological conditions to learn from, not likely to be found outside of its walls, autopsy facilities which allowed them to verify their diagnoses and acquire confidence in their bedside judgments, and a collegial atmosphere that eased the burden of learning the new physical, chemical, and microscopical signs of disease. The best way to train a practitioner was said to be for him "to pass his time amongst the sick in the wards of an hospital, and follow to the dead-house the bodies of those who die there. If he does this faithfully, he cannot fail to lay the best foundation for his own practice."[2] The English physician James Clark reported, in 1820, that in France a central office would even dispatch patients with a particular affliction to a hospital where physicians had a special interest in that disease.[3]

Thus pathological anatomy, auscultation, and the techniques of mechanical and laboratory diagnosis that followed had laid the foundation for the centralized system within which contemporary medicine is practiced – a system dependent upon the geographic proximity of doctors to each other, to patients, and to the implements of technology.

While the centralized system has prospered and enlarged for

more than a century, inventions have appeared which may, one day, change the organization of medical practice back again to a decentralized state. The earliest of these decentralizing inventions was the electric telegraph. In 1835, the American Samuel Morse built a crude working model of the telegraph, and in 1843 sent over a wire strung between Baltimore and Washington the famous message, "What hath God wrought," which helped to inaugurate the era of telegraphic communication. Physicians used the invention to transmit oral data to each other, and to evaluate absent patients more quickly and over greater distances than ever before possible. For example, U.S. Senator Charles Sumner was treated for years by the eminent physician Charles Brown–Séquard through the telegraph.[4] But for transmission of verbal data, the telephone was more convenient.

After a patent for the instrument was issued, in 1876, to Alexander Graham Bell, physicians quickly seized upon the invention for use in practice. Like the letter of consultation, the telephone was a substitute for face–to–face dialogue. In July 1878, an advertisement appeared in a California newspaper that a certain doctor "wishes to inform his patients and the public that he may be summoned or consulted through the telephone either by night or day. The communication is made through the American Speaking Telephone Company, and is absolutely private and confidential."[5] In Cincinnati in 1879, a doctor told of being called late one night by a worried parent whose child was coughing severely. Since the patient's house was several miles away and the doctor was tired, he asked to hear the child's cough through the telephone. The sound convinced the physician that the cough was not serious. He gave some therapeutic directions to the parent, visited the child in the morning, and found him well.[6]

During the 1880s physicians increasingly used the telephone to manage medical practices that covered large areas and the telegraph to prescribe in emergencies, but not without trouble. One doctor who made recommendations for his patient over the phone, instead of acceding to a request for a visit, reported that his patient later switched to another doctor. Further, as telephones spread amongst the population, physicians became increasingly vulnerable to the patient's anxieties; patients could freely call physicians whenever it entered their minds to do so. By the start of the twentieth century, the physician was described as "a slave to the peremptory call of the instrument, and must constantly be ready to answer it, as in many cases no one can answer it for him."[7]

A number of doctors protested their concern about diagnosis by telephone. In the age of physical diagnosis not to see a patient seemed "not in accord with the true ideal of professional duty."[8] But soon after the invention of the telephone, physicians began to speculate that physical diagnosis itself might be conducted over long distances, "that even such feeble sounds as those produced by the heart and lungs might be transmitted for many miles and be correctly interpreted by an educated ear," thereby allowing a physician in his consulting room to "listen to the heart or the pulse of a patient lying in bed (speaking modestly as to distance) a mile or two away."[9] Enthusiasts envisioned a future in which practitioners would nest themselves down in the center of a web of wires and auscultate patients far away. In 1877, investigators conducted one of the first experiments that attempted to telephonically monitor sounds from the chest and transmit the sounds to a receiver 800 feet away; only faint thuds were heard.[10] Other efforts to detect chest sounds with early telephonic receivers also ended in failure. Because of the susceptibility of telephonic transmission to external electric currents, and its tendency to pick up extraneous sounds (such as those produced by the contact of receiver and skin), it appeared unsuitable to convey the subtle nuances of heart and lung sounds.

The invention of the microphone in 1878 raised hopes that the device could improve telephonic auscultation. But the assumption proved premature. When the sounds heard by telephone were augmented by the microphone, tones low in pitch were not transmitted, and the sensitivity to slight disturbance generated by the contact of microphone and body surface enhanced extraneous noises.[11]

Nineteenth–century physicians had also sought to transmit objective data (such as numbers and graphs) over long distances, to transcend the need for the patient to be physically present for examination, and also to ensure that the facts of the case were similarly understood by all physicians concerned. As early as 1835, Julius Hérisson had appreciated the possibility of improving long–distance diagnosis by changing the form in which medical data were sent;[12] he believed that when a physician wrote a colleague, asking his opinion about a patient's pulse, numerical characterization was more informative than a verbal description of the pulse.

In 1860, the telegraph was again pressed into medical service to transmit medical data. A Boston physician, J. B. Upham, conducted an experiment with a device that translated the heart's motion into currents which he sent over a telegraph wire from Boston to Cambridge, three and a half miles away.[13] A decade later, the clinician Edouard Seguin sharply criticized the care given to Napoleon III during his fatal illness while staying on the Island of Chiselhurst. Instead of Napoleon's doctors traveling by steamboat to his bedside to gain diagnostic evidence, they could have received by wire numerical data about the illness, such as temperature readings; tracings of body activity such as those produced by the sphygmograph could also have been sent through the telegraph, by rigging a strip of ruled paper to the receiving end. With such evidence, the physicians could have prescribed immediately, by wire.[14]

In 1905, Willem Einthoven exploited the potential of long-distance broadcast of graphic data, in the manner Seguin had urged. Perplexed by the problem of bringing seriously ill patients to his laboratory to use the delicate, nontransportable electrocardiograph, Einthoven reasoned that since electric currents carrying messages could be sent to all corners of the world, "why should not the currents originating in the heart be conducted from the hospital to the laboratory?"[15] By making minor alterations of the telephone wire that spanned the 1.5 kilometers between his laboratory and the Leyden Hospital, Einthoven secured long–distance electrocardiograph records from patients in the wards, and renamed them "telecardiograms." This achievement attracted attention, and at the Presbyterian Hospital of New York in 1910 the wards were connected to the electrocardiograph in its laboratory by wire.[16] In 1910, S. G. Brown in London perfected an electric magnifying stethoscope by means of which long–distance auscultation became possible. His invention permitted the heart sounds of a London patient to be heard distinctly over telephone wires by doctors 100 miles away in the Isle of Wight.[17]

None of these advances however attracted a substantial following. As physicians clustered together in hospitals and urban areas in ever greater numbers, they felt no great need to exploit long–distance transmission of medical signs. Only the telephone was widely used for patient and doctor to verbally consult, but neither physician nor patient regarded this dialogue as anything but an expedient when person–to–person consultation was difficult.

Experiments in the long–distance transmission of data resumed after World War II. In 1947, a successful telephonic transmission of X-ray pictures occurred between doctors in Chester, Pennsylvania, and experts in Philadelphia, twenty miles away;[18] and in 1952 trials at sending electrocardiograms through telephone wires began again.[19] Both efforts reflected concern about the growing isolation of rural doctors from current medical technology and specialists housed in urban centers. The problems facing the Kansas State Tuberculosis Sanitarium were typical. The sanitarium was located in a town whose population of 3,000 could not attract a full–time heart specialist. The sanitarium had been mailing its electrocardiograms to the nearest city, Emporia, for interpretation, but the round trip by mail consumed four days. The installation of an apparatus in 1954 that transmitted the tracings over telephone wires to Emporia allowed a physician to receive an interpretation in only one hour.[20]

In 1967, it had become possible to make a long–distance analysis of an electrocardiogram from almost anywhere in the world. An electrocardiogram of a patient in Tours, France, was sent by telephone line and a communications satellite to a computer in Washington, D.C., which analyzed the data in 15 seconds and immediately sent back its interpretation to France.[21]

The use of television in long–distance diagnosis was another recent innovation. In 1968 the American physician Kenneth Bird opened a medical station at Logan Airport in Boston, which was visually linked with the Massachusetts General Hospital, three miles away. Physicians at the hospital took the patient's history. The nurse on duty at the airport applied electronic instruments to the patient's body which transmitted to the doctor blood pressure, heart and lung sounds, EKG, and X-ray. The television camera, controlled by the physician, monitored the nonverbal communication of facial expression, the fine details of surface anatomy, and even transmitted a magnified image of any part or product of the body.[22]

The introduction of the computer into medicine during the 1960s also stirred hopes that it could serve as a long–distance general consultant for physicians who were geographically separated from specialists. Devices were developed that converted the physician's telephone into a computer terminal through which he could send diagnostic questions and data to the computer and receive answers. In one experiment, a general practitioner located in a remote town in Missouri was linked electronically to a computer and medical specialists 130 miles away: "It's a fantastic set–up," the doctor commented. "It's the same as having the whole staff and library of the University of Missouri School of Medicine right here in my office."[23]

Such developments made the possibility seem real that the forces drawing physicians into the technological core of the hospital might be resisted – that one day a decentralization could occur that would allow a highly scientific medicine to be practiced in regions distant from specialists and the technology of modern hospitals.

The computer was the most promising of a group of machines that physicians, especially in the United States, hoped would extricate them from a deluge of information about patients, which threatened to undermine their traditional methods of organizing and using medical data. The idea for a machine having many characteristics now associated with the computer had occurred to the English mathematician–engineer Charles Babbage in the 1830s, when he developed plans for a device he called the "analytical engine." Although it was never built, Babbage had designed it to excel in three actions: performing mathematical calculations, segregating and ordering masses of data to demonstrate associations within them, and determining future courses of action based upon the analyses it had performed. Babbage's analytical engine would not only have a memory that stored the data, but would also respond to instructions from a program specified by holes punched in cards inserted into it.

Little more than a century later, in the early 1940s, separate advances in all of these areas were finally brought together in the electronic digital computer. The essential breakthrough was the notion of the stored program conceived by the American mathematician John von Neumann. This idea, the historian of science I. Bernard Cohen explains, "gave the computer the capability of treating its regulatory instructions in the same fashion as the numerical data of the input, so that the computer could alter its program and make such logical decisions as might be required from moment to moment in the course of its operation."[24] In 1951 the U.S. Census Bureau purchased the first computer to come off a production line.

By the mid-1950s, although some biomedical scientists began to use the computer to analyze the complicated data generated by their laboratory experiments, most clinicians still ignored the computer. They treated the notion of using it in medical practice as a prospect reserved for posterity, and a fitting idea to parody:

The waiting room of the future will serve eight doctors; it will be completely soundproof. The furniture will consist of contour chairs with built–in gentle massage. Color television will delight the eye, and soft music will allay anxiety. . .History taking will be painless. A group of preferential questions will be asked by tape, and the answers punched on a card. Nothing will be left to chance, and by cybernetics, the card will be quickly deposited in a slot which will provide the three most probable historical diagnoses. Thence, on a moving floor, the patient will be transported to the lab. All laboratory procedures will be done by machine – a single electronic brain which will draw blood, do all blood work, including chemistries. . .The information will be presented on [another] card, again with the three most probable diagnoses.[25]

At the same time as this appeared a cadre of physicians, scientists, and engineers were beginning to explore clinical applications for the computer.[26] The progress achieved was displayed at the Conference on Diagnostic Data Processing held in New York at the Rockefeller Institute in January, 1959 – the first major scientific meeting devoted to the prospects of using the computer in medical care. The participants raised most of the issues that were to dominate discussion during the decade ahead; at the close of the conference they unanimously and confidently adopted a resolution which stated that in medicine, electronic data processing was "ready to assume the attitudes and responsibilities of a mature field of endeavor."[27]

Two features of the computer particularly captivated physicians: its capacity to store a prodigious amount of data in a little space; and, with dispatch, to search for and to establish complicated associations that existed within the data. The computers available in 1960 could store 100 items of information on each of 50,000 patients on one reel of magnetic tape small enough to carry in a brief case; the machine could then scan all of this material and compile any requested statistics in less than an hour. The computer thus became the center of conceptual and technological developments in the 1960s that produced significant reassessments of the processes by which medical data were gathered, ordered, analyzed, and stored. In some instances, this caused a change in the conduct of medical diagnosis and the organization of men and machines that furnished medical care. The computer generated change not only through its own capabilities but, equally important, it helped to remove cobwebs of tradition covering many concepts and practices in medicine, and made physicians more receptive to other innovations to automate medical tasks.

As computer experts applied their knowledge of data–handling to medicine, they demonstrated that medical diagnosis and decision making often occurred in the face of incomplete evidence; that because of limits on the amount of data the mind could hold, the memory could recall, and the intellect could analyze, giving more pertinent information to the doctor did not necessarily diminish the uncertainty under which he acted. These were disquieting conclusions for three reasons. First, there was an expanding fund of knowledge necessary to incorporate into medical diagnosis. So many diseases and syndromes had been described by 1960, numbering in the thousands, that physicians could not recall all their names, much less the symptoms that identified them. For example, over 1,000 illnesses and about 200 symptoms were associated with the cornea of the eye alone.[28] By 1960, more than 15,000 papers pertinent to medicine appeared each year, any one of which might shed light on the illness of a patient.[29] Second, there was the doctor's inability to determine with precision, at his first encounter with a patient, which of all the kinds of data he could collect about the patient would be most useful.[30] Given this problem, doctors usually assembled all data it was possible to gather in the initial encounter with the patient, an amount limited only by discomfort, danger, or expense to the patient. Third, a growing demand for medical services threatened to flood physicians with yet more data to analyze. This demand stemmed from public pressure on physicians to discover illness in its earliest possible stages in well people, from the increasing number of older people in the population whose incidence of illness was higher than average, and from the growth of private and governmental insurance plans that removed doctor and hospital fees as barriers to obtaining care. How could physicians such as general practitioners, who usually spent seven minutes or less with each patient during office visits, or hospital interns, whose daily visit to each patient usually lasted less than ten minutes, reasonably cope with the expanding volume of patients and clinical evidence being thrust at them?[31]

To bridge the gap between the limited memory and analytic ability of the doctor, and the mass of knowledge he could now acquire through a growing armory of technology, physicians earlier in the twentieth century had turned to two agencies: specialization, and enlargement of the document in which they stored and ordered the growing cache of data generated by specialty examinations – the medical record. But by the 1960s both agencies seemed more and more inadequate to deal with this problem.

As for specialization, the recent information explosion in medicine implied such increasingly narrow focus that future specialists, even in closely related fields, might have difficulty understanding one other. And further, the information explosion foreshadowed significant problems even in organizing these experts so that their information could be efficiently united in a comprehensive diagnosis and plan of therapy for the whole patient.[32] The need for a more cohesive organization of medical practice to accommodate the multiplication of specialties also implied a greater drain of medical talent from rural communities to cities where technology, money, and large hospitals attracted doctors.

As for the medical record, it had become dinosaurlike by the 1960s, and seemed fatally encumbered by proportions grown too large during its long history. Systematic notes describing events in a patient's illness are prominent in early medical writings such as the Hippocratic school of medicine that existed in the fifth century B.C. The main organizing feature of the Hippocratic records, and those that followed in later centuries, is chronological – early aspects of illness precede later ones. Doctors have kept such records through the centuries to sustain their memory of clinical events, to teach students, and to preserve knowledge, but they sometimes wrote only brief histories, or carried the facts in their heads. A London physician in 1861 had to urge his colleagues to "take notes, not of your diagnosis, but of the *grounds on which you base it.* It is of no use to yourself, your patient, or to science to remember that on such a day you thought that there was pneumonia or tubercle, but it is of great use to all to remember why you thought so."[33]

Studies of private medical practice in the United States by Allon Peebles in 1929[34] and by Osler Peterson in 1956 revealed that fewer than one–fifth of the physicians evaluated regularly maintained complete records of the patients' symptoms and illness, diagnosis, and therapy. A few kept no records – most kept sketchy ones. The story of one doctor seemed typical. When he began practicing he kept complete records on his patients, as he had been instructed in medical school. As demands of his practice increased, he adopted a printed outline to gather data. As his practice grew still larger, filling in the outline took too much time, and he finally resorted to a small filing card on which he noted minimal data about the patient, his illness, and the therapy.[35]

Evidence was accumulated in the Peterson study which disputed the common wisdom that the personal physician's intimate knowledge of his patient made medical–record keeping unnecessary. The research found, for example, that in small towns the doctor "was likely to know a patient by his first name, that he had a backward child, how many relatives resided in his home, that his brother was in jail, etc. However, it was frequently discovered that the physicians could not recall many medical details about their regular patients. . . To expect a physician to remember all or even most of the facts about three or four thousand patients whom he has seen a variable number of times in the preceding year or two is to expect prodigies of memory beyond human capacity."[36]

Record keeping in hospitals, until well into the twentieth century, was as irregular as in private practice. Medical records written between 1885–1907 by physicians working with the Mayo brothers at St. Mary's Hospital in Rochester, Minnesota, gave scant attention to physical findings; even the diagnosis and therapy were left out half the time. It was quite unusual to find direct statements such as " 'Goes to hospital' or 'Operated on next week.' " Often the only evidence that the patient had been to surgery was inferential: a note written in the margin saying " 'Died six months after operation,' or 'It was appendix.' " The record of many patients only contained data such as name, date, age, residence, and terse statements about their illness: " 'Complains of sciatic rheumatism,' 'Wants to know the cause of her sterility,' 'Gas on the stomach and poor sleep,' or 'Night terrors – wetting bed.' "[37] In 1919, when the American College of Surgeons surveyed 617 general hospitals in the United States of 100 beds or more, fewer than one–third met their standards for acceptable records on patients.[38] Hospitals often stored records in bundles and only the better institutions, such as the Massachusetts General Hospital, bound them in volumes and ordered them chronologically.

Since its opening in 1821, the Massachusetts General has maintained detailed accounts of patient care, a record equaled by few other American hospitals. In 1837 the regulations of the hospital declared it the special duty of the house physician and surgeon "to keep a daily record of every important fact in the history of the patient and as soon as possible to enter it in a handsome manner in the case book of the department."[39] This was done not only for the purpose of improving medical care, but also to furnish data for medical research. In his letter to the hospital's Board of Trustees, written in 1837, the Boston physician James Jackson urged "that the practice be always continued of keeping full and exact records that may be resorted to as a means of promoting medical science in all future times. It may be needless to add that such records will also furnish the best security for a faithful attention to the welfare of those who are the subjects of them."[40] Although these records were bound in volumes, the case of any given patient might be written on widely separated pages in one or several of these volumes, according to the date he visited the hospital. However, physicians were referred to the volume and page on which observations continued by notations at breaks in the patient's record, and by name indices at the end of each volume. Medical, surgical, and outpatient department records, even on the same patient, were separately maintained. In 1848 an index volume was completed containing the names and diagnoses for all patients previously admitted. In 1892, an updated, alphabetical card index replaced it. In 1897 the hospital hired Mrs. Grace Meyers as custodian for the records, a rare appointment for a hospital of this period, to deal with the accumulation of information in the records. The data on patients treated on the wards filled 1,730 folio volumes (each about 250 pages) by 1914, but these volumes did not contain records of outpatient visits, over 223,000 in number, which were unbound and stacked in drawers.[41]

The files of the Massachusetts General Hospital also provide insight into the methods used in the nineteenth and twentieth centuries to organize facts within medical records.[42] From the 1820s to 1860s, the story of the patient's complaint generally came first (occasionally interspersed with comments about past illnesses or habits) followed by the physician's observations and examinations. A new feature that helped to organize the data in the medical record appeared in 1870, a chart on which the daily temperature was recorded graphically, along with a daily tabular record of the pulse and respiration rate denoted numerically.

During the 1880s, the graphic method also came into use at Massachusetts General, as a means of indicating the location of physical signs and injuries. An outline of the body's trunk was stamped onto records, and places in which pathology existed noted on them.[43] The record was frequently divided into explicitly labeled categories: the patient's family history (usually brief), his habits (e.g., did he drink), his past history, his present illness, and last, the doctor's examinations. In the 1890s, a growing number of laboratory results were written into the record, and in the decade of the 1900s, photographs, consultant notes, laboratory and X-ray reports were pasted in page margins; sometimes they overlapped and obscured the page notes themselves. By 1910, the record of a patient was not only scattered, as in the past, within one volume, or among many volumes, but the randomly pasted comments and technical results created a confusing mass of facts for the doctor consulting any given page.

Beginning about 1915, pressure developed in the United States to improve data storage in the medical record. It came from many sources: newly created professional associations, such as the American College of Surgeons who hoped to elevate hospital standards; a growing cadre of investigators who sought to use the records for research; litigants in need of medical records as legal evidence; clinicians who hoped that a more orderly arrangement of the facts would improve their understanding of the patient's illness; hospital review boards wanting to evaluate the efficiency of a physician's medical practices.[44] Two basic approaches for organizing the hospital record better were suggested: standardization of the collection of data; and a single unified record – bringing together in one place data about the patient that were scattered among different departments of the hospital and among the volumes of records maintained in each department.

Some critics of the record believed that if physicians noted the facts of an illness on a preprinted, standardized form, several major faults might be remedied – neglect of significant observations, omission of negative findings, or even of elementary facts such as the patient's age or sex. Foremost among these critics was the Johns Hopkins medical statistician Raymond Pearl, who in 1921 noted disapprovingly that "the general scheme or outline which a history is to follow resides, far too often, in the head of the history writer, and there only. And heads, especially of human beings, do vary so! The remedy is patent. . .Have printed a series of *standard* history forms, which will cover not merely general routine facts common to all diseased conditions, but special forms as well, for at least all of the more frequently occurring conditions."[45] The suggested standard forms required the physician to check one of several choices when asking patients questions that permitted qualitative responses. For example, the inquiry "Hears tick of watch in right ear?" could be answered on the form only with a yes or no; but the standard form also allowed physicians to write in clinical facts that could be quantitatively expressed, such as blood pressure.

Opponents in turn argued that standardized data forms would stifle the individuality of the physician, who required freedom to broadly comment on his patient's illness, and would create a Procrustean rigidity in case writing, since patients varied, as data forms did not. However, advocates of the form contended there was nothing against having essential features of the patient's illness recorded in a standard manner, and allowing the physician to write the rest in his own style. Recording clinical data in a uniform way would only "inordinately cramp such portion of [the doctor's] individuality as finds its expression in carelessness, inaccuracy, forgetfulness, and inattentive observation. In so far as it is desirable to foster and preserve these intellectual qualities, and embalm their results in the permanent archives of a hospital, clinicians and surgeons should be encouraged to go on writing histories in the old way."[46] Standardized records, their advocates believed, helped ensure that the important aspects of an illness would be observed and recorded. By 1950, many hospitals had adopted this recommendation, and provided their house staff with printed forms to gather information about newly admitted patients.[47]

The second major response to remedying the faults in medical data collection was to provide a single unit record for a patient. This was probably first established in 1907 at the St. Mary's Hospital run by the Mayo brothers,[48] but extensively explored and refined at the Presbyterian Hospital in New York City in 1916.[49] Under this scheme, data for every patient were kept in a single folder, no matter in what division of the hospital the patient may have received care. This concept curtailed the dispersal of medical data, and made physicians believe their observations would be more effectively used. Hospitals gradually adopted this method of assembling information: the Massachusetts General Hospital, for example, had its record keeping changed to the unit system by 1937.[50]

In spite of such efforts to organize the data in the medical record, in most hospitals by 1960 the record remained a pastiche of laboratory reports, X-ray reports, nurses' notes, social workers' notes, statements by patients, objective facts, and subjective narratives. Sometimes over 100 pages long, it was the repository of the findings of all the specialized people and techniques that medicine

209

could assemble; a crucial device for organizing and centralizing medical care, the endpoint of the network of communications that bound together the specialties dividing medicine. But the sheer bulk of information increasingly strained the doctors' capacity to integrate the material in any orderly fashion, as well as the financial capacity of hospitals, some of which devoted over a quarter of their budgets to record keeping. Moreover, the record possessed by any given hospital or physician was usually but a segment of the patient's total medical history. Visits of the patient to different hospitals and doctors' offices had created a fragmented almanac of his total medical experiences.

Burgeoning data about patients themselves were being matched during the twentieth century with an equally expanding volume of new facts about illness. Even the books that helped medicine to extend memory of accumulated knowledge, seemed to some physicians no longer an efficient device to store medical knowledge in a way useful to diagnosis. Handbooks of differential diagnosis were the best texts for the clinician confronted by symptoms he could not match to a disease. He looked up his patient's most salient symptoms and beneath each entry found a list of diseases commonly associated with the symptoms. The forerunner of these handbooks for modern medicine was Morgagni's *On the Seats and Causes of Diseases* (1761) whose major feature was tables linking symptoms with anatomical disorders in which they appeared. Given one or two conspicuous symptoms, modern handbooks of differential diagnosis were helpful; but when illnesses that had many prominent symptoms appeared, the large number of possible disorders to be evaluated hopelessly complicated the task of diagnosis. This situation worsened as the number of diseases uncovered through research grew. The pages of the handbook, and the resultant data, could not be rearranged to fit the problem for which physicians consulted the book. There was a call to "inaugurate the *era of the thought – saving* devices. In this era *human knowledge will be arranged in processable, i.e., manipulable form.*"[51]

Several mechanical expedients had appeared in the 1950s to free medical knowledge from the imprisonment created by a book's structure. One was F. A. Nash's logoscope, which he described in 1954. Resembling a slide rule, the device had a list of diseases inscribed upon its face. Under the list was a grooved space into which could be slipped as many as five narrow slides. Each slide represented one symptom and had cross–stripes linking the symptom to diseases in which it appeared, which were inscribed on the face of the logoscope. The patient's most likely illness was the one under which were aligned the largest number of cross–stripes. The logoscope could be used by physicians with greater speed than a book, but its inventor warned that "metaphorically, the device can be described as a diagnostic bus or street–car, not as a diagnostic taxi–cab. The user must realize that it will often take him somewhere near his diagnostic destination, and so save him much effort; but he will not usually be taken from door to door."[52]

A second effort to release medical knowledge from the confines of books and journals was a special card and needle system developed in 1955 by Martin Lipkin and James Hardy. They selected 26 blood diseases, and represented the most characteristic symptoms of each by holes punched on cards, every disease having its own card. They used the patient's symptoms to needle the cards, and to isolate the most likely illnesses.[53] This card system attracted little attention; it lacked storage capacity, speed, and flexibility – qualities that emerged only with the appearance of the computer.

Stirred by the enormous information–processing power of the computer, experts from medicine and other branches of science banded together during the 1960s to exploit the full potential of the machine for medicine and to relieve hospitals and physicians overburdened by too many data and too many patients. These efforts were particularly vigorous in the United States. The experts tried to devise sets of instructions that would allow computers to replace physicians in the diagnosis of disease. They thereby subjected the processes of logic and reasoning underlying the act of diagnosis to the most intensive examination in medical history. Two schools of thought emerged whose advocates debated the best way of realizing their common goal, computer diagnosis: one school attempted to duplicate with a computer program the mental steps that physicians used to reach a diagnosis; the other developed diagnostic strategies particularly suited to the strengths of the computer, without the requirement that they mimic human logic.

Pursuit of the first course required intensive study of how physicians obtained and processed information to reach a diagnostic decision. The model that most investigators adopted assumed that the doctor, when confronted with a large number of symptoms, designated several as most crucial and used these selected symptoms to draw up a list of diseases in which they appeared. He compared, essentially, the clinical picture of the patient with descriptions of disease that he had memorized. Further study demonstrated that the physician's reasoning was considerably more complex than this behavioristic model assumed. Physicians differed markedly in the way they used even the most common signs of illness to distinguish the healthy from the ill. The frequent disregard of clear abnormalities on the road to reaching judgments suggested that physicians measured the significance of a defect against yardsticks fashioned from their experience with illness and their values as human beings, in ways that neither they nor anyone yet fully understood.

A number of doctors believed that this indefinable aspect of decision making was a component of the art of medicine, while others maintained that it was separate and could be analyzed. They argued that the speed with which the mind processed data in the making of decisions encouraged the erroneous belief that the decision was reached in some intuitive manner, neither definable nor logical; they believed that the mind operated in obedience to definable, logical laws which they were determined to learn, and that mathematical techniques, such as symbolic logic, could be used in reaching a diagnosis. According to this view, the observations of the brain and of the computer were based on four activities which could be studied: memory, comparison, computation, decision.[54]

By the mid–1960s investigators had not precisely determined how physicians interpreted data, and many turned to a second approach to enlist computers in diagnosis. Since the beginning of the decade, modes of thinking with machines had been examined in ways never before attempted by the human mind: "There is no reason to make the machine act the same way the human brain does, anymore than to construct a car with legs to move from place to place."[55] Without the restraint of having machines reason as people did, experts explored with computers many patterns of data analysis and systematic approaches to disease diagnosis, and thereby exercised the full capabilities of the machine. By the late 1960s these efforts had produced several sets of computer instructions, each of which mobilized the power of the computer to diagnose disease in a different part of the body – the heart, blood, glands, bones, and mind – in patients who were already being overseen by a specialist. In each case, the computer's diagnostic accuracy nearly equalled the specialist's.[56]

As such computer instructions however were designed to consider only a small number of diseases, skeptics doubted whether the computer could deal fully with two major problems that faced a doctor meeting a patient for the first time: data selection, or choosing from all the information presented by the patient the most fruitful evidence to explore; and differential diagnosis, or producing a list of disorders that explained the patient's symptoms and picking one as the tentative diagnosis. Implicit in the first problem was the abundance of information that could be collected about the patient. The physician dealt with it by heeding some facts and disregarding others, through a process that computer experts could not reproduce, and used the information selected to develop hypotheses about the cause of the illness. However, it was impossible at this time to design a computer large and fast enough to store and quickly retrieve all the evidence about a patient, or to design a set of instructions for the computer that would guide it in analyzing all the collected evidence – deciding which to use, which to ignore. At best, a physician first had to examine the patient to decide which data to feed into the computer. Thus "diagnosis from scratch" remained the prerogative of the human being, not the machine.

To meet the second problem – constructing a list of diseases and choosing one as the diagnosis – the computer provided physicians with the mathematical odds for each disease on the list. The set of instructions that guided analysis were usually based on the mathematical theorem developed in 1763 by the Reverend Thomas Bayes. Using Bayes' Theorem to establish a patient's diagnosis however required two conditions frequently absent in cases of illness: mutually exclusive categories of disease – if a patient had one disease he could not also have another; and mutually independent symptoms – the onset or intensity of one symptom could not influence the onset or intensity of any other symptom. Several other conditions assumed in probability computations about the existence of diseases were often not met: that the patient come from the same population as the people used to furnish statistics about the disease; and that all the evidence required to make the diagnosis be available.

Doubts also lingered about whether probabilities furnished an adequate basis for medical judgments. If the most likely diagnosis also entailed the most perilous therapy, for instance, a factor other than mathematical odds would be introduced into the final choice of therapy. The criteria physicians used to make decisions depended on the total clinical situation; different decisions were often made for patients who presented similar signs of diseases.[57]

Some participants in this debate recognized nevertheless that future improvements in computers, and in human ability to construct better rules for handling data, might overcome some of these barriers. Research is continuing.

As controversy persisted over the computer's capacity to replace the physician in diagnosis, investigators attempted to overcome the difficulties of processing in the computer the various kinds of evidence generated by old and new diagnostic techniques. The computer accepted only data that could be encoded in a defined vocabulary, systematically organized, manipulated through rules developed by the computer expert, and then programed – or put into a computer language.

Efforts to process medical information contained in pictures and graphs in computers were inaugurated in the mid-1950s, with the invention of the Cytoanalyzer.[58] It scanned human cells and transmitted data about them to a computer, which used characteristics such as the size of nuclei and the composition of cytoplasm to distinguish normal from abnormal cells. Other computer programs were developed that converted into numbers the electronic impulses generated by the scan of X-ray pictures. In one variation of the method, investigators divided the X-ray into a lattice of tiny squares. They matched the average density of each square to one of 64 gradations of gray, and transformed the picture into a pattern of numbers. The computer compared the patterns with patterns stored in its memory bank to determine whether those being studied were normal or pathological.

In one experiment, in 1972, a group of ten radiologists was pitted against the computer. The problem: to find rheumatic heart disease. The computer won with an accuracy of 73 percent, compared with the doctors' 62 percent. Moreover, the computer's overall score was higher than any physician's.[59] Some radiologists had come to believe that their discipline was more suitable for computer analysis than any other in medicine. Electrocardiograms and heart sounds were also being successfully converted into forms of evidence that permitted computer analysis.

Those doing research on such machines have always been optimistic about the future: "We are no longer surprised when a mechanical device is contrived to perform almost any task formerly done by man."[60] It was such confidence that investigators applied to the largest of their efforts to analyze evidence with the computer – the storage and evaluation of the patient's history.

Doctors of the 1960s found gathering historical data a time–consuming and increasingly arduous task, given the growing demand for their services and their own doubts about the value of the data. After the work of Raymond Pearl in the 1920s, who had considered ways of organizing all kinds of clinical data in a standardized form, the most notable effort to systematize and simplify the method of learning about the patient's illness was the Cornell Medical Index, developed in the United States during World War II to expedite the medical processing of military recruits. It was a questionnaire self–administered by the patient, which brought problems to the physician's attention that he could immediately focus upon. The questionnaire was designed to eliminate the physician's need to take a comprehensive history. Studies showed that it brought as many facts to light as the doctor could elicit by taking the history himself, and even found out more about the patient's emotional problems than the doctor. Moreover, its standardized format provided legible records and historical data on patients that were readily comparable for purposes of medical research. The document had several drawbacks: the patient had to be literate, and its format was inflexible – it asked the same questions of everyone, regardless of their responses.[61] Thus it failed to attract much attention among physicians in the 1940s or 1950s.

The automated computer history overcame some of the inflexibility of the written questionnaire. Either through typewritten phrases or through flashed messages on a cathode–ray tube, it presented questions that had several alternative answers. The patient's answer determined the next question given him. All answers were stored in the computer's memory bank and could be quickly retrieved. Comparison revealed that the computer often found a number of significant symptoms of illness that equaled or surpassed the number found by the physician during interviews. Many patients preferred the computer history–taking to the physician's history–taking.[62] The computer gave patients a chance to think unhurriedly about their problems, as they could not do in the brief time allowed them in a busy doctor's office. Patients believed the computer husbanded the physician's time and hoped this would permit the physician to evaluate their complaints more thoroughly. Physicians also praised the computer history, for it allowed comparison of data from different patients by removing the variability when several physicians obtained and organized data. The computer history eliminated the effort sometimes needed to decipher

215

the hasty scrawl of the physician; it provided a neutral setting for questions about mental problems, questions that might embarrass doctor or patient when face to face. It allowed a parallel set of questions to be asked of relatives of the patient, which could be compared readily with the patient's answers and so added a new dimension to the clinical portrait. It provided fruitful avenues which doctors could explore with further questions, and made possible frequent reevaluations of the patient: unlike the doctor, the computer was a tireless interviewer.[63] But few doctors used it.

Much doubt persisted in the 1960s that the computer history could perform several crucial functions of the dialogue history. The physician taking a history could constantly evaluate the data he was receiving; and he could construct an almost infinite number of related questions to clarify or broaden his inquiry. In contrast, the largest computers available by the end of the decade could ask at most about 1000 ten–word questions, each of which had to be imbedded in a hierarchial or branching computer program. This meant the physician who constructed a computer questionnaire had to anticipate the most likely response of doctor and patient to any given problem: for the computer could not respond to a patient's answers if they were at all atypical. Standardization of the clinical history required specificity – consequently some things had to be left out. Also lost in the computer history were all the nonverbal cues about illness – the implied meanings as distinct from the logical content of words that physicians might detect. For the doctor shared some of the patient's hopes and fears during the historical dialogue. Both doctor and patient needed to think about the problems of the illness in the human perspective, and some believed that the best time for this activity was during history–taking.[64]

In spite of these doubts, the computer–analyzed history became a key aspect of a multiple, automated testing process designed to separate persons who probably had a disease from those who probably did not. This process located suspects, who then received more definitive diagnostic study for the disorders found.

The idea of using tests to sort the probably well from the probably sick had attracted much public and medical attention following World War I. Of the three million men examined for service in the United States between 1917–18, almost a third were partially or totally disqualified because of physical and mental illness that either was hidden from its victims, or was apparent and remediable but not acted upon, conditions such as venereal disease, tuberculosis, and defective vision.[65] The army draft was the first national physical examination conducted in the United States. The results, characterized often as "the horrible example,"[66] convinced the public and many doctors that annual medical examinations of the population to detect such problems were essential. During the 1920s many campaigns were launched to promote this idea, which used slogans such as "Have a Health Examination on your Birthday,"[67] and posters carrying such messages as "Your body is a wonderful machine. You own and operate it. You can't buy new lungs and heart when your own are worn out. Let a doctor overhaul you once a year."[68]

Efforts to popularize the comprehensive health examination were paralleled by campaigns to induce the public to submit to tests for specific diseases. The first major effort began in 1912 when people were urged to get "precautionary" X-rays to detect early signs of tuberculosis.[69] This campaign was soon joined by one that employed a blood test to detect syphilis. In the period between the world wars, many people volunteered for these procedures because they were quick, inexpensive or free, easy to administer, and the diseases they detected usually serious.

A new concept to locate illness in apparently well people – multiphasic screening – developed in the late 1940s. It used a battery of tests to evaluate people for a number of diseases, and was aided by new advances, such as the technique of photofluoroscopy that speeded up the taking of X-rays, and a vacuum–based hypodermic syringe that speeded up the drawing of blood samples. In contrast to single screening tests, the multiple approach saved administrative agencies the expense of directing several campaigns, furnished a more comprehensive health survey of each patient, and led to greater efficiency in contacting those with positive findings. It did not rely on anxiety about illness to attract people, and provided a greater yield of pathology from efforts and expenditures that were little more than those for single tests.[70]

With the development of automated diagnostic machines, use of the screening concept spread beyond the public health agencies and started to become an integral part of the clinical examination. The results of a battery of procedures, such as a self–administered patient history, electrocardiogram, and laboratory tests performed with an automatic analyzer, were fed into a computer, and a provisional diagnosis printed out which required follow–up work by the physician. Some American doctors began to hope that, as such ex-

217

aminations became more comprehensive, quantitative, and precise, automated, computer-analyzed multiphasic screening would one day become automated diagnosis.[71]

The computer also helped to integrate into medical practice a new set of machines that continuously monitored physiological changes taking place within the body. These devices were the product of a substantive effort begun in the late 1930s to introduce the techniques of physical science into medical research. As has been noted, by the early years of the twentieth century, the exploration of body chemistry was a dominant theme in medical research. The chemist and biologist were becoming closely allied, as evidenced by the remark of one doctor in 1912: "I struck a hybrid the other day, a bio–chemist!"[72] In 1935, the British physician Sir Henry Dale could still write that if he "were asked to name a prevailing tendency of the present time, in medical, and indeed in a wider range of biological research. . .the rapidly increasing dominance of chemical methods and chemical ideas" would be his response.[73] But indications of an impending change appeared in 1938. Karl Compton, president of the Massachusetts Institute of Technology, in an address delivered to the American College of Physicians, proposed that a knowledge of physics, chemistry, and electrical engineering be systematically applied to biology to create the "useful art of biological engineering."[74]

The working together of investigators from different disciplines, who sought to solve scientific problems engendered by World War II, increased collaboration between physical scientists and physicians. By the war's end, the number of articles and books written on physical phenomena in disease had increased appreciably. The new research involved a quantitative study of how living organisms were affected by physical phenomena, such as X-rays and the minute voltages called action potentials produced by the biological activity of the heart, brain, and other parts of the body. The detection, amplification, and analysis of this electrical activity in the body had already resulted, at the start of the twentieth century, in the development of the electrocardiograph to measure heart function and, during the 1920s, had led the pioneering German physician Hans Berger to invent the electroencephalograph that measured the electrical activity of the brain graphically.[75] Investigators now hoped that research in electrical activity in other organs would create new diagnostic techniques and improve older ones. One such technique, for example, resulted when the electric currents generated by muscle tissue (a phenomenon that was the subject of much laboratory investigation throughout the nineteenth and early twentieth centuries) became increasingly exploited to diagnose muscular disorders.[76]

Another major focus of biophysical research was radioactive isotopes: atoms or molecules whose radioactivity allowed investigators to trace the actual route of metabolic activities in the human body. To apply the tracer techniques a substance containing radioactive atoms was fed to the human subject, and subsequently the blood, tissues, and secretions were tested with a Geiger counter, to determine the path taken by the molecules. As early as 1923, George Hevesy studied plant and animal physiology using the naturally occurring radioactive isotope of lead. Since few naturally occurring isotopes existed, tracer techniques could not be widely used until Frédéric Joliot and his wife Irène Curie discovered in 1934 that atoms could be made radioactive by bombarding atomic nuclei; then Ernest Lawrence and his colleagues in 1936 completed work on the "cyclotron," which facilitated the production of radioactive isotopes. Isotopic techniques could test such activities as the function of the thyroid gland by measuring the amount and places of concentration of radioactive iodine it absorbed, and the pumping capacity of the heart by measuring the flow of blood into and out of the organ. The use of radioactive isotopes in diagnosis burgeoned after World War II, a part of the great interest in finding peaceful uses for atomic energy. In 1950, a scanner was designed that recorded in dots the beats of the scintillation counter that detected radiation. The density of the dots indicated where, in the area of the body being examined, the greatest amount of radioactive isotope had accumulated.[77]

Some hospitals recognized that the conduct of such research required the presence of physicists on their staff; after the war a few hospitals not only hired them but installed biophysical laboratories, analogous to the existing, biochemical laboratories. The large number of requests received by the Massachusetts Institute of Technology from hospitals seeking physicists to work on biological problems prompted the Institute to initiate a special training program for physicists, and also one for engineers interested in designing medical instruments. In 1952, a professional organization devoted to the study of medical electronics was formed in the United States, whose membership had expanded to over 1000 three years later.[78] At this time, investigators were beginning to develop machines that continuously monitored body functions, such as the blood pressure.[79]

Physicians in the past had relied on random observation of body functions, both to diagnose disease and to follow its course, but this had two crucial shortcomings. First, minute–to–minute changes in the patient's condition went unnoticed. Second, since body functions tended to hover around certain normal points, they exhibited significant departures from the normal at different times of the day. Hence, a random sample often failed to detect rhythmic changes in body physiology. It was thought too, that relying on overburdened nurses to continually chart the physiological changes in the patient, through the periodic measurement of body functions such as pulse, temperature, and respiration, led to many errors.

The possibility of tracking such changes through machines was appreciably advanced by the invention of sophisticated equipment to observe physiological changes in animals and astronauts during the space exploration program that grew during the 1960s. As one enthusiast commented, "If monkeys 100 miles in the air can be monitored, there is no reason why patients cannot be monitored."[80] Experiments began in which miniature transmitters were placed on people engaged in the daily activities of life, to study normal heart function and find better ways to diagnose and follow patients with heart disease.[81] Even more important was the trial of monitoring devices to continually evaluate the condition of hospitalized patients.

A crucial problem remained however. Even if clinically applicable machines to perform continuous readings of body function were perfected, doctors lacked the time to evaluate the mass of data thus produced. One solution was the linking of physiological measuring devices to computers which analyzed and stored the data and, in some designs, even caused an alarm to ring when dangerous changes in body function occurred or were imminent.[82]

A number of criticisms of the monitoring concept were made: the equipment's constant sound created physical and psychological disturbances in some patients; nurses and other medical personnel tended to focus on supervising the machines more than caring for the patient. Doubts were raised that the continuous stream of data provided by the machines, in most cases of illness, was more valuable than the random data obtained by people using their own senses or simple instruments such as thermometers. Several studies showed that patients who suffered serious heart attacks had no better rate of recovery, when hooked up to these machines, than when cared for without them. But a strong belief in the overall benefits of the monitoring concept prevailed and the use of monitoring equipment in hospitals grew during the 1960s and 1970s.[83]

The medical workers who ran such machines and others who performed a multitude of patient–care activities, but were not physicians, began to play a more important role in medicine: they took histories, conducted physical examinations, and monitored the technology of medicine. In 1900, physicians had accounted for approximately three in five (60 percent) of the nearly 200,000 professionally educated persons who delivered medical care in the United States (included in this group were nurses, pharmacists, dietitians, technicians, etc.). By 1950, the number of professionally educated people in medicine had climbed to almost 900,000, of whom only one in four (25 percent) was a physician. By 1969, of nearly 1.7 million professionally educated medical personnel, fewer than one in five (20 percent) was a physician.[84] A new category of health workers was emerging – the physician assistant – specially educated to assume some of the diagnostic and therapeutic duties of physicians, who supervised their activities. Physicians in several hospital outpatient departments in the United States were encouraging some nurses to leave their traditional role as the doctor's subordinate. Although they frequently consulted with physicians, these nurses assumed the principal responsibility for the evaluation and care of patients. The transformation from doctor's assistant to doctor's colleague occurred because physicians recognized that a mutual overlap in training and experience allowed them to enlarge the nurse's diagnostic and therapeutic responsibilities.

Some fears were expressed that delegating too much medical authority to nonphysicians would encourage them to perform medical acts for which they were improperly trained. Minority groups worried that a cadre of health workers was being created to provide care exclusively to poor people – a cut–rate medicine. Physicians who oversaw allied health workers were concerned lest their mistakes increase the doctors' liability to malpractice suits. Yet the pressure of patient demand encouraged the movement toward accepting their help; aided by machines, they relieved the physician of routine tasks that were readily definable and easily supervised. Physicians even suggested that some of these nonphysician health workers might be trained to assume direct responsibility for general medical care if they were assisted by automated devices for diagnosis, taught the techniques of physical examination, and were to keep in touch with consultant physicians through communication devices. Modern technology made it easier than in the past to specify medical assignments for the allied health worker, who seemed to hold the key to increasing the supply of care in response to growing demand. Such people provided an alternative to the training of more doctors to counteract the shortage of health providers.[85]

A number of physicians in the 1960s and 1970s also saw in the alliance of machines and technological assistants, a means of freeing themselves to devote more time to understand and interact with their patients.[86] Yet one study showed that the time freed for physicians in group practice by the delegation of clinical tasks to machines and assistants which groups (unlike individual practitioners) could readily purchase, was usually not spent with the patients.[87]

The computer clearly towered in prestige and performance above all other automated machines. By the middle of the 1960s, a single computer could perform 1,000 operations a second for up to 1,000 people using it simultaneously. But those who believed that the use of computers in daily medical practice was at hand harbored unrealistic expectations. By the end of the decade the average practitioner was almost as far from using computers to evaluate medical evidence as when the decade began. A principal cause was conflict between the physical scientists who built computers, and the doctors who used them. Doctors feared these scientific experts would invade their domain of professional competence: "The physician thinks that the computer engineer is out to get him with an all–knowing diagnostic computer."[88] And some computer scientists, emboldened by the success of computers in solving business problems, indeed sometimes acted as if they believed they could show the doctor how to diagnose.

Another major obstacle was the difference in languages and problem–solving techniques between the medical and engineering professions. The physician rarely had the training in mathematics and physical science that enabled him to understand the computer scientist; he, in turn, could not understand the medical vocabulary of the physician. The two groups not only lacked a common language, but evaluated problems in different ways, each using the concepts mastered during separate training. Although both groups

222

might learn enough of the other's vocabulary to converse, their different conceptual approaches to problem solving seemed a formidable obstacle to surmount.[89]

Many physicians who resisted computers feared that the machines might push them even farther away from an interest in human relationships, and convert them to analysts who cared more about measuring than understanding patients. This possibility deeply troubled those physicians who were convinced that only by preserving a deep interest in their patients as persons could they retain mastery of their medical art. Concern also existed that computers would undermine the physician's authoritative role in evaluating the facts in an illness and in making final judgments about what action was to be taken. The *British Medical Journal* expressed these anxieties in speculating whether the physician who lived in the modern technological environment would become "a sort of machine–minder? or someone controlling the machine in the human interests of a patient he must from time to time remember is more than mechanism?"[90] There was even concern that the physician who closely allied himself to computers might himself become machinelike: "How will he prevent his own conversion to automation? What will keep him a human being, a person, a self?" asked one doctor.[91]

At the turn of the twentieth century, fears of domination by machines had already begun to surface in the medical literature. When machines for testing eyesight turned up in English railroad stations and drugstores in 1895, the *British Medical Journal* was driven to comment:

In everything else machinery is used, why not in medicine? So the public drops in its penny and receives its prescription. It is not difficult to foresee the time when the prescribing chemist [pharmacist] will be a thing of the past. There will, in fact, be no need for him; his shop will be crowded with penny–in–the–slot machines, by the use of which the patient's weight will be taken, his eyesight tested, his urine examined, his vital capacity ascertained, his muscle power measured, his knee–jerks recorded, his pulse trace taken, and ultimately his prescription written plainly by a typewriter, so that it can be made up by an assistant at a mere living wage, while the chemist, free from all responsibility, will take the fee and flourish exceedingly.[92]

This satire on the apothecary had clear implications for physicians. When computer scientists in the 1960s enthusiastically predicted that the computer would eventually be more intelligent than man,

223

and would one day manage medicine by itself, a more widespread anxiety was felt than physicians had felt about machines earlier in the century. Doctors spoke of the creeping amoeba of automation, of the electronic brain that threatened their status, even their livelihood. The jacket of one book on the computer portrayed a twined serpent, the symbol of medicine, peering through a window in the center of the machine. An American reviewer wondered whether the serpent had not become a prisoner: "He is certainly encircled, and the embrace is not that of love. Am I over–interpreting? Likely. Projecting? Certainly. But not idiosyncratically so. My prejudices are shared, if not by the artist who drew the picture, by many physicians."[93] Scenarios of medical futures envisioned an environment in which physical contact between doctor and patient had disappeared:

Sir, can you tell me the meaning of an obsolete word? I know medical history is a hobby of yours.

I'll try. What word?

Auscultation. It meant listening.

Listening to what, Sir?

Sounds made by the human body. . .I thought you'd be puzzled. Doctors used to listen to patients' bodies, and palpate them directly, too.

Directly? You mean they used some simpler kind of palpating machine than ours?

No, really directly. . .I see I'll have to demonstrate. Come here. Put your hand on my wrist – right on it, skin to skin.

May I really, Sir?

Yes, yes: no–one's looking.[94]

The laboratory specialist also suffered in this vision of the future. He was pictured peering through an obsolete light microscope in an obscure cubicle in the hospital basement: "No one sent Dr. Zbin current material for microscopical study. In the new, brightly lighted portions of the tremendous multistory laboratory the automated gizmos burbled, bubbled, rotated and transmitted test results (to the sixth decimal place) to the battery of computers. . .A meager pension awaited him. For decades he had been without assistants or residents. He would not be replaced. His position was being abolished."[95]

In another envisioned future, even the personal physician had become unnecessary:

For several days you have not been feeling well and you call your local health center for an appointment. You can remember when you used to call your doctor, but it's been many years since he's bothered with initial diagnoses and he would be the first to admit he could not be as thorough or accurate as the health center. At the center you give all the necessary information to a medical secretary whose typewriter feeds it into a computer system. . .On the basis of the information given so far and a comparison with your previous history the computer may venture an immediate diagnosis, – but if it has any doubts – and it is a highly conservative computer – it recommends one or several diagnostic tests. . .In a matter of seconds, after the tests are completed, the system presents its full diagnosis. At the same time it also makes recommendation for treatment, perhaps printing out a prescription which can be filled before you leave the center. Fortunately, in your case only medication was recommended, and you go home not only with the proper medication but confident that your case was given the best medical attention, even though you never saw a doctor during the entire visit. The health center efficiently adds the day's information to your medical history and sends your doctor a copy just for the record. By the way, you do get to see your doctor – on the weekend when you play bridge with him.[96]

This sort of medical future was endorsed by an American physician in 1976 as a "feasible, probable, and desirable" model to provide future health services. He predicted that by about the first quarter of the twenty–first century, "doctors would be rendered obsolete," replaced by a "medic–computer symbiosis." His model assigned to computers most diagnostic and therapeutic decisions now made by doctors "while *medics*, a hitherto unknown type of health care professional," would provide "the supportive and some of the technical tasks" now carried out by doctors.[97]

A common response within medicine to fears of computer dominance was to depict the machine as an intellectual beast of burden. The computer was only a brain; it lacked the ability to gather data or to act upon its own decisions, depended wholly on the facts received from a human being, and like other technological servants, extended man's power but did not control him: "Computers are not monsters; they have no black magic; they do not 'think.' It should be apparent that a computer is in fact incredibly stupid, doing only what it has been directed to do."[98] But more significant to the defenders of the computer was the hope that it would restore attention to the patient as a whole person. Twentieth–century technology with all its progress had tended to push the human dilemmas of illness out of the doctor's thoughts, and replace them with laboratory facts derived from tests on the patient's body. With its capac-

225

ity to remember and sort facts, the computer might give new meaning to evidence found by questioning and examining the patient, and thereby, reestablish the patient's experiences, as well as the senses of the physician, as a main focus of evidence in clinical medicine.[99]

More than any other automated diagnostic instrument, the computer has raised anxieties among physicians that many of their functions might one day become replaced by machines. The computer is remarkably humanlike in some respects, utterly machinelike in other respects – an amalgam that at the same time awes and alarms physicians. Many physicians appreciate that medicine requires its tremendous capacity to store, classify, and integrate data; for current medical practice is splitting into larger and larger numbers of smaller and smaller units of specialization in response to the exponential growth of medical knowledge and techniques. The complexity of the interrelationships between the new evidence being generated within medicine, and the personnel who apply the evidence, requires a higher level of coordination than was needed in the days when individual practitioners carried out most medical tasks by themselves. The computer seems destined to become an essential factor in achieving such coordination.

In broad terms technology can influence the structure in which medical resources will be combined in the future. For example, the capacity of the computer to handle prodigious amounts of data can encourage the development of a medical–care system composed, basically, of large centralized facilities in which specialists and machines of all kinds will be in close physical proximity to each other. Conversely, the technology which permits many types of medical evidence to be transmitted over long distances can encourage a decentralized form of organization having, basically, many individual practitioners and small units linked by telecommunications to each other and to a number of large centralized facilities.

11 *Conclusion*

Since the nineteenth century, physicians have moved through a series of stages: from direct communication with their patients' experiences, based upon a verbal technique of information gathering, to direct connection with their patients' bodies through techniques of physical examination, to indirect connection with both the experiences and bodies of their patients through machines and technical experts. After each move to a new stage and new techniques, skills in using the old techniques have declined, with the resulting sacrifice of the unique insights they provided.

Different kinds of facts are revealed through the various methods of collecting data that have evolved during medicine's history. Each fact–gathering technique uncovers a particular component of the disease picture, different in some ways from that revealed by another such technique, and so presents the physician with a particular view of his patient and the patient's illness. However, the technique chosen does more than generate a particular kind of fact – it influences human attitudes and relationships. Techniques influence the relationship of the patient with the physician; they influence the doctor's image of himself as a decision maker; they influence the association of physicians with each other, and thus the manner in which the institutions of medical practice are organized. Attitudinal and relational changes such as these are often not recognized but they are crucial, and physicians should consider them in evaluating the benefits and harm of different fact–gathering techniques.

Illness is best treated when the facts and relationships developed through several techniques are brought together. The creative juxtaposition of different, yet equally well–documented views of the same event – for example, a disturbance of respiration evidenced by certain sensations, sounds, X-ray appearance, chemistry, and outside influences on the life of the patient – provides a synthesis that brings insights the observer cannot acquire by focusing primarily on any one view.

Yet the ability of physicians to maintain competence in several

227

techniques is limited by events that accompany the acceptance of an innovation. Innovations transform the perceptual experiences and the social relationships of those who use them. To appreciate the new dimension of a phenomenon, which each innovation reveals, the physician undergoes what may be a painful change in his habitual way of thinking about that phenomenon, as well as in the vocabulary he uses to speak about it. Thus, caught in a time of transition between different ways of seeing illness, the physician my find it difficult to learn the new view and at the same time retain his former degree of skill with old techniques. Moreover, in getting a new technique accepted, its advocates dwell on the defects of old techniques and inevitably obscure and debase their virtues. Once established, an innovation influences power relationships in medicine. Developed expertness in new and accepted techniques enhances professional status. The old guard, wedded to their proficiency in the old ways, find themselves gradually dominated by physicians who are expert in the new. This further reduces the incentive to maintain earlier skills.

Appreciating the unreliability of memory and the inadequacies of an ordinary vocabulary to describe the effects of illness, physicians of the early nineteenth century gradually turned away from relying on the patient's verbal evidence, to adopt in its place the evidence obtained from physical examination. Using the manual techniques and simple instruments available, they found themselves in the strongest position they have ever held as individualists and masters of the facts they obtained. Dependent only upon their own sensory and expert impressions, they dispensed truly personal judgments to patients and colleagues. But gradually there grew in medicine a distrust of the accuracy with which sense impressions gained at the bedside were engraved on the memory of the doctor, a distrust of his ability to accurately describe and recall these impressions, and to attain full insight into the facts that he had acquired. The word descriptions of the doctor were challenged just as the word descriptions of the patient had been.

Physicians then began to look for medical evidence with two essential qualities: reproducibility – or the capacity of a technique to accurately and permanently transcribe the exact character of a finding; and standardization – the degree to which a finding represented the same thing to different observers. Inventions appeared that converted subjective sensory events into numbers, graphs, and pictures whose immutability eliminated controversial evaluations of illness, by producing records that could be readily checked and trusted as measures of change. Such numerical and visual depictions did not simply provide more precise, limited definitions of a medical fact – fundamentally they were agencies to dependably store information. Inventors of instruments that expressed evidence in these forms sought to equalize medical competence by making excellence less a matter of heredity or of sensory training than the ability to know from which technology or specialist to request assistance. Yet the fact that many of these instruments seemed to run themselves made the physician in a sense more steward than master.

Technologies can develop identities of their own. Human ingenuity, anxiety, and fantasy can transform technologies into independent creatures, which are supposed to operate according to unvarying automatic procedures and to produce uniformly trustworthy evidence. The numbers generated by the thermometer, the graphs drawn by the electrocardiograph, the pictures created by the X-ray machine, the images captured by the microscope, the diagnostic judgments rendered by the computer – all are generally assumed to be free of the flaws and biases that admittedly distort facts gathered by human beings through their natural senses. Such evidence, it is further assumed, is therefore the most valuable in diagnosing and treating disease. Neither belief is true. The evidence produced by such instruments, though valuable, is inevitably influenced by the human hand that operates them and the human mind that evaluates the results. Furthermore, the machines are denied complete access to a whole range of nonmeasurable facts about a human being that a physician can obtain only through his own senses – questioning, observing, making judgments.

If physicians in general come to accept a fundamentally mechanical view of human beings, in a world that is more and more enamored of technology, the prospect for the future of medicine is extremely disquieting. To counter the fears of such a prospect, a myth has arisen in contemporary medicine that the more the machines can take over the performing of medical functions, the more the doctor will have time to deal with his patient as a human being. Thus reliance on technology is supposed to improve the doctor–patient relationship, to the benefit of both.

These are illusions. Machines inexorably direct the attention of both doctor and patient to the measurable aspects of illness, but away from the "human" factors that are at least equally important.

Insofar as technological evidence occupies the time and commands the chief allegiance of both doctor and patient, it diminishes the possibility that a close personal relationship will develop between the two. So, without realizing what has happened, the physician in the last two centuries has gradually relinquished his unsatisfactory attachment to subjective evidence – what the patient says – only to substitute a devotion to technological evidence – what the machine says. He has thus exchanged one partial view of disease for another. As the physician makes greater use of the technology of diagnosis, he perceives his patient more and more indirectly through a screen of machines and specialists; he also relinquishes his control over more and more of the diagnostic process. These circumstances tend to estrange him from his patient and from his own judgment.

The separation that has developed between the physician as healer and the patient as human being continues to be viewed with concern in many quarters of medicine and of society. Medical experts interested in emotional and social factors that contribute to illness keep up the appeal they have been making to colleagues since the twentieth century began: that the healing of illness requires more than healing parts of the body; it also requires intensive efforts to communicate with patients – to gain their trust and to understand their needs and hopes. In the 1970s this appeal has been joined by new demands that physicians listen more to patients, tell them more about the circumstances of their illness, and do the listening and telling with more candor and skill. These new demands are part of the broad reconsideration of the moral dimensions of medical care that began in large part as individuals' responses to the insecurity and powerlessness they felt as patients in modern medical institutions. This examination of medical ethics focuses on the patient as a person, not as an object, with rights and a dignity he is not made to forfeit because he is ill and dependent.

These events may be more than isolated humanist responses to the impersonality of the technological atmosphere permeating the relation of doctor and patient. They may express a broadly emerging conviction: that the problems of illness hatched from beliefs, illusions, values, and other facets of cultural and mental life – and best approached through dialogue with the patient and with humanist learning – are as forceful and significant as the biological problems of illness approached through technology and scientific learning. And if this conviction is sustained in the future, perhaps the gap that technology has helped to create between physician and patient might lessen.

Technological developments of the future may also improve the situation. If communications technology can give a physician prompt access to the knowledge of specialists and to the analytic capacity of modern diagnostic instruments, a larger number of physicians might pursue their work outside of the physical and psychological confines of medical institutions. While the proximity of machines and specialists in such institutions allows the physician to use medical resources efficiently, and makes him feel secure in his medical judgments, the environment of medical institutions can also encourage a dependence on machines and specialists that erodes a physician's self–confidence, and distracts him from considering the patient as a whole person. In a decentralized medical environment he might well exercise and trust his own judgment more, conduct a more personalized practice in which he was really mindful of his patients' human needs, and even settle his practice in regions shunned because of their isolation from medical centers.

Technologies that improve accuracy, and centralized organizations that enhance efficiency and provide security, are essential factors in modern medicine. Yet accuracy, efficiency, and security are purchased at a high price when that price is impersonal medical care and undermining the physician's belief in his own medical powers. To be free to develop his medical skills to their highest point, to increase what is despite these problems a positive balance of benefits over harms, today's physician must rebel. He can use his strongest weapon – a refusal to accept bondage to any one technique, no matter how useful it may be in a particular instance. He must regard them all with detachment, as mere tools, to be chosen as necessary for a particular task. He must accept the patient as a human being, and regain and reassert his faith in his own medical judgment.

Notes

CHAPTER 1. EXAMINATION OF THE PATIENT IN THE
SEVENTEENTH AND EIGHTEENTH CENTURIES

1 Several modern authors have examined the techniques used by physicians to evaluate their patients and the consequences for medicine of changes in these techniques. Notable works are: Charles Newman, *The Evolution of Medical Education in the Nineteenth Century* (London: Oxford University Press, 1957); Charles Newman, "Diagnostic Investigation before Laennec," *Med. Hist.*, vol. 4 (1960), pp. 322–9; Michel Foucault, *The Birth of the Clinic: An Archeology of Medical Perception*, trans. A. M. Sheridan Smith (New York: Pantheon, 1973); Kenneth D. Keele, *The Evolution of Clinical Methods in Medicine* (Springfield: Thomas, 1963); Iago Galdston, "Diagnosis in Historical Perspective," *Bull. Hist. Med.*, vol. 9 (1941), pp. 367–84; P. Lain Entralgo, *Doctor and Patient*, trans. Frances Partridge (New York: McGraw-Hill, 1969); I. Snapper, *Meditations on Medicine and Medical Education, Past and Present* (New York: Grune and Stratton, 1956); Ralph L. Engle, Jr., and B. J. Davis, "Medical Diagnosis: Present, Past, and Future," *Arch. Intern. Med.*, vol. 112 (1963), pp. 512–43.

2 James Mackenzie, *Symptoms and Their Interpretation* (London: Shaw and Sons, 1920), p. 14. The distinction between symptoms and signs in medical history has been skillfully analyzed by Lester S. King, "Signs and Symptoms," *J.A.M.A.*, vol. 206 (1968), pp. 1063–5, and by Foucault, *Birth of the Clinic*, pp. 90–4.

3 F. N. L. Poynter and W. J. Bishop, *A Seventeenth-Century Country Doctor and his Patients: John Symcotts, 1592?–1662*, Bedfordshire Historical Record Society, vol. 31 (Luton: Bedfordshire Historical Record Society, 1951), p. 59.

4 For an excellent discussion of this point, consult Newman, "Diagnostic Investigation before Laennec," pp. 322–9 and Newman, *Evolution of Medical Education*, pp. 25–31.

5 Poynter and Bishop, *Seventeenth-Century Country Doctor*, pp. 62–3.

6 Andrew Duncan, *Medical Cases, selected from the records of the public dispensary at Edinburgh . . .*, 2nd ed. (Edinburgh: C. Elliot, 1781), pp. 166–7.

7 Poynter and Bishop, *Seventeenth-Century Country Doctor*, p. 14.

8 Hermann Boerhaave, *Medical Correspondence . . .* (London: John Nourse, 1745), p. 107. The noted eighteenth-century Scottish physician William Cullen also conducted a wide medical practice by letter. See Guenter B. Risse, "Doctor William Cullen, Physician, Edinburgh: A Consultation Practice in the Eighteenth Century," *Bull. Hist. Med.*, vol. 48 (1974), pp. 338–51. For accounts of the setting of medical practice in the seventeenth and eighteenth centuries consult: R. M. S. McConaghey, "The History of Rural Medical Practice," in F. N. L. Poynter, ed., *The Evolution of Medical Practice in Britain* (London: Pitman Medical Publishing, 1961), pp. 131–3; Brian Abel-Smith, *The Hospitals in*

England and Wales: 1800–1948 (Cambridge, Mass.: Harvard University Press, 1964), pp. 2–4; Barnes Riznik, "Medicine in New England, 1790–1840" (A report prepared by the department of research of Old Sturbridge Village, Sturbridge, Massachusetts, 1963), pp. 82–5.

9 John Morgan, *A Discourse Upon the Institution of Medical Schools in America* (Philadelphia: William Bradford, 1765), p. ii. See also Richard Harrison Shryock, *Medicine and Society in America: 1660–1860* (New York: New York University Press, 1960), p. 8.

10 "Is There Any Certainty in Medical Science?" *Edinb. Med. Surg. J.*, vol. 1 (1805), p. 425.

11 Caleb Crowther, "Case of Abscess in the Abdominal Muscles, which Terminated Fatally," *Edinb. Med. Surg. J.*, vol. 2 (1806), p. 129.

12 Ibid., p. 132.

13 John Forbes, in translator's preface, R. T. H. Laennec, *A Treatise on Diseases of the Chest. . .* , 1st ed. (London: T. and G. Underwood, 1821), p. xvi.

14 Shryock, *Medicine and Society in America*, p. 50.

15 L. J. Rather, "Towards a Philosophical Study of Disease," in *The Historical Development of Physiological Thought*, ed. Chandler McC. Brooks and Paul Cranefield (New York: Macmillan (Hafner Press), 1959), p. 353.

16 Walter Pagel, *Paracelsus: An Introduction to Philosophical Medicine in the Era of the Renaissance* (Basel: S. Karger, 1958), pp. 128–31.

17 Thomas Sydenham, "Medical Observations Concerning the History and Cure of Acute Diseases," in *The Works of Thomas Sydenham, M.D.*, trans. R. G. Latham, vol. 1 (London: Sydenham Society, 1848–50), p. 19.

18 Ibid., p. 15.

19 Sydenham, "On Gout," in *Works of Thomas Sydenham*, vol. 2, pp. 123–5.

20 Knud Faber, "Nosography in Modern Internal Medicine," *Ann. Med. Hist.*, vol. 4 (1922), pp. 8–9.

21 Ibid., pp. 7–8. See also Lester S. King, "Boissier de Sauvages and 18th Century Nosology," *Bull. Hist. Med.*, vol. 40 (1960), pp. 43–51.

22 William Cullen, *A Synopsis of Methodical Nosology . . .* 4th ed., trans. Henry Wilkins (Philadelphia: Parry Hall, 1793), p. x.

23 Ibid., pp. v–vi.

24 Thomas Sydenham, "Anatomie," in *Dr. Thomas Sydenham (1624–1689): His Life and Original Writings*, ed. Kenneth Dewhurst (Berkeley: University of California Press, 1966), p. 86.

25 Ibid. Sydenham's views on anatomy are also discussed by David E. Wolfe, "Sydenham and Locke on the Limits of Anatomy," *Bull. Hist. Med.*, vol. 35 (1961), pp. 193–200, and Kenneth Dewhurst, "Locke and Sydenham on the Teaching of Anatomy," *Med. Hist.*, vol. 2 (1958), pp. 1–12.

26 Mondino de' Luzzi, *Anothomia*, in *The Fasciculo Di Medicina, Venice 1493*, trans. and introduced by Charles Singer (Florence: R. Lier and Co., 1925), pp. 71, 76, 83, 93–4. For further commentary on Mondino, see Charles Singer, *A Short History of Anatomy and Physiology from the Greeks to Harvey* (New York: Dover, 1957), pp. 74–86; and George W. Corner, *Anatomy* (New York: Macmillan (Hafner Press), 1964), pp. 14–16.

27 Charles Talbot, "Medical Education in the Middle Ages," in C. D. O'Malley, ed., *The History of Medical Education* (Berkeley: University of California Press, 1970), p. 78.

28 Ibid., p. 83.
29 C. D. O'Malley, "Translations from the *Fabrica* (1543)" in *Andreas Vesalius of Brussels: 1514–1564* (Berkeley: University of California Press, 1965), p. 319.
30 Ibid., pp. 319–20.
31 O'Malley, *Vesalius of Brussels*, p. 183.
32 O'Malley, "Translations from the *Fabrica*," p. 321.
33 Lester S. King, *The Growth of Medical Thought* (Chicago: University of Chicago Press, 1963), p. 148.
34 Esmond R. Long, *A History of Pathology* (New York: Dover, 1965), pp. 38–41.
35 Ibid., p. 42.
36 Ibid., pp. 59–62.
37 John Baptist Morgagni, *The Seats and Causes of Diseases Investigated by Anatomy*, trans. Benjamin Alexander, with a Preface, Introduction, and a new Translation of five letters by Paul Klemperer (New York: Macmillan (Hafner Press) 1960). Valuable essays on the influence of Morgagni on anatomy are Rudolph Virchow, "Morgagni and the Anatomic Concept," trans. Robert E. Schlueter, *Bull. Hist. Med.*, vol. 7 (1939), pp. 975–89; Saul Jarcho, "Morgagni and Auenbrugger in the Retrospect of Two Hundred Years," *Bull. Hist. Med.*, vol. 35 (1961), pp. 489–96; Paul Klemperer, "Pathological Anatomy at the End of the Eighteenth Century," *J. Mt. Sinai Hosp.*, vol. 24 (1957), pp. 589–603; Paul Klemperer, "The Pathology of Morgagni and Virchow," *Bull. Hist. Med.*, vol. 32 (1958), pp. 24–38.
38 Morgagni, *Seats and Causes of Diseases*, author's preface, vol. 1, p. xxx.
39 Book review, *Br. Foreign Med. Rev.*, vol. 6 (1838), pp. 293–307.
40 Morgagni, *Seats and Causes of Diseases*, introduction, vol. 1, p. xiii.
41 Ibid., p. xxx.
42 Ibid., p. xxiv.
43 Matthew Baillie, *The Morbid Anatomy of Some of the Most Important Parts of the Human Body*, 2nd ed. (London: J. Johnson, 1797), pp. i–xviii.
44 Xavier Bichat, *General Anatomy, applied to Physiology and Medicine*, trans. George Hayward (Boston: Richardson and Lord, 1822), vol. 1, p. 60.
45 Owsei Temkin, "The Role of Surgery in the Rise of Modern Medical Thought," *Bull. Hist. Med.*, vol. 25 (1951), pp. 255, 259.
46 Leopold Auenbrugger, "On Percussion of the Chest," trans. John Forbes from 1761 Latin edition, *Bull. Hist. Med.*, vol. 4 (1936), pp. 373–403.
47 Ibid., p. 379.
48 John Forbes, *Original Cases with Dissections and Observations Illustrating the Use of the Stethoscope and Percussion* (London: T. and G. Underwood, 1824), pp. xi–xii; James B. Herrick, "A Note Concerning the Long Neglect of Auenbrugger's 'Inventum Novum,' " *Arch. Intern. Med.*, vol 71 (1943), pp. 741–8.
49 Auenbrugger, "On Percussion of the Chest," p. 383.
50 Rozière de la Chassagne observed, in his 1770 translation of Auenbrugger's work into French: "Mr. Auenbrugger has not the merit of inventing the method of which I speak. . .Hippocrates had used it in the course of his practice." Cited by George Dock, "Rozière de la Chassagne and the Early History of Percussion of the Thorax," *Ann. Med. Hist.*, vol. 7 (1935), p. 445.
51 In one view, this was the principal reason for the delayed recognition of percussion. Consult Henry E. Sigerist, "Science and History" in Felix Marti-Ibañez, ed., *Henry E. Sigerist on the History of Medicine* (New York: MD Publica-

tions, 1960), pp. 88–9. See also Saul Jarcho, "Observation on the History of Physical Diagnosis: Hippocrates, Auenbrugger, Laennec," *J. Intern. Coll. Surg.*, vol. 31 (1959), p. 722.
52 Herrick, "Long Neglect of Auenbrugger's 'Inventum Novum,' " p. 741.
53 Auenbrugger, "On Percussion of the Chest," p. 379.

CHAPTER 2. THE STETHOSCOPE AND THE DETECTION OF PATHOLOGY BY SOUND

1 R. T. H. Laennec, *A Treatise on the Diseases of the Chest. . .* , 2nd ed., p. 23. [Each of the successive editions translated in English has a somewhat different title and publisher: see Bibliography.]
2 William Harvey, *Exercitatio Anatomica de Motu Cordis et Sanguinis in Animalibus*, trans. Chauncey D. Leake (Springfield: Thomas, 1928), Part 2, p. 29.
3 Robert Hooke, "A General Scheme, or Idea of the Present State of Natural Philosophy . . . ," in *The Posthumous Works of Robert Hooke*, ed. Richard Waller (London: Samuel Smith and Benjamin Walford, 1705), pp. 39–40.
4 James Douglass, "Ventriculus cordis sinister stupendae magnitudinis, lately communicated to the Royal–Society," *Philo. Trans. R. Soc*, vol. 29, tract. no. 345 (1715), p. 326.
5 Edward Augustus Holyoke, "An Account of an Uncommon Case of Emphysema; and of an external Abscess whose Contents were discharged by coughing," *Memoirs of the American Academy of Arts and Sciences*, vol. 2, part 1 (1793), pp. 189–90.
6 Laennec, *Diseases of the Chest*, 2nd ed., p. 23.
7 J. N. Corvisart, *An Essay on the Organic Diseases and Lesions of the Heart and Great Vessels*, trans. Jacob Gates (Boston: Bradford and Read, 1812), p. 284.
8 Laennec, *Diseases of the Chest*, 1st ed., p. 285.
9 Laennec experimented with stethoscopes made of material having a low density, such as gold-beaters skin, inflated with air. He also experimented with stethoscopes constructed from dense materials such as metal or glass. But he found that stethoscopes fashioned from materials of moderate density, such as wood or paper, transmitted chest sounds most distinctly (Laennec, *Diseases of the Chest*, 2nd ed., p. 6). Accounts of Laennec's life and the discovery of the stethoscope can be found in Roger Kervan, *Laennec: His Life and Times*, trans. D. C. Abrahams-Curiel (New York: Pergamon Press, 1960); William Pearce Coues, "Laennec, the Man – 1781–1826," *Boston Med. Surg. J.*, vol. 195 (1926), pp. 208–17; Warfield T. Longscope, "A Note on Laennec's Invention of the Stethoscope," *Am. Rev. Tubercul.*, vol. 19 (1929), pp. 1–8; and Alfred Hudson, "Laennec: His Labors and their Influence in Medicine," *Br. Med. J.*, vol. 2 (1879), pp. 204–9.
10 Laennec, *Diseases of the Chest*, 1st ed., p. xxxii. However, a year prior to the publication of his treatise, Laennec explained the technique before a meeting of the French Academy of Sciences. A committee of the academy wrote favorably about auscultation in its report published several months later. For the full text of the academy's report see R. T. H. Laennec, *De l'auscultation médiate . . .* (Paris: J. A. Brosson et J. S. Chaudé, 1819), xi–xiv.
11 Laennec, *Diseases of the Chest*, 1st ed., pp. xxxii, 283–7, 367–8.

12 Ibid., p. xxxiii.
13 Leopold Auenbrugger, *Nouvelle méthode pour reconnaître les maladies internes de la poitrine par la percussion de cette cavité*, trans. J. N. Corvisart (Paris: Migneret, 1808).
14 Luther V. Bell, "How far are the external means of exploring the condition of the internal organs to be considered useful and important in medical practice?" (Boylston Prize Dissertations for 1836), Library of Practical Medicine, vol. 7 (Boston: Perkins & Marvin, 1836), p. 42. See also John Bell, "Some general remarks on the use of the Stethoscope, as an aid in forming a correct diagnosis of Diseases of the Lungs . . . ," *N.Y. Med. Phys. J.*, vol. 3 (1824), pp. 270–1; John Forbes, in translator's preface, Laennec, *Diseases of the Chest*, 1st ed., p. xxiii.
15 Laennec, *Diseases of the Chest*, 1st ed., pp. 389–90.
16 There have been a number of interesting accounts of the introduction of auscultation into medicine: Edward I. Bluth, "James Hope and the Acceptance of Auscultation," *J. Hist. Med.*, vol. 25 (1970), pp. 202–10; Harold N. Segall, "Introduction of the Stethoscope and Clinical Auscultation in Canada," *J. Hist. Med.*, vol. 22 (1967), pp. 414–17; Victor A. McKusick, "The History of Methods for the Diagnosis of Heart Disease," *Bull. Hist. Med.*, vol. 34 (1960), pp. 16–18; Robert Coope, "Mr. Bampton's Prize, or the Tale of an Old Stethoscope," *Lancet*, vol. 2 (1952), pp. 577–80; James B. Herrick, *A Short History of Cardiology* (Springfield: Thomas, 1942); Lawrason Brown, *The Story of Clinical Pulmonary Tuberculosis* (Baltimore: Williams & Wilkins, 1941); James J. Waring, "The Vicissitudes of Auscultation," *Am. J. Tuberc.*, vol. 34 (1936), pp. 1–9; George W. Balfour, "On the Evolution of Cardiac Diagnosis from Harvey's Days Till Now," *Edinb. Med. J.*, vol. 32 (1887), part 2, pp. 1065–81; James T. Whittaker, "The History of Auscultation," *Med. Rec.*, vol. 16 (1879), pp. 411–14; G. Peyraud, "A History of the Improvements which Practical Medicine has Derived from Auscultation," *West. J. Med. Surg.*, vol. 6 (1842), pp. 1–58, 80–142.
17 Laennec, *Diseases of the Chest*, 1st ed., p. 300.
18 Robert J. Graves, *Clinical Lectures . . .* (Philadelphia: Adam Waldie, 1838), p. 4.
19 P. M. Latham, "Lectures on Subjects Connected with Clinical Medicine," *Lond. Med. G.*, vol. 17 (1835–36), p. 280.
20 John Forbes, in translator's preface, Laennec, *Diseases of the Chest*, 1st ed., p. xiv. See also Lester S. King, "Auscultation in England, 1821–1837," *Bull. Hist. Med.*, vol. 33 (1959), pp. 446–7.
21 John Taylor, "Introductory Lecture on the Opening of the Medical Session of 1841–1842, in University College," *Lancet*, vol. 1 (1841–42), p. 106.
22 F. Magendie, "On Abnormal Sounds in Different Parts of the Human Body," *Boston Med. Surg. J.*, vol. 12 (1835), p. 182.
23 John Turnbull, "Value of Auscultation in Diseases of the Chest," *Boston Med. Surg. J.*, vol. 34 (1846), p. 232. See also John E. Elliotson, *The Principles and Practice of Medicine . . .* (London: Joseph Butler, 1839), p. xiii; Luther V. Bell, "Exploring the condition of the internal organs," pp. 40–1.
24 Laennec, *Diseases of the Chest*, 1st ed., p. xvii.
25 J.–B.–P. Barth and Henri Roger, *A Practical Treatise on Auscultation*, trans. Patrick Newbigging (Lexington, Kentucky: Scrugham & Dunlop, 1847), p. 1. See

also Taylor, "Introductory Lecture," p. 106; book review, *Lancet*, vol. 9 (1826), p. 471.

26 Grant Klein, ed., *Memoir of the Late James Hope, by Mrs. Hope . . .* , 4th ed. (London: J. Hatchard and Son, 1848), pp. 75–6.

27 Book review, *Med.–Chir. Rev.*, vol. 8 (1828), pp. 112–13; H. M. Hughes, "Illustrations of the Alleged Fallacies of Auscultation," *Lond. Med. G.*, vol. 32 (1842–43), p. 418; book review, *Edinb. Med. J.*, vol. 23 (1825), p. 407; "Auscultation and Thoracic Diseases," *Med.–Chir. Rev.*, vol. 4 (1826), p. 449.

28 P. Ch. A. Louis, *An Essay on Clinical Instruction*, trans. Peter Martin (London: S. Highley, 1834), p. 28.

29 William Corrigan, "Aneurism of the Aorta," *Lancet*, vol. 1 (1828–29), p. 588. This view was also expressed in a book review, *Med.–Chir. Rev.*, vol. 2 (1825), p. 62; and in James Clark, *Medical Notes on Climate, Diseases, Hospitals, and Medical Schools . . .* (London: T. and G. Underwood, 1820), pp. 155–6.

30 James Jackson, *Memoir of James Jackson Jr. . . .* (Boston: I. R. Butts, 1835), p. 177. Similar views are found in Robert Spittal, *A Treatise on Auscultation, Illustrated by Cases and Dissertations* (Edinburgh: R. Grant & Sons, 1830), pp. 12–13.

31 John Forbes, in translator's preface, Laennec, *Diseases of the Chest*, 1st ed., p. xix. For similar views, see also Thomas Addison, "On the Difficulties and Fallacies Attending Physical Diagnosis in Diseases of the Chest," *Guy's Hosp. Rep.*, vol. 4 (1846), p. 3; Charles J. B. Williams, *Lectures on the Physiology and Diseases of the Chest* (Philadelphia: Haswell, Barrington, and Haswell, 1839), p. 12.

32 Oliver Wendell Holmes, "The Stethoscope Song: A Professional Ballad," *Poems* (Boston: Ticknor, Reed & Fields, 1850), pp. 272–7. See also "The Stethoscope," *Lond. Med. G.*, vol. 1 (1828), p. 473; Klein, *Memoir of the Late James Hope*, p. 74; Robert Martin, ed., *The Collected Works of P. M. Latham*, vol. 1 (London: New Sydenham Society, 1876), p. 49.

33 Book review, *Br. Foreign Med. Rev.*, vol. 9 (1840), p. 299. See also book review, *Br. Foreign Med.–Chir. Rev.*, vol. 9 (1852), p. 486.

34 Laennec, *Diseases of the Chest*, 3rd ed., pp. 226–7, and footnote.

35 "One of the New School," *Lond. Med. G.*, vol. 1 (1827–28), pp. 408–9. For other examples of the public's fascination with the idea of listening to disease, see the poem "To the Stethoscope," *Blackwood's Edinb. Mag.*, vol. 61 (1847), p. 361; and also George Rosen, "A Note on the Reception of the Stethoscope in England," *Bull. Hist. Med.*, vol. 7 (1939), pp. 93–4.

36 Hospital Reports, *Med.–Chir. Rev.*, vol. 8 (1828), pp. 131–2. See also book review, *Med.–Chir. Rev.*, vol. 28 (1838), p. 33.

37 Laennec, *Diseases of the Chest*, 2nd ed., pp. 23–4.

38 Charles J. B. Williams, *Memoirs of Life and Work* (London: Smith, Elder and Co., 1884), p. 48.

39 H. Veale, "The Medical Officer's Stethoscope," *Lancet*, vol. 2 (1879), p. 819. See also Laennec, *Diseases of the Chest*, 2nd ed., p. 24; Jacob Bigelow, "Brief Rules for the Exploration of the Chest, in Diseases of the Lungs and Heart," *Boston Med. Surg. J.*, vol. 20 (1839), p. 373.

40 John Forbes, in translator's preface, Laennec, *Diseases of the Chest*, 1st ed., p. xix.

41 Book review, *Lancet*, vol. 2 (1831–32), p. 121. See also Laennec, *Diseases of the Chest*, 2nd ed., p. 24, and 3rd ed., p. 32.

42 David Riesman, "The Oral and Written Traditions," in *Explorations in Communication*, ed. Edmund Carpenter and Marshall McLuhan (Boston: Beacon Press, 1960), p. 110.

43 Sir William Gull, "Some Guiding Thoughts to the Study of Medicine," (delivered at Guy's Hospital at the opening of the 1855–56 session), in *A Collection of the Published Writings of William Withey Gull: Memoir and Addresses*, ed. Theodore Dyke Acland (London: New Sydenham Society, 1896), p. 8.

44 William Markham, in translator's preface, Joseph Skoda, *A Treatise on Auscultation and Percussion* (London: Highley and Son, 1853), p. x.

45 Ibid., p. iii.

46 Book review, *Br. Foreign Med.–Chir. Rev.*, vol. 9 (1852), p. 487.

47 Skoda, *Treatise on Auscultation*, p. 60.

48 Ibid., p. 7.

49 Herbert C. Clapp, *A Tabular Handbook of Auscultation and Percussion for Students and Physicians* (Boston: Houghton, Osgood and Co., 1879), p. xi.

50 Several interesting essays have been written on the history of the changes in stethoscope design: D. M. Cammann, "An Historical Sketch of the Stethoscope," *N. Y. Med. J.*, vol. 43 (1886), pp. 465–6; Samuel Wilks, "Evolution of the Stethoscope," *Lancet*, vol. 2 (1882), pp. 882–3; Theodore C. Williams, "Laennec and the Evolution of the Stethoscope," *Brit. Med. J.*, vol. 2 (1907), pp. 6–8; Paul B. Sheldon and Janet Doe, "The Development of the Stethoscope: An Exhibition," *Bull. N.Y. Acad. Med.*, vol. 11 (1935), pp. 608–26; Stephen Morris, "The Advent and Development of the Binaural Stethoscope," *Practitioner*, vol. 199 (1968), pp. 674–80.

51 N. P. Comins, "New Stethoscope," *Lond. Med. G.*, vol. 4 (1829), p. 429. See also Golding Bird, "Observations on the Advantages Presented by the Employment of a Stethoscope with a Flexible Tube," *Lond. Med. G.*, vol. 1 (1840–41), pp. 440–2.

52 Arthur Leared, "On the Self-Adjusting Double Stethoscope," *Lancet*, vol. 2 (1856), p. 202. Dr. Landouzy of Paris, M. B. Marsh of Cincinnati, Arthur Leared of London in 1851, and George Cammann in 1852, all reported making flexible binaural devices. But Leared displayed his at the Great Exhibition of London in 1851 and claimed priority for the invention (Cammann, "Historical Sketch," p. 465).

53 Comins, "New Stethoscope," p. 430; Charles J. B. Williams, "On the Acoustic Principles and Construction of Stethoscopes and Ear-Trumpets," *Lancet*, vol. 2 (1873), p. 665.

54 For physicians' reaction to Alison's stethoscope see book review, *Edinb. Med. J.*, vol. 7 (1861–62), p. 835. For a description of the differential stethoscope and its functions, see Somerville Scott Alison, *The Physical Examination of the Chest in Pulmonary Consumption. . .*(London: John Churchill, 1861), pp. 6–7, 21–3.

55 "The Microphone in Diagnosis," *Lancet*, vol. 1 (1878), p. 766.

56 Book review, *Br. Foreign Med.–Chir. Rev.*, vol. 28 (1861), p. 47. See also, Hyde Salter, "On the Stethoscope," *Brit. Med. J.*, vol. 1 (1863), p. 107.

57 James E. Pollock, "On a Self-Adjusting Double Stethoscope," *Lancet*, vol. 1 (1856), p. 398. See also W. H. Spencer, "On a New Form of Stethoscope in its Relations to the Theory and Practice of Auscultation," *Brit. Med. J.*, vol. 1 (1874), p. 409.

CHAPTER 3. VISUAL TECHNOLOGY AND THE
ANATOMIZATION OF THE LIVING

1 William Thau, "Purkyně: A Pioneer in Ophthalmoscopy," *Arch. Ophthalmol.*, n.s., vol. 27 (1942), pp. 303–4. An alternative, more literal rendering of this quoted passage, as well as a translation of Purkyně's treatise in which it appears, *A Physiological Examination of the Organ of Vision and the Integumentary System*, can be found in Henry J. John, *Jan Evangelista Purkyně* (Philadelphia: American Philosophical Society, 1959), p. 61. See also Daniel M. Albert and William H. Miller, "Jan Purkinje and the Ophthalmoscope," *J. Ophthalmol.*, vol. 76 (1973), pp. 494–9.
2 Hermann von Helmholtz, "The History of the Discovery of the Ophthalmoscope," *Med. Rec.*, vol. 44 (1893), p. 771. See also Hermann von Helmholtz, *Treatise on Physiological Optics*, ed. and trans. from the 3rd German edition by James P. C. Southall (Menasha, Wis.: Optical Society of America, 1924), vol. 1, p. 257. William Cumming's investigations are recorded in "On a Luminous Appearance of the Human Eye, and Its Application to the Detection of Disease of the Retina and Posterior Part of the Eye," *Med. Chir. Trans.*, vol. 29 (1846), pp. 283–96. Two other scientists had experimented with lenses to see into the eye before Helmholtz. In 1845, Adolf Kussmaul, the German physician, attempted to use a concave and a convex lens, each mounted at the end of a tube, to peer into the eye. He subsequently wrote: "My ophthalmoscope was the best in the world for there existed only one – mine, its only disadvantage being that one could not see with it." Henry H. Mark, "The First Ophthalmoscope? Adolf Kussmaul 1845," *Arch. Ophthalmol.*, vol. 84 (1970), p. 521. In 1847 the English inventor Charles Babbage was reported to have designed an ophthalmoscope. But the first account of it was published in 1854 by T. Wharton Jones, "Report on the Ophthalmoscope," *Br. Foreign Med.–Chir. Rev.*, vol. 14 (1854), p. 551.
3 W. R. Sanders, "On Helmholtz's Speculum for Examining the Retina in the Living Eye," *Mon. J. Med. Sci.*, vol. 15 (1852), p. 44.
4 Adolf Zander, *The Ophthalmoscope, Its Varieties and Its Use*, trans. Robert Brundenell Carter (London: Robert Hardwicke, 1864), p. 4.
5 Hasket Derby, "The Relations of the Ophthalmoscope to Legal Medicine," *Boston Med. Surg. J.*, vol. 66 (1862), pp. 525–7.
6 A. E. Ewing, "Test Objects for the Illiterate," *J. Ophthalmol.*, vol. 3 (1920), pp. 5–22. For an excellent study of the origin of eyeglasses see Edward Rosen, "The Invention of Eyeglasses," *J. Hist. Med.*, vol. 11 (1956), pp. 18–46, 183–218.
7 A. Edward Davis, *The Refraction of the Eye* (New York: Macmillan, 1900), pp. 1–2.
8 Edward Jackson, et al., "Report on the Value of Objective Tests for the Determination of Ametropia, Ophthalmoscopy, Ophthalmometry, Skiascopy," *J.A.M.A.*, vol. 23 (1894), pp. 337–9.
9 H. V. Würdemann, "The Status of Skiascopy," *J.A.M.A.*, vol. 23 (1894), p. 341. Other papers and comments presented on this subject at the American Medical Association meeting were Alexander Randall, "Retinoscopy as a Crucial Test in Measuring Errors of Refraction," ibid., pp. 340–1; Edward Jack-

son, "The Visual Zone of the Dioptic Media and Its Study by Skiascopy," ibid., pp. 342–3; "Discussion," ibid., pp. 343–5.

10 Montrose A. Pallen, "Vision, and Some of its Anomalies, as Revealed by the Ophthalmoscope," *Trans. Am. Med. Assoc.*, vol. 11 (1858), p. 908. See also Jabez Hogg, "The Speculum Oculi, or Ophthalmoscope," *Lancet*, vol. 1 (1857), p. 400.

11 Laurence Turnbull, "The Clinical Use of the Ophthalmoscope in Diseases of the Eye," *Med. Surg. Rep.*, vol. 2 (1859), p. 262; Wharton T. Jones, "Report on the Ophthalmoscope," *Br. Foreign Med.–Chir. Rev.*, vol. 14 (1854), p. 554. This Hippocratic moral principle is found in "Epidemics I"; see W. H. S. Jones, *Hippocrates* (Cambridge: Harvard University Press, 1923), vol. 1, p. 165.

12 "A New Ophthalmoscope," *Med. Times Gaz.*, vol. 7 (1853), pp. 379–80; D. Argyll Robertson, "The Progress of Ophthalmology, a Sketch," *Edinb. Med. J.*, vol. 8, part 1 (1862), pp. 47–8; John H. Dix, "On the Ophthalmoscope – Its Uses and Methods of Application," *Boston Med. Surg. J.*, vol. 54 (1856), pp. 419–20.

13 John H. Dix, "Dangers and Uses of the Ophthalmoscope," *Boston Med. Surg. J.*, vol. 51 (1855), p. 436; "Value of the Ophthalmoscope in Eye Diseases," *Am. J. Med. Sci.*, vol. 33 (1857), p. 261; "Medical Ophthalmoscopy," *Lancet*, vol. 1 (1868), p. 57; Zander, *The Ophthalmoscope*, p. 76.

14 E. Williams, "The Ophthalmoscope . . . ," *Med. Times Gaz.*, vol. 9 (1854), p. 31; "On the Employment of the Ophthalmoscope in the Investigation of Deep-Seated Disease of the Eye," *Am. J. Med. Sci.*, vol. 34 (1854), p. 261.

15 "On the Importance of the Ophthalmoscope as an Aid in General Practice," *Boston Med. Surg. J.*, vol. 84 (1871), pp. 205–7; J. Hughlings Jackson, "Ophthalmology in its Relation to General Medicine," *Br. Med. J.*, vol. 1 (1877), pp. 575–7.

16 Philipp Bozzini, "The Light Conductor . . . ," trans. L. B. Murdoch, in *Quar. Bull. Northwest. Univ. Med. Sch.*, vol. 23 (1949), pp. 332–54.

17 Morell Mackenzie, *The Use of the Laryngoscope in Diseases of the Throat, with an Appendix on Rhinoscopy* (Philadelphia: Lindsay and Blakiston, 1865), pp. 14, 20–35.

18 Antoine Ruppaner, "The Practice of Laryngoscopy and Rhinoscopy," *N.Y. Med. J.*, vol. 6 (1867), pp. 2–4.

19 Manuel Garcia, "Physiological Observations on the Human Voice," *Proc. R. Soc.*, vol. 7 (1854–55), pp. 399–410.

20 Johann Czermak's treatise, *On the Laryngoscope and its Employment in Physiology and Medicine*, trans. George D. Gibb (London: New Sydenham Society, 1861), pp. 1–10; and Ruppaner, "Practice of Laryngoscopy," pp. 5–13, provide good accounts of these events.

21 George D. Gibb, "The Laryngoscope: Its Value in Healthy and Diseased Conditions of the Throat and Windpipe," *Lancet*, vol. 2 (1860), p. 307. See also book review, *Br. Foreign Med. Rev.*, vol. 36 (1865), p. 310; "Laryngoscopy," *Lancet*, vol. 1 (1862), p. 580.

22 Thomas J. Walker, "Report of a Case of Polypoid Growth of the Larynx Diagnosed and Removed by Aid of the Laryngoscope," *Lancet*, vol. 2 (1861), p. 444.

23 Eben Watson, "Laryngoscopy and its Revelations," [part 2] *Lancet*, vol. 2 (1865), pp. 6–8.

24 "The Laryngoscope," *Lancet*, vol. 1 (1860), p. 454. See also Ephraim Cutter, "On the Laryngoscope and Rhinoscope," *Boston Med. Surg. J.*, vol. 69 (1863), p.

396; George Johnson, "Two Lectures on the Laryngoscope," *Lancet*, vol. 1 (1864), pp. 573–5, 603–5.
25 Watson, "Laryngoscopy and its Revelations," [part 1] *Lancet*, vol. 1 (1865), p. 589.
26 "New Inventions in Aid of the Practice of Medicine and Surgery. Professor Czermak's Laryngoscope," *Lancet*, vol. 2 (1860), pp. 516–7; Francis Mason, "Description of a Laryngoscope," *Lancet*, vol. 2 (1863), p. 159; Ephraim Cutter, "Remarks on Laryngoscopy," *Med. Surg. Rep.*, vol. 13 (1865), p. 375.
27 "The Laryngoscope," *Lancet*, vol. 1 (1860), p. 454; Cutter, "On the Laryngoscope and Rhinoscope," p. 397.
28 Book review, *Br. Foreign Med. – Chir. Rev.*, vol. 59 (1862), p. 346. See also E. H. Sieveking, "Lecture on the Use of the Laryngoscope," *Lancet*, vol. 1 (1865), pp. 359–62.
29 "The Laryngoscope," *Boston Med. Surg. J.*, vol. 62 (1860), p. 489.
30 Book review, *N.Y. Med. J.*, vol. 4 (1866–67), p. 229; Henry Thompson, "Lecture on the Diagnosis of Surgical Diseases of the Urinary Organs especially in Connexion with the Use of the 'Nietze-Lietner' Endoscope," *Lancet*, vol. 2 (1879), p. 823. An excellent historical examination of the introduction of the gastroscope has been written by Audrey B. Davis, "Rudolf Schindler's Role in the Development of Gastroscopy," *Bull. Hist. Med.*, vol. 46 (1972), pp. 150–70.
31 Alfred Meadows, "Description of Two New Vaginal Specula," *Lancet*, vol. 1 (1870), p. 692. An excellent discussion of gynecological examination and the use of the speculum in the nineteenth century is found in James V. Ricci, *The Development of Gynecological Surgery and Instruments* (Philadelphia: Blakiston Co., 1949), pp. 294–319.
32 "Electric Illumination of the Male Bladder and Urethra," *Lancet*, vol. 1 (1888), p. 305; Reginald Harrison, "Remarks on Endoscopy with the Electric Light," *Lancet*, vol. 1 (1888), p. 1021; "Apparatus for Examining the Cavities of the Face by Electric Light," *Lancet*, vol. 1 (1892), p. 1195.
33 See for example, Hugo J. Loebinger, "Description of a 'Pelvescope,' " *N.Y. Med. J.*, vol. 53 (1891), pp. 399–400.
34 "Photography in Medical Science," *Lancet*, vol. 1 (1859), p. 89.
35 "Animal Locomotion and Instantaneous Photography," *Lancet*, vol. 1 (1889), p. 645. See also "Photographing the Larynx," *N.Y. Med. J.*, vol. 44 (1886), p. 520.
36 Francis Galton and F. A. Mahomed, "The Physiognomy of Phthisis by the Method of 'Composite Portraiture,' " *Guy's Hosp. Rep.*, vol. 25 (1881), pp. 474–95.
37 "Clinical Photography," *Br. Med. J.*, vol. 1 (1895), p. 1402; A. L. Benedict, "Auscultatory Percussion and Allied Methods of Physical Diagnosis," *Med. Surg. Rep.*, vol. 72 (1895), p. 586.
38 The most authoritative version of this generally accepted account of the discovery of X-rays is given by Roentgen's principal biographer Otto Glasser in *Wilhelm Conrad Röntgen and the Early History of the Roentgen Rays* (Springfield: Thomas, 1934), and in his shorter biography, *Dr. W. C. Röntgen*, 2nd ed. rev. (Springfield: Thomas, 1958). See also G. L'E. Turner, "Wilhelm Conrad Röntgen (Roentgen)," *Dictionary of Scientific Biography*, ed. Charles C. Gillespie (New York: Scribners, 1975), vol. 11, pp. 529–31. The exact date and exact circumstances of Roentgen's discovery, as given in the above account, have been questioned by Herbert S. Klickstein in his *Wilhelm Conrad Röntgen on a New*

Kind of Rays, Mallinckrodt Classics of Radiology, vol. 1 (St. Louis: Mallinckrodt Chemical Works, 1966), pp. 16–21.
39 W. C. Röntgen, "On a New Kind of Rays," *Nature*, vol. 53 (1895–96), p. 274.
40 D. W. Hering, "A Year of the X-Rays," *Pop. Sci. Mon.*, vol. 50 (1896), p. 654.
41 *New York Times*, January 16, 1896, p. 9.
42 G. E. M. Jauncey, "The Birth and Early Infancy of X-rays," *Am J. Phys.*, vol. 13 (1945), p. 365.
43 "The Photography of the Invisible," *Q. Rev.*, vol. 183 (1896), p. 496.
44 *New York Times*, February 9, 1896, p. 9.
45 "Possibilities of the Roentgen Ray in Medicine," *Medical News*, vol. 68 (1896), p. 210.
46 C. H. T. Crosthwaite, "Röntgen's Curse," *Longman's Mag.*, vol. 28 (1896), pp. 469–84.
47 "The New Photography," *Punch*, January 25, 1896, p. 45.
48 "Her Latest Photograph," *New York Times*, May 29, 1898, p. 14.
49 Ibid.
50 Ibid.
51 "Cakes Under X-ray," *Lancet*, vol. 1 (1897), p. 289.
52 "Possibilities of the Roentgen Ray in Medicine," p. 211.
53 "Death of President McKinley," *J.A.M.A.*, vol. 37 (1901), p. 781.
54 Henry Cattell, "Roentgen's Discovery – Its Application in Medicine," *Med. News*, vol. 68 (1896), p. 170.
55 M. Goltman, "The History of the X-Rays: their Medical and Surgical Application," *Memphis Med. Mon.*, vol. 17 (1897), pp. 289, 293. See also Dayton C. Miller, "Roentgen X-Rays and their Application in Medicine and Surgery," *Cleve. Med. G.*, vol. 2 (1896), p. 332; James Burry, "A Preliminary Report on the Roentgen or X Rays," *J.A.M.A.*, vol. 26 (1896), p. 402; "The New Photographic Discovery," *Lancet*, vol. 1 (1896), p. 310.
56 H. W. van Allen, "Dangers from the 'X-Ray Atmosphere' to the Operator. Their Prevention," *Boston Med. Surg. J.*, vol. 152 (1905), p. 273. See also "A Notable Demonstration of the X-Rays," *Boston Med. Surg. J.*, vol. 134 (1896), pp. 448–9; Francis H. Williams, "A Method for More Fully Determining the Outline of the Heart by Means of the Fluoroscope Together with Other Uses of This Instrument in Medicine," *Boston Med. Surg. J.*, vol. 135 (1896), p. 337; "Important Improvements in the Application of the 'X' Rays to Medicine," *Lancet*, vol. 2 (1896), p. 47.
57 "The New Photography," *Lancet*, vol. 1 (1896), pp. 1159–60. See also George R. Fowler, "A Preliminary Note upon the Possibilities of the Application of Photography of Unseen Substances to Surgical Diagnosis," *Brooklyn Med. J.*, vol. 10 (1896), pp. 137–8; Robert Jones and Oliver Lodge, "The Discovery of a Bullet Lost in the Wrist by Means of the Roentgen Rays," *Lancet*, vol. 1 (1896), pp. 476–7.
58 Charles Lester Leonard, "The Application of the Roentgen Rays to Medical Diagnosis," *J.A.M.A.*, vol. 29 (1897), pp. 1157–8.
59 "Outline of the Clinical Uses of the X-rays," *Boston Med. Surg. J.*, vol. 139 (1898), p. 526.
60 Philip Mills Jones, "X-Rays and X-Ray Diagnosis," *J.A.M.A.*, vol. 29 (1897), p. 947. See also Francis H. Williams, "The Roentgen Rays in Thoracic Dis-

eases," *Trans. Assoc. Am. Physicians*, vol. 12 (1897), pp. 322–34; H. Campbell Thomson, "The Roentgen Rays in Medical Diagnosis," *Lancet*, vol. 2 (1897), pp. 710–11; "Skiagraphic Diagnosis Applied to Soft Parts," *Br. Med. J.*, vol. 1 (1897), p. 99.

61 "Our Limited Vision and the New Photography," *Lancet*, vol. 1 (1896), p. 499.
62 Walter B. Cannon, "The Movements of the Stomach Studied by Means of the Röntgen Rays," *Am. J. Physiol.*, vol. 1 (1898), pp. 359–82. The first published record of Cannon's work in X-raying the stomach appears in the brief report by H. P. Bowditch, "Movements of the Alimentary Canal," *Science*, n.s., vol. 5 (1897), pp. 901–2.
63 G. E. Pfahler, "Physiologic and Clinical Observations on the Alimentary Canal by Means of the Roentgen Rays," *J.A.M.A.*, vol. 49 (1907), p. 2069; Frederick Taylor, "Examination of Stomach by X-Rays and Tube Filled with Subnitrate of Bismuth," *Br. Med. J.*, vol. 1 (1905), p. 720.
64 W. W. Keen, "The Clinical Application of the Röntgen Rays in Surgical Diagnosis," *Am. J. Med. Sci.*, vol. 111 (1896), p. 259; H. E. Safford, "The Present Status of the X-Ray in Diagnosis," *Physician & Surg.*, vol. 20 (1898), p. 540; C. Mansell Moullin, "The Application of the Roentgen Rays to Medicine and Surgery," *Lancet*, vol. 2 (1899), p. 475.
65 "About X-Ray Photography," *N.Y. Times Mag.*, September 6, 1896, p. 12.
66 "X ray Photographs as Evidence," *J.A.M.A.*, vol. 29 (1897), p. 870.
67 "An X-Ray Danger," *J.A.M.A.*, vol. 32 (1899), p. 1122.
68 Harvey R. Reed, "The X-Ray from a Medico-Legal Standpoint," *J.A.M.A.*, vol. 30 (1898), p. 1016. See also "Roentgen Rays and Forensic Medicine," *Lancet*, vol. 2 (1899), p. 1682; Edward A. Tracy, "The Fallacies of X-Ray Pictures," *J. Electro. Ther.*, vol. 16 (1898), pp. 238–43.
69 "Report of the Committee of the American Surgical Association on the Medico-Legal Relations of the X-Rays," *Am. J. Med. Sci.*, vol. 120 (1900), p. 32.
70 Reed, "X-Ray from a Medico-Legal Standpoint," p. 1017.
71 Charles Lester Leonard, "The Past, Present and Future of the X-Ray," *Am. Med.*, vol. 10 (1905), p. 1082; "Report of the Committee of the American Surgical Association," p. 32; Sidney Lange, "The Present Status of the Roentgen Ray," *Lancet-Clin.*, vol. 58 (1907), p. 83.
72 Reed, "X-Ray from a Medico-Legal Standpoint," pp. 1013–17; "Possibilities of the Roentgen Ray in Medicine," *Med. News*, vol. 68 (1896), p. 210. In the first several years after the X-ray's discovery, medical journals, as well as newspapers and magazines, often referred to X-rays as photographs. For example, the excellent series of commentaries on developments in radiology written in 1896 by Sidney Rowland for the *Br. Med. J.* was entitled "Report on the Application of the New Photography . . ."
73 E. A. Codman, "No Practical Danger from X-ray," *Boston Med. Surg. J.*, vol. 144 (1901), p. 197.
74 Carl Beck, "Errors Caused by the False Interpretation of the Roentgen Rays, and Their Medico-Legal Aspects," *Med. Rec.*, vol. 58 (1900), p. 281.
75 "Untoward Effects of X-rays," *Boston Med. Surg. J.*, vol. 152 (1905), p. 173; "The Legal Conditions of the Medical Use of the Roentgen Rays," *Br. Med. J.*, vol. 1 (1906), p. 231.
76 "Edison and X-Ray Injuries," *J.A.M.A.*, vol. 41 (1903), p. 499.
77 David L. Edsall, "The Attitude of the Clinician in Regard to Exposing Patients

to the X-Ray," *J.A.M.A.*, vol. 47 (1906), pp. 1425–9. See also Walter J. Dodd, "The Public and the Medical Profession: The Use of the X-ray in Medicine and Surgery," *Boston Journal*, April 15, 1913.

78 In the modern period, the radiation hazards of nuclear explosions helped to refocus attention on the dangers of X-ray use. See "The Responsibilities of the Medical Profession in the Use of X-rays and other Ionising Radiation. Statement by the United Nations Scientific Committee on the Effects of Atomic Radiation," *Lancet*, vol. 1 (1957), pp. 467–8; Hanson Blatz, "Common Causes of Excessive Patient Exposure in Diagnostic Radiology," *New Engl. J. Med.*, vol. 271 (1964), pp. 1184–8; International Commission on Radiological Protection, "Patient Exposure in Diagnostic Radiology: Protection Problems of Current Concern," *Br. J. Radiol.*, vol. 46 (1973), pp. 1086–8; J. Thomas Payne and Merle K. Loken, "A Survey of the Benefits and Risks in the Practice of Radiology," *Crit. Rev. Clin. Radiol. Nucl. Med.*, vol. 6 (1975), pp. 425–37.

79 A. L. Benedict, "The Art of Diagnosis," *Med. Age*, vol. 17 (1899), p. 684. See also Zander, *The Ophthalmoscope*, p. 5.

CHAPTER 4. THE MICROSCOPE AND THE REVELATION OF A CELLULAR UNIVERSE

1 Charles Singer, "Notes on the Early History of Microscopy," *Proc. R. Soc. Med.*, vol. 7 (1913), pp. 247–8; Reginald S. Clay and Thomas H. Court, *The History of the Microscope* (London: Charles Griffen and Co., 1932), pp. 1–5; S. Bradbury, *The Evolution of the Microscope* (Oxford: Pergamon Press, 1967), pp. 2–7.

2 Alfred N. Disney, "An Historical Survey on the Early Progress of Optical Science," in Alfred N. Disney, Cyril F. Hill, and Wilfred E. Watson, eds., *Origin and Development of the Microscope, As Illustrated by Catalogues . . . of the Royal Microscopical Society* (London: The Royal Microscopical Society, 1928), p. 89; M. Rooseboom, "The History of the Microscope," *Proc. R. Microsc. Soc.*, vol. 2 (1967), p. 266; Silvio A. Bedini and Derek J. De Solla Price, "Instrumentation," in Melvin Kranzberg and Carroll W. Pursell, Jr., eds., *Technology in Western Civilization*, vol. 1 (New York: Oxford University Press, 1967), p. 168; Bradbury, *Evolution of the Microscope*, pp. 15, 21.

3 Rooseboom, "History of the Microscope," pp. 267–8; Disney, "Early Progress of Optical Science," pp. 90–2, 97, 101; Clay and Court, *History of the Microscope*, p. 12.

4 Fielding H. Harrison, *An Introduction to the History of Medicine* (reprinted, Philadelphia: Saunders, 1966), pp. 255–6; Bradbury, *History of the Microscope*, pp. 56–7.

5 R. Hooke, *Micrographia: or Some Physiological Descriptions of Minute Bodies Made by Magnifying Glasses with Observations and Inquiries Thereupon* (London: Jo. Martyn and Ja. Allestry, 1665), p. 113. For an excellent biography of Hooke see Margaret 'Espinasse, *Robert Hooke* (Berkeley: University of California Press, 1962).

6 It is conceivable that Leeuwenhoek also ground lenses with a magnifying power of 500 diameters. See A. Shierbeek, *Measuring the Invisible World: The*

Life and Works of Antoni van Leeuwenhoek FRS (London: Abelard-Schuman, 1959), pp. 48–52; Clay and Court, *History of the Microscope*, p. 9.

7 Bradbury, *Evolution of the Microscope*, p. 73. See also Rooseboom, "History of the Microscope," pp. 273–4.

8 Schierbeek, *Measuring the Invisible World*, p. 65.

9 Ibid., p. 69.

10 Clifford Dobbell, *Antony van Leeuwenhoek and his 'Little Animals'* (New York: Russell & Russell, 1958), pp. 222–30.

11 John E. Lane, "Bonomo's Letter to Redi: An Important Document in the History of Scabies," *Arch. Dermatol. Syphilol.*, vol. 18 (1928), pp. 22–4. This article contains facsimiles of Bonomo's original letter and an English translation of a portion by Richard Mead.

12 David E. Wolfe, "Sydenham and Locke on the Limits of Anatomy," *Bull. Hist. Med.*, vol. 35 (1961), pp. 193–200. See also William Addison, *On Healthy and Diseased Structure* . . . (London: John Churchill, 1849), p. 4.

13 Rooseboom, "History of the Microscope," p. 273.

14 William Hewson and Magnus Falconar, *A Description of the Red Particles of the Blood* (London, 1777), in *The Works of William Hewson*, ed. George Gulliver (London: Sydenham Society, 1846), p. 214.

15 Bradbury, *Evolution of the Microscope*, pp. 71–2.

16 Hewson, *Description of the Red Particles*, p. 215.

17 Ibid.

18 Henry Baker, *The Microscope Made Easy* . . . (London: R. Dodsley, M. Cooper, and J. Coff, 1744), p. iii. See also Bradbury, *Evolution of the Microscope*, pp. 59–60, 105–6.

19 Book review, *Edinb. Med. Surg. J.*, vol. 73 (1850), p. 173.

20 Thomas Bell, "Observations on the Use of the Microscope . . . ," *Trans. Med. Soc. London*, vol. 1 (1846), p. 1.

21 Alfred Hudson, "Laennec, His Labours and Their Influence in Medicine," *Br. Med. J.*, vol. 2 (1879), p. 205.

22 Bradbury, *Evolution of the Microscope*, pp. 179–88.

23 William Hyde Wollaston, "A description of a microscopic doublet," *Philos. Trans. Roy. Soc.*, vol. 119 (1829), p. 9.

24 Joseph Jackson Lister, "On some properties in achromatic object-glasses applicable to the improvement of the microscope," *Philos. Trans. Roy. Soc.*, vol. 120 (1830), pp. 187–200.

25 S. Bradbury, "The Quality of the Image Produced by the Compound Microscope: 1700–1840," *Proc. Roy. Soc. Microscop.*, vol. 2 (1967), p. 163.

26 For an examination of the development of test-objects, see G. L'E. Turner, "The Microscope as a Technical Frontier in Science," *Proc. Roy. Soc. Microscop.*, vol. 2 (1967), pp. 178–97.

27 John Hughes Bennett, "Introductory Address to a Course of Lectures on Histology, and the Use of the Microscope," *Lancet*, vol. 1 (1845), p. 520. See also John Quekett, *A Practical Treatise on the Use of the Microscope* (London: H. Baillière, 1848), p. vii.

28 Thomas Williams, "On the Pathology of Cells," *Guy's Hosp. Rep.*, vol. 1 (1843), p. 424. See also F. Gerber, *Elements of the General and Minute Anatomy of Man and the Mammalia* . . . (London: H. Baillière, 1842), pp. v–vi; F. J. Gant,

"What has Pathological Anatomy Done for Medicine and Surgery?" *Lancet*, vol. 2 (1857), p. 437; book review, *Dublin J. Med. Sci.*, vol. 26 (1845), pp. 323–33.

29 Williams, "Pathology of Cells," p. 426.
30 Book review, *Am. J. Med. Sci.*, vol. 25 (1853), pp. 48–9; "Use of the Microscope in the Diagnosis of Cancer," *Am. Med. Mon.*, vol. 3 (1855), p. 141; Addison, *Healthy and Diseased Structure*, pp. 185–95.
31 "American Microscopes," *Boston Med. Surg. J.*, vol. 60 (1859), p. 47; Professor Bennett, "The Microscope as a Means of Diagnosis," *Month. J. Med. Sci.*, vol. 11 (1850), pp. 548–52; Bradbury, *Evolution of the Microscope*, pp. 229–49. It was still common to examine fresh tissues in microscopic work during the 1830s and 1840s. The use of stains to outline structures in tissues is a product of the late 1850s. For the use of staining procedures, see Lionel Beale, *How to Work with the Microscope*, 3rd ed. (London: Harrison, 1865), pp. 189–94, and W. H. McMenemey, "Cellular Pathology, with Special Reference to the Influence of Virchow's Teachings on Medical Thought and Practice," in *Medicine and Science in the 1860s*, ed. F. N. L. Poynter (London: Wellcome Institute of the History of Medicine, 1968), pp. 19–20.
32 Rudolf Virchow, "Atoms and Individuals," in *Disease, Life, and Man: Selected Essays by Rudolf Virchow*, trans. and introduced by Lelland J. Rather (Stanford: Stanford University Press, 1958), p. 129. See also Erwin H. Ackerknecht, *Rudolf Virchow* (Madison: University of Wisconsin Press, 1953), pp. 71–2.
33 Garrison, *Introduction to the History of Medicine*, pp. 454–5.
34 Williams, "Pathology of Cells," pp. 426–7.
35 Rudolf Virchow, *Cellular Pathology as based upon Physiological and Pathological Histology*, 2nd ed., trans. Frank Chance (London: John Churchill, 1860).
36 Ibid., pp. 9–16, 25–8, 60.
37 Rudolf Virchow, "The Influence of Morgagni on Anatomical Thought," *Lancet*, vol. 1 (1894), p. 846.
38 Ibid.
39 Rudolf Virchow, "Cellular Pathology," in Rather, *Disease, Life, and Man*, p. 84.
40 Ibid., p. 85.
41 Williams, "Pathology of Cells," p. 425. See also George Owen Rees, "Observations on the Blood, with Reference to its Peculiar Condition in the Morbus Brightii," *Guy's Hos. Rep.*, vol. 1 (1843), p. 317.
42 H. Bence Jones, "A Course of Lectures on Animal Chemistry Specially Illustrating the Diagnosis and Treatment of Stomach and Renal Diseases," *Lancet*, vol. 1 (1850), p. 2. See also William B. Carpenter, *The Microscope and its Revelations* (London: John Churchill, 1856), p. 8.
43 Bell, "Use of the Microscope," p. 22.
44 Lionel S. Beale, *How to Work with the Microscope* (London: John Churchill, 1857), p. 3.
45 J. Marion Sims, "On the Microscope, as an Aid in the Diagnosis and Treatment of Sterility," *N. Y. Med. J.*, vol. 8 (1869), p. 397.
46 Ibid., p. 413.
47 James Tyson, "Some Reasons Why the Microscope Should Be Used by Every Physician," *Med. Surg. Rep.*, vol. 39 (1878), pp. 45–8. See also "The Microscope," *Lancet*, vol. 2 (1876), p. 208; "Virchow on the Diagnosis and Prognosis of Cancer," *Br. Med. J.*, vol. 1 (1888), p. 142.

48 Jacob Henle, "On Miasmata and Contagia," trans. George Rosen, *Bull. Hist. Med.*, vol. 6 (1938), p. 942.
49 Baron Justus von Liebig, "On the Mutual Relations between Physiology and Pathology, Chemistry and Physics," *Lancet*, vol. 2 (1846), p. 420.
50 John Simon, "A Course of Lectures in General Pathology: Lecture XII, Morbid Poisons," *Lancet*, vol. 2 (1850), p. 230.
51 W. D. Foster, *A History of Medical Bacteriology and Immunology* (London: William Heinemann, 1970), p. 10.
52 "Minutes of the Medical Society of London," *Lancet*, vol. 1 (1849), p. 99.
53 J. K. Crellin, "The Dawn of the Germ Theory: Particles, Infection and Biology," in Poynter, *Medicine and Science in the 1860s*, p. 58.
54 Joseph Lister, "On the Antiseptic Principle in the Practice of Surgery," *Lancet*, vol. 2 (1867), pp. 353–6.
55 Foster, *History of Medical Bacteriology*, p. 17.
56 Ibid., p. 18.
57 Ibid., p. 51.
58 "Koch's Investigations on Tuberculosis," *Br. Med. J.*, vol. 1 (1882), p. 707.
59 Robert Koch, "The Etiology of Tuberculosis," in *Recent Essays by Various Authors on Bacteria in Relation to Disease*, ed. W. Watson Cheyne (London: New Sydenham Society, 1886), pp. 70–3.
60 Robert Koch, "On the Investigation of Pathogenic Organisms," in Cheyne, *Bacteria in Relation to Disease*, pp. 7–18.
61 "How to Detect the Tubercle Bacillus," *Med. Surg. Rep.*, vol. 49 (1883), p. 671. See also "Staining Microscopic Organisms," *Br. Med. J.*, vol. 2 (1880), p. 873; Henry S. Gabbett, "The Diagnostic Value of the Discovery of Koch's Bacilli in Sputum," *Br. Med. J.*, vol. 1 (1884), p. 805.
62 Koch, "Investigation of Pathogenic Organisms," pp. 37–53.
63 "Bacterial Cultures," *Med. Surg. Rep.*, vol. 57 (1887), p. 542.
64 Koch, "Investigation of Pathogenic Organisms," pp. 26–32.
65 Ibid., p. 19.
66 Ibid., pp. 18–25. See also for an examination of the techniques and problems of photomicrography, George M. Sternberg, *Photo-Micrographs and How to Make Them* (Boston: James R. Osgood, 1884), pp. 17–23.
67 G. A. Heron, "Observations, Clinical and Sanitary, Concerning the Bacillus of Tubercle," *Lancet*, vol. 1 (1883), p. 189.
68 Solomon Charles Smith, "Modern Study of Micro-organisms, and Its Influence on Medical Thought," *Lancet*, vol. 2 (1882), pp. 309–11.
69 "The Age of Bacilli," *Med. Surg. Rep.*, vol. 46 (1882), p. 682. See also "The Practical Value of the Tubercle Bacillus," *Lancet*, vol. 1 (1883), p. 67.
70 J. Dreschfeld, "On the Diagnostic Value of the Tubercle Bacillus," *Br. Med. J.*, vol. 1 (1883), p. 305. See also "On the Colouring of the Bacillus of Koch, and on its Semeiotic Importance," *Edinb. Med. J.*, vol. 30, part 1 (1884), pp. 186–7; "Bacteriological Test for Surgical Tuberculosis," *Br. Med. J.*, vol. 1 (1888), p. 1246.
71 "The Diagnosis of Asiatic Cholera," *J.A.M.A.*, vol. 20 (1893), pp. 537–8; "The Early Diagnosis of Diphtheria and the Physician's Duty when Confronted with Cases of Doubtful Character, Presenting Symptoms of Diphtheria," *J.A.M.A.*, vol. 25 (1895), pp. 118–19.
72 Alfred Stengel, "Chemical and Biological Methods in Diagnosis," *Trans. Cong.*

Am. Surg., vol. 7 (1907), pp. 34–6; Richard C. Cabot, "The Relation of Bacteriology to Medicine," *Boston Med. Surg. J.*, vol. 142 (1900), pp. 479–82.

73 Rudolf Virchow, "Value of Pathological Experiment," *Lancet*, vol. 2 (1881), pp. 212–13; "Is Medicine a Science or an Art?" *Med. Surg. Rep.*, vol. 43 (1880), p. 477.

74 Sir Dyce Duckworth, "The Prognosis of Disease," *Br. Med. J.*, vol. 2 (1896), pp. 251–2.

CHAPTER 5. THE TRANSLATION OF PHYSIOLOGICAL ACTIONS INTO THE LANGUAGES OF MACHINES

1 John Hutchinson, "On the Capacity of the Lungs, and on the Respiratory Functions, with a View of Establishing a Precise and Easy Method of Detecting Disease by the Spirometer," *Med.-Chir. Trans.*, vol. 29 (1846), pp. 137–252. See also Hutchinson's later work, *The Spirometer, the Stethoscope and the Scale Balance. . .*(London: John Churchill, 1852).

2 Stephen Hales, *Statical Essays: Containing Hemastaticks* (London: W. Innys and R. Manby, 1733), p. 229; Humphrey Davy, *Researches, Chemical and Philosophical . . .* (London: J. Johansen, 1800), pp. 410–11.

3 Hutchinson, "Capacity of the Lungs," p. 236. At this period, weighing a patient was not common in clinical examinations. Knowledge of normal weight for different ages was scanty, and the diagnostic significance of its increase and decline was unclear to most physicians. Yet Hutchinson declared that if he could only make one observation to estimate a person's general health he would select the weight. It was a measure of the person's total constitution and vigor, and also was a test that did not depend on the patient's memory or veracity – "gravitation never 'changes'." See Hutchinson, *The Spirometer, the Stethoscope and the Scale Balance*, p. 53.

4 Hutchinson, "Capacity of the Lungs," p. 219.

5 M. Mattson, "On the Curability of Consumption," *Boston Med. Surg. J.*, vol. 43 (1851), pp. 449–53.

6 Hutchinson, "Capacity of the Lungs," p. 223.

7 Friedrich Oesterlen, *Medical Logic*, trans. G. Whitley (London: Sydenham Society, 1855), pp. 233–5.

8 Henry M. Hughes, *A Clinical Introduction to the Practice of Auscultation. . .*(London: Longman, Brown, Green and Longman, 1854), p. 288. See also Herbert Davies, "A Course of Lectures on the Physical Diagnosis of Diseases of the Chest," *Lancet*, vol. 1 (1850), p. 40.

9 Francis Adams, trans., *The Seven Books of Paulus Aegineta*, vol. 1 (London: Sydenham Society, 1844), pp. 202–22. Excellent historical accounts of pulse feeling are found in W. H. Broadbent, *The Pulse* (Philadelphia: Lea Brothers & Co., 1887), 6–11; D. Evan Bedford, "The Ancient Art of Feeling the Pulse," *Br. Heart J.*, vol. 13 (1951), pp. 423–37.

10 Richard H. Shryock, "The History of Quantification in Medical Science," *Isis*, vol. 52 (1961), pp. 218–19.

11 James J. Walsh, *Old Time Makers of Medicine* (New York: Fordham University Press, 1911), p. 341.

12 S. Weir Mitchell, *The Early History of Instrumental Precision in Medicine* (New Haven: Tuttle, Morehouse and Taylor, 1892), p. 40. For an interesting ac-

count of Galileo's instruments, consult S. A. Bedini, "The Instruments of Galileo," in Ernan McMullin, ed., *Galileo, Man of Sience* (New York: Basic Books, 1967). Several other good essays also exist on the development of a quantitative approach to medical problems: Sir Henry Dale, "Measurement in Medicine," *Br. Med. Bull.*, vol. 7 (1951), pp. 261–4; E. Ashworth Underwood, "The History of the Quantitative Approach in Medicine," *Br. Med. Bull.*, vol. 7 (1951), pp. 265–74; Hebbel E. Hoff, "Nicolaus of Cusa, van Helmont, and Boyle: The First Experiment of the Renaissance in Quantitative Biology and Medicine," *J. Hist. Med. Allied Sci.*, vol. 19 (1964), pp. 99–117; Logan Clendening, "The History of Certain Medical Instruments," *Ann. Intern. Med.*, vol. 4 (1930–31), pp. 176–89.

13 Mitchell, *Early History of Instrumental Precision*, p. 36.

14 Sir John Floyer, *The Physician's Pulse–Watch . . .* (London: Sam. Smith and Benj. Walford, 1707), A4–A9. There are several good historical essays about Floyer: Gary L. Townsend, "Sir John Floyer (1649–1734) and His Study of Pulse and Respiration," *J. Hist. Med.*, vol. 22 (1967), pp. 286–316; Lilian Lindsay, "Sir John Floyer (1649–1734)," *Proc. R. Soc. Med.*, vol. 44 (1951), pp. 43–8; Jacob Rosenbloom, "The History of Pulse Timing with Some Remarks on Sir John Floyer and his Physician's Pulse Watch," *Ann. Med. Hist.*, vol. 4 (1922), pp. 97–9.

15 Théophile de Bordeu, *Inquiries Concerning the Varieties of the Pulse. . .* (London: T. Lewis and G. Kearsly, 1764), pp. 9–16.

16 Townsend, "Sir John Floyer," p. 314.

17 William Heberden, "Remarks on the Pulse," *Med. Trans. R. Coll. Physicians*, vol. 2 (1772), p. 20.

18 W. Falconer, *Observations Respecting the Pulse . . .* (London: T. Cadell, Jr. and W. Davis, 1796), pp. 1–5.

19. An examination of the medical records of the Massachusetts General Hospital (M.G.H.), Boston, reveals pulse counts were not routinely taken on patients. Consult the case of William Stewart, *M.G.H. Rec.*, vol. 3 (1823), pp. 9–16, 22–6, and compare the case of Ebenezer Saule, *M.G.H. Rec.*, vol. 100 (1840), pp. 1–4, 81–2, 161–2. See also Milo North, "The Proper Influence of the Pulse in its Application to the Diagnosis and Prognosis of Diseases," *New Engl. J. Med. Surg.*, vol. 15 (1826), pp. 339–41.

20 R. T. H. Laennec, *A Treatise on Diseases of the Chest*, trans. John Forbes, 1st ed. (London: T. and G. Underwood, 1821), pp. 364–8.

21 Hales, *Hemastaticks*, pp. 1–9.

22 Ralph Major, "The History of Taking the Blood Pressure," *Ann. Med. Hist.*, vol. 2 (1930), p. 50.

23 Julius Hérisson, *The Sphygmometer, an Instrument which Renders the Action of Arteries Apparent to the Eye . . .* , trans. E. W. Blundell (London: Longman, Rees, Orme, Brown, Green, and Longman, 1835), p. 14.

24 David Badham, "A Few Remarks on the Sphygmometer," *Lond. Med. Gaz.*, vol. 16 (1834–35), pp. 265–7. See also Hérisson, *Sphygmometer*, pp. xiii–xiv, 40–1.

25 Major, "History of Taking the Blood Pressure," p. 30. See also Kenneth Keele, *The Evolution of Clinical Methods in Medicine* (Springfield: Thomas, 1963), pp. 75–9.

26 Alexander Wood and Frank Oldham, *Thomas Young: Natural Philosopher, 1773–1829* (Cambridge: Cambridge University Press, 1954), pp. 136–7.

27 William Harvey, *Exercitatio Anatomica De Motu Cordis et Sanguinis in Animalibus*, trans. Chauncey Leake (Springfield: Thomas, 1928), Part 2, p. 25.

28 Alonzo T. Keyt, *Sphygmography and Cardiography.* . .(New York: Putnam & Son, 1887), p. 2. See also Edgar Holden, *The Sphygmograph and the Physiology of the Circulation* (New York: W. Wood and Co., 1871), p. 17.

29 E.-J. Marey, *Researches sur le pouls au moyen d'un nouvel appareil enregistreur, le sphygmographe* (Paris: E. Thunot et Cie, 1860).

30 Francis E. Anstie, "Lectures on the Prognosis and Treatment of Certain Acute Diseases, with Special Reference to the Indications Afforded by the Graphic Study of the Pulse," *Lancet*, vol. 2 (1867), p. 387.

31 Ibid., p. 124.

32 Book review, *Br. Foreign Med.-Chir. Rev.*, vol. 42 (1868), pp. 5–8.

33 An example of this is J. Burdon-Sanderson's *Handbook of the Sphygmograph* (London: Robert Hardwicke, 1867). See also the comments of Bedford, "Ancient Art of Feeling the Pulse," p. 435.

34 W. H. Broadbent, "A Clinical Lecture on the Pulse: Its Diagnostic Prognostic, and Therapeutic Implications," *Lancet*, vol. 2 (1875), p. 549; W. H. Broadbent, "The Croonian Lectures on the Pulse," *Br. Med. J.*, vol. 1 (1887), p. 657; "The Sphygmograph," *Med. Surg. Rep.*, vol. 46 (1882), pp. 378–9.

35 Book review, *Br. Foreign Med.-Chir. Rev.*, vol. 42 (1868), p. 4.

36 J. Burdon-Sanderson, "Characteristics of the Arterial Pulse . . . ," *Br. Med. J.*, vol. 2 (1867), p. 39. See also William Aitken, *The Science and Practice of Medicine* (London: Griffin, 1868), pp. 571–3.

37 Furneaux Jordan, "Shock After Surgical Operations and Injuries," *Br. Med. J.*, vol. 1 (1867), p. 193; book review, *Edinb. Med. J.*, vol. 13, part 2 (1868), p. 1051; Anstie, "Prognosis and Treatment," p. 35. For more general comments on the superiority of machines over the human senses, see John S. Billings, "Our Medical Literature," *Lancet*, vol. 2 (1881), p. 269.

38 W. T. Gairdner, "A Short Account of Cardiac Murmurs," *Edinb. Med. J.*, vol. 7 (1861–62), pp. 442–50. In the twentieth century, Harold N. Segall suggested a code of symbols and rules for the graphic depiction of heart sounds and murmurs. He hoped its use would eliminate the failings of memory and verbal description as means of recording and retrieving information obtained from heart sounds (Harold N. Segall, "A Simple Method for Graphic Description of Cardiac Auscultatory Signs," *Am. Heart J.*, vol. 8 (1933), pp. 533–6).

39 Hyde Salter, "Lectures on Dyspnoea," *Lancet*, vol. 2 (1865), pp. 465–78.

40 F. A. Mahomed, "Some of the Clinical Aspects of Chronic Bright's Disease," *Guy's Hosp. Rep.*, vol. 24 (1879), pp. 364–80.

41 Theodore C. Janeway, *The Clinical Study of the Blood-Pressure* (New York: D. Appleton and Co., 1907), pp. 46–8, 54–5, 77. For good historical essays on the measurement of the blood pressure see William Hall Lewis, "The Evolution of Clinical Sphygmomanometry," *Bull. N. Y. Acad. Med.*, vol. 17 (1941), pp. 871–81; Major, "History of Taking the Blood Pressure," p. 47–55.

42 Harold N. Segall, "Dr. N. C. Korotkoff: Discovery of the Auscultatory Method for Measuring Arterial Pressure," *Ann. Intern. Med.*, vol. 63 (1965), pp. 147–9; John C. da Costa, Jr., *Principles and Practices of Physical Diagnosis* (Philadelphia: Saunders, 1919), p. 33.

43 Harvey Cushing, "On Routine Determinations of Arterial Tension in Operating Room and Clinic," *Boston Med. Surg. J.*, vol. 148 (1903), pp. 250–2. See

also "Blood Pressure Observations in Surgical Cases: Report of the Committee on Research for the Division of Surgery, Harvard Medical School," *Boston Med. Surg. J.*, vol. 150 (1904), pp. 264–6.

44 Frederic A. Washburn, *The Massachusetts General Hospital: Its Development, 1900–1935* (Boston: Houghton Mifflin, 1939), p. 376.

45 Augustus D. Waller, "A Demonstration on Man of Electromotive Changes Accompanying the Heart's Beat," *J. Physiol.*, vol. 8 (1887), p. 229. See also Augustus D. Waller, "The Electromotive Properties of the Human Heart," *Br. Med. J.*, vol. 2 (1888), pp. 751–4.

46 Thomas E. Sattethwaite, "Electrocardiograms and their Significance," *Med. Rec.*, vol. 79 (1911), pp. 189–90.

47 Ibid., p. 192. For an interesting discussion of the cost of making an early electrocardiograph see Alfred E. Cohn and Horatio B. Williams, "Recollections Concerning Early Electrocardiography in the United States," *Bull. Hist. Med.*, vol. 29 (1955), pp. 469–74.

48 Sattethwaite, "Electrocardiograms and their Significance," pp. 192–3.

49 S. Calvin Smith, "The Clinical Value of Electrocardiography," *Pa. Med. J.*, vol. 21 (1917), pp. 10–18; James E. Talley, "The Electrocardiograph as a Clinical Instrument," *Am. J. Med. Sci.*, vol. 147 (1914), pp. 692–8; Walter B. James and Horatio B. Williams, "The Electrocardiogram in Clinical Medicine: I. The String Galvanometer and Electrocardiogram in Health," *Am. J. Med. Sci.*, vol. 140 (1910), pp. 408–15.

50 Thomas Lewis, "Electro-cardiography and its Importance in the Clinical Examination of Heart Affections: Part III–The Analysis of Cardiac Irregularities," *Br. Med. J.*, vol. 2 (1912), p. 67. Good commentaries on the history of cardiology can be found in George E. Burch, "Developments in Clinical Electrocardiography since Einthoven," *Am. Heart J.*, vol. 61 (1961), p. 330; George E. Burch and Nicholas P. De Pasquale, *A History of Electrocardiography* (Chicago: Year Book Medical Publishers, 1964); A. L. Flint, *The Heart* (New York: P. B. Hoeber, 1921).

51 Wilhelm [or Willem] Einthoven, "The Different Forms of the Human Electrocardiogram and Their Signification," *Lancet*, vol. 1 (1912), p. 854.

52 Thomas Lewis, *The Mechanism of the Heart Beat* (London: Shaw and Sons, 1911), p. ix. See also J. F. Halls Dally, "Electro-cardiography and its Clinical Application," *West Lond. Med. J.*, vol. 19 (1914), p. 266; Hugo A. Freund, "Clinical and Instrumental Methods of Estimating the Efficiency of the Heart," *J. Mich. State Med. Soc.*, vol. 11 (1912), pp. 571–3.

53 James B. Herrick, "Thrombosis of the Coronary Arteries," *J.A.M.A.*, vol. 72 (1919), p. 390. Two other works by Herrick contain interesting reflections on this subject. See his *Memoirs of Eighty Years* (Chicago: University of Chicago Press, 1949), p. 196, and "An Intimate Account of My Early Experiences with Coronary Thrombosis," *Am. Heart J.*, vol. 27 (1944), pp. 10, 13.

54 Henry Carrington Bolton, *Evolution of the Thermometer, 1592–1743* (Easton, Pa.: Chemical Publishing Co., 1900), p. 18.

55 Mitchell, *Early History of Instrumental Precision*, p. 13.

56 Robert Boyle, *New Experiments and Observations Touching Cold* (London: Richard Davis, 1683), p. 1.

57 Bolton, *Evolution of the Thermometer*, pp. 35–8. See also Mitchell, *Early History of Instrumental Precision*, pp. 30–1.

58 George Martine, *Essays on the Construction and Graduation of Thermometers and on the Heating and Cooling of Bodies* (Edinburgh: William Creech, 1792), pp. 20–7.
59 Boyle, *Observations Touching Cold*, p. 15. The English scientist Edmund Halley had similar complaints about how the lack of common standards made thermometers incomparable. See his essay, "The Divisions of the Thermometer," *Philosophical Transactions and Collections to the End of the Year MDCC. Abridged and Disposed under General Heads.* Adapted by John Lowthrop, vol. 2, 5th ed. (London: W. Innys et al., 1749), p. 36.
60 Halley, "Divisions of the Thermometer," p. 35.
61 Martine, *Construction and Graduation of Thermometers*, p. 8.
62 Ibid., pp. 11–12.
63 Ibid., pp. 16–17.
64 Bolton, *Evolution of the Thermometer*, pp. 65–6.
65 G. A. Lindeboom, *Herman Boerhaave: The Man and his Work* (London: Methuen & Co., 1968), pp. 294–7.
66 C. A. Wunderlich, *On the Temperature in Diseases: A Manual of Medical Thermometry*, trans. W. Bathurst Woodman (London: New Sydenham Society, 1871), pp. 21–3.
67 Martine, *Construction and Graduation of Thermometers*, pp. 38–51, 95–181.
68 James Currie, *Medical Reports on the Effects of Water, Cold and Warm, as a Remedy in Fever and Febrile Diseases* (Liverpool: Cadell & Davies, 1797).
69 Martine, *Construction and Graduation of Thermometers*, p. 34.
70 Wunderlich, *On the Temperature*, p. 21.
71 Michel Foucault, *The Birth of the Clinic* (New York: Pantheon Books, 1973), p. 180.
72 Wunderlich, *On the Temperature*, p. 20.
73 Ibid., p. 30.
74 Ibid.
75 Ibid., p. 32.
76 Ibid., pp. 32–3.
77 Ibid., pp. 37–8.
78 Ibid., pp. 39, 46.
79 Austin Flint, "Remarks on the Use of the Thermometer in Diagnosis and Prognosis," *N. Y. Med. J.*, vol. 4 (1866–67), p. 82. See also "The Thermometer in Acute Disease . . . ," *Lancet*, vol. 2 (1865), p. 512; John Southey Warter, "An Inquiry into the Practical Value of the Thermometer in the Diagnosis and Prognosis of Acute Diseases," *Br. Med. J.*, vol. 2 (1865), p. 57.
80 Book review, *Lancet*, vol. 1 (1872), p. 544. See also J. F. Goodhart, "Thermometric Observations in Clinical Medicine," *Guy's Hosp. Rep.*, vol. 15 (1869), pp. 365–6; T. J. Maclagan, "Thermometrical Observations," *Edinb. Med. J.*, vol. 13 (1868), p. 601.
81 Wunderlich, *On the Temperature*, pp. 58–60.
82 Ibid., p. 75.
83 Edwyn Andrew, "The Thermometer in Practice," *Br. Med. J.*, vol. 2 (1868), p. 83.
84 A further example of this belief is the book written by the physician Edouard Seguin, *Family Thermometry: A Manual of Thermometry for Mothers, Nurses, Hospitalers, Etc., and All Those Who Have Charge of the Sick and of the Young* (New York: Putnam, 1873).

85 Wunderlich, *On the Tmperature*, p. 52.
86 James Sawyer, "Clinical Thermometry," *Birm. Med. Rev.*, vol. 4 (1875), p. 116.
87 "The Force of Imagination," *Br. Med. J.*, vol. 1 (1876), p. 139.
88 Edouard Seguin, *Medical Thermometry and Human Temperature* (New York: William Wood & Co., 1876), pp. 258–9. See also W. O. Johnson, *Modern Medicine* (Boston: James R. Osgood, 1873), p. 27; Elliott Richardson, "The Thermometer in Disease," *Med. Surg. Rep.*, vol. 25 (1871), p. 247.
89 Seguin, *Medical Thermometry*, pp. 258–9; F. C. Curtis, "Thermometry in Health and Disease," *N.Y. Med. J.*, vol. 16 (1872), p. 618.
90 J. W. Carhart, "The Clinical Thermometer," *Med. Surg. Rep.*, vol. 72 (1895), p. 120.
91 Ibid., pp. 120–1.
92 "A Few Thoughts on the Clinical Thermometer," *Med. Surg. Rep.*, vol. 54 (1886), p. 602.
93 "The Thermometric Bureau of Yale College," *N. Y. Med. J.*, vol. 36 (1882), pp. 221–3.
94 Moritz Immisch, "Comparison Between Mercurial and Avitreous Thermometers," *N. Y. Med. J.*, vol. 50 (1889), p. 313. See also "Verification and Correction of Thermometers," *Boston Med. Surg. J.*, vol. 103 (1880), p. 185; W. B. Kesteven, "Clinical Thermometers and their Deviations," *Lancet*, vol. 1 (1873), p. 824.

CHAPTER 6. CHEMICAL SIGNPOSTS OF DISEASE AND THE BIRTH OF THE DIAGNOSTIC LABORATORY

1 Henry E. Sigerist, trans., "The Treatise *De Cautelis Medicorum* Attributed to Arnald of Villanova," *Q. Bull. Northwest. Univ. Med. Sch.*, vol. 20 (1946–47), pp. 136–43; Thomas Brian, *The pisse-prophet* (London: S. and B. Griffen, 1679); Joseph H. Kiefer, "Uroscopy: the Clinical Laboratory of the Past," *Trans. Am. Assoc. Genito-Urin Surg.*, vol. 50 (1958), pp. 161–72; Theodore W. Schaffer, "A Brief Historical Retrospect of the Examination of the Urine in Ancient and Modern Times," *Boston Med. Surg. J.*, vol. 136 (1897), pp. 623–6.
2 Walter Pagel, *Paracelsus: An Introduction to Philosophical Medicine in the Era of the Renaissance* (Basel: S. Karger, 1958), p. 192. See also Allen G. Debus, *The English Paracelsians* (New York: Franklin Watts, 1965), pp. 157–8.
3 Thomas Willis, "Of Urines," in *Practice of Physick, Being the whole Works of that Renowned and Famous Physician . . .* , trans. S. Pordage (London: J. Dring, C. Harper and J. Leigh, 1684), p. 17.
4 Ibid., p. 18.
5 Robert Boyle, *Memoirs for the Natural History of Humane Blood* (London: Samuel Smith, 1683/4), preface (n.p.).
6 Raymond Vieussens, "The Constituent Parts of Human Blood," *Philosophical Transactions and Collections to the End of the Year MDCC. Abridged and Disposed under General Heads.* Adapted by John Lowthorp, vol. 3, 5th ed. (London, W. Innys et al., 1749), p. 235.
7 Ibid., p. 238.
8 J. Maria Lanius, "The Opinion of the College of Physicians at Rome, concerning Dr. Vieusion's [sic] Analysis of Human Blood," *Philosophical Transactions*

and Collections to the End of the Year MDCC. Abridged and Disposed under General Heads. Adapted by John Lowthorp, vol. 3, 5th ed. (London, W. Innys et al., 1749;, p. 244.

9 Browne Langrish, *The Modern Theory and Practice of Physic*. . . , 2nd ed. (London: A. Bettesworth and C. Hitch, 1738), p. 91.

10 Ibid., pp. 79–80.

11 Henry M. Leicester, *The Historical Background of Chemistry* (New York: Wiley, 1965), p. 231.

12 William Hewson, *An Inquiry into the Properties of the Blood* (London, 1772) in George Gulliver, ed., *The Works of William Hewson* (London: Sydenham Society, 1846).

13 Willis, "Pharmaceutice Rationalis," in *Practice of Physick*, p. 76. Aretaeus in naming diabetes observed: "The epithet diabetes has been assigned to the disorder, being something like the passing of water by a siphon"; see Henry Alan Skinner, *The Origin of Medical Terms* (Baltimore: Williams & Wilkins, 1961), p. 139. For the statements of Maimonides on diabetic urine see Fred Rosner and Sussman Munter, "Moses Maimonides' Aphorisms Regarding Analysis of Urine," *Ann. Intern. Med.*, vol. 71 (1969), p. 217.

14 John Rollo, *Cases of the Diabetes Mellitus*. . . , 2nd ed. (London: C. Dilly, 1798), p. 95. Rollo's commentary on previous European physicians who advanced medical knowledge of diabetes is found in ibid., pp. 356–79. For Matthew Dobson's work on the connection of sugar with diabetes see his essay, "Experiments and Observations on the Urine in a Diabetes," *Med. Obs. Inq.*, vol. 5 (1776), pp. 298–316.

15 William Cruikshank, "Experiments on Urine and Sugar," in Rollo, *Cases of Diabetes Mellitus*, p. 451.

16 W. B. Johnson, *History of the Progress and Present State of Animal Chemistry*, vol. 1 (London: J. Johnson, 1803), pp. 2–3. See also D. M. Raine, "Medical Chemistry and Chemical Medicine in the Nineteenth Century," in F. N. L. Poynter, ed., *Medicine and Science in the 1860s*, (London: Wellcome Institute of the History of Medicine, 1968), p. 119.

17 Richard Bright, *Reports of Medical Cases, selected with a view of illustrating the Symptoms and Cure of Diseases by a reference to Morbid Anatomy* (London: Longman, Rees, Orme, Brown and Green, 1827).

18 William Cruikshank in Rollo, *Cases of Diabetes Mellitus*, pp. 447–8; William C. Wells, "On the presence of the red Matter and Serum of Blood in the Urine of Dropsy, which has not originated from Scarlet Fever," *Trans. Soc. Improve Med. Chirur. Knowl.*, vol. 3 (1812), p. 194; John Blackall, *Observations on the Nature and Cure of Dropsies and particularly on the Presence of the Coagulable Part of the Blood in Dropsical Urine* (London: Longman, Hurst, Rees, Orme and Brown, 1818), pp. 83–9.

19 James Crawford Gregory, "On Diseased States of the Kidney connected during Life with Albuminous Urine; illustrated by cases," Part 1, *Edinb. Med. Surg. J.*, vol. 36 (1831), pp. 318–20; ibid., Part 2, *Edinb. Med. Surg. J.*, vol. 37 (1832), pp. 86–90.

20 Bright, *Reports of Medical Cases*, p. 2.

21 John Bostock, "Observations of the Chemical Properties of the Urine in the Foregoing Cases," in *Original Papers of Richard Bright on Renal Disease*, ed. A. Arnold Osman (London: Oxford University Press, 1937), p. 83. See also Richard

Bright, "Cases and Observations Illustrative of Renal Disease Accompanied with the Secretion of Albuminous Urine," *Guy's Hosp. Rep.*, vol. 1 (1836), p. 342.

22 Editorial, *Lancet*, vol. 2 (1889), p. 545. See also Richard Bright, "On the Functions of the Abdomen, and some of the Diagnostic Marks of its Disease," *Lond. Med. Gaz.*, vol. 12 (1833), pp. 381–2.

23 W. Bowman, "Observations on the Minute Anatomy of Fatty Degeneration of the Liver," *Lancet*, vol. 1 (1841–42), p. 561. See also John Hughes Bennett, "Pathological and Clinical Researches into the Nature and Treatment of Scrofulous and Tubercular Diseases," *North J. Med.*, vol. 24 (1846), pp. 211, 284; François Magendie, *Lectures on the blood and changes it undergoes during disease* (Philadelphia: Haswell, Barrington, and Haswell, 1839), p. 9.

24 Book review, *Med.-Chir. Rev.*, vol. 35 (1841), p. 178. See also William Addison, *On Healthy and Diseased Structure and the True Principles of Treatment for the Cure of Disease, especially Consumption and Scrofula, Founded on Microscopical Analysis* (London: John Churchill, 1849), p. 5.

25 Alfred B. Garrod, "Lectures on the Chemistry of Pathology and Therapeutics, Showing the Application of the Science of Chemistry to the Discovery, Treatment and Cure of Disease," *Lancet*, vol. 1 (1848), p. 353; Louis–Alfred Becquerel and Marie–Jean–Alexandre Rodier, *Pathological Chemistry in its Application to the Practice of Medicine*, trans. Stanhope Templeman Speer (London: John Churchill, 1857), p. 18; book review, *Lancet*, vol. 1 (1854), pp. 546–8.

26 Book review, *Am. J. Med. Sci.*, vol. 3 (1842), p. 155. See also book review, *Med.-Chir. Rev.*, vol. 43 (1843), p. 35; George Owen Rees, *On the Analysis of the Blood and Urine in Health and Disease and on the Treatment of Urinary Diseases* (London: Longman, Rees, Orme, Brown, Green and Longman, 1845), p. iii.

27 Book review, *Dublin J. Med. Sci.*, vol. 23 (1843), pp. 290–2; "Dr. Mandl on the Clinical Analysis of the Blood in a Pathological State," *Med.-Chir. Rev.*, vol. 35 (1841), p. 179.

28 G. Andral, *Pathological Hematology: An Essay on the Blood in Disease* (Philadelphia: Lea and Blanchard, 1844), particularly pp. 13–18, 46–7, 57–9. See also G. Andral and J. Gavarret, *Recherches sur les Modifications de proportion de quelques principes du Sang* (Paris: Fortin, Masson, 1842), pp. 3–4.

29 Book review, *Br. Foreign Med. Rev.*, vol. 17 (1844), p. 137.

30 Alfred B. Garrod, "Observations on Certain Pathological Conditions of the Blood and Urine in Gout, Rheumatism and Bright's Disease," *Med.-Chir. Trans.*, vol. 31 (1848), pp. 83–97; book review, *Med.-Chir. Rev.*, vol. 19 (1834), pp. 190–1; G. O. Rees, "On Diabetic Blood," *Guy's Hosp. Rep.*, vol. 3 (1838), pp. 398–9.

31 Book review, *Med.-Chir. Rev.*, vol. 34 (1841), p. 196.

32 Book review, *Am. J. Med. Sci.*, vol. 3 (1842), p. 159. See also book review, *Br. Foreign Med. Rev.*, vol. 13 (1842), pp. 435–45. The English physician Golding Bird conducted studies similar to Becquerel's. He found 23 deposits that could be identified in the urine and discussed their significance in his book *Urinary Deposits, Their Diagnosis, Pathology, and Therapeutical Indications* (London: John Churchill, 1844). Henry Bence Jones explores the basic mechanisms that account for normal and disordered body chemistry in *On Animal Chemistry in its Application to Stomach and Renal Diseases* (London: John Churchill, 1850), particularly pp. 2–12, 40–51, 260–3. An interesting evaluation of the use of chemis-

try in diagnosis, pessimistic in tone, is F. J. Gant, "What Has Pathological Anatomy done for Medicine and Surgery," *Lancet*, vol. 2 (1857), pp. 335–6, 359–60, 385–7.

33 J. Burdon-Sanderson, "Address on Appliances used in Biological Investigation," *Lancet*, vol. 1 (1876), p. 766; M. L. Verso, "The Evolution of Blood Counting Techniques," *Med. Hist.*, vol. 8 (1964), pp. 149–58.

34 W. R. Gowers, "On the Numeration of Blood-Corpuscles," *Lancet*, vol. 2 (1877), pp. 797–8.

35 Joseph W. Hunt, "Notes on the Use of the Haemacytometer in Anaemia," *Lancet*, vol. 1 (1879), pp. 661–2.

36 "New York Academy of Medicine: Section in General Medicine," *N. Y. Med. J.*, vol. 59 (1894), p. 151. See also Frederick P. Henry and Chas. B. Nancrede, "Blood-Cell Counting: A Series of Observations with the Hématimètre of Mm. Hayem and Nachet and the Haemacytometer of Dr. Gowers," *Boston Med. Surg. J.*, vol. 100 (1879), pp. 494–5.

37 Judson Daland, "A Volumetric Study of the Red and White Corpuscles of Human Blood in Health and Disease by Aid of the Hematokrit," *Univ. Med. Mag.*, vol. 4 (1891), p. 99.

38 Henry L. Elsner and Hiram B. Hawley, "On the Clinical Value of the Centrifuge," *N. Y. Med. J.*, vol. 60 (1894), pp. 526–9; Frederick E. Sondern, "The Value of the Centrifugal Apparatus for Diagnostic Purposes," *N. Y. Med. J.*, vol. 57 (1893), pp. 218–20; "Centrifugal Force in the Examination of Sputum," *Lancet*, vol. 2 (1894), pp. 1362–3.

39 W. R. Gowers, "An Apparatus for the Clinical Estimation of Hemoglobin," *Clin. Soc. Trans.*, vol. 12 (1879), pp. 64–7; Joseph W. Hunt, "Observations on the Blood in Anemia," *Lancet*, vol. 2 (1880), pp. 89–91.

40 E. Buchanan Baxter and Frederick Willcocks, "A Contribution to Clinical Haemometry," *Lancet*, vol. 1 (1880), pp. 361–2; Sidney Coupland, "Anemia," *Br. Med. J.*, vol. 1 (1881), pp. 419–21. For an exploration of the problems resulting from lack of good standards to evaluate constituents in urine, consult William Robert's "Lectures on Certain Points in the Clinical Examination of the Urine," *Lancet*, vol. 1 (1862), p. 480.

41 Coupland, "Anemia," p. 419.

42 Julius Vogel, *A Guide to the Qualitative and Quantitative Analysis of the Urine* . . . , trans. William Orlando Markham (London: New Sydenham Society, 1863), pp. 272–3, 351–78.

43 Prof. Oppolzer, "The Tests for Sugar in the Urine," trans. Alfred L. Haskins, *Half-Yearly Abstract of the Medical Sciences*, vol. 48 (1868), pp. 129–31. See also Roberts, "Clinical Examination of the Urine," p. 508; W. R. Basham, "A Sediment Tube for the more Readily Collecting from the Urine Tube-Casts and other Objects for Microscopic Examination," *Lancet*, vol. 1 (1867), pp. 269–70; Henry William Fuller, "On Excess of Urea in the Urine as a Guide to the Diagnosis and Treatment of Certain Forms of Dyspepsia and Nervousness," *Lancet*, vol. 2 (1867), p. 705.

44 Rees, *Analysis of the Blood and Urine*, p. 35.

45 Roberts, "Clinical Examination of the Urine," pp. 507–10, 535–6; Felix Hoppe-Seyler, "On the Development of Physiological Chemistry and its Significance for Medicine," *N. Y. Med. J.*, vol. 40 (1884), p. 171; Daniel Hooper,

"On Fehling's Test and the Significance of Sugar in the Urine," *Lancet*, vol. 1 (1873), p. 360.

46 J. M. Da Costa, *Modern Medicine* (Philadelphia: J. B. Lippincott, 1872), p. 16.

47 Julius Friedenwald, "The Diazo Reaction of Ehrlich," *N. Y. Med. J.*, vol. 58 (1893), pp. 745–8.

48 B. J. A. Charrin and G. E. H. Roger, "Note sur le Développement des Microbes Pathogènes dans le Sérum des Animaux Vaccinés," *Compt. Rend. de la Soc. de Biol.*, n. s., vol. 1 (1889), pp. 667–9.

49 Richard C. Cabot, *The Serum Diagnosis of Disease* (New York: William Wood and Co., 1899); Richard C. Cabot, "The Relation of Bacteriology to Medicine," *Boston Med. Surg. J.*, vol. 142 (1900), pp. 479–82; William H. Welch, "Principles Underlying the Serum Diagnosis of Typhoid Fever and the Methods of Its Application," *J.A.M.A.*, vol. 29 (1897), pp. 301–9.

50 Thomas S. Southworth, "The Technique and Diagnostic Value of Ehrlich's Method of Staining the White Blood-Corpuscles," *N. Y. Med. J.*, vol. 57 (1893), pp. 2–7; Richard C. Cabot, "The Diagnostic and Prognostic Importance of Leucocytosis," *Boston Med. Surg. J.*, vol. 130 (1894), pp. 277–82; James Ewing, "A Study of the Leucocytosis of Lobar Pneumonia," *N. Y. Med. J.*, vol. 58 (1893), pp. 713–18; John M. Wyeth, "The Value of Clinical Microscopy, Bacteriology and Chemistry in Surgical Practice," *Boston Med. Surg. J.*, vol. 144 (1901), pp. 541–7; Jean Captain Sabine, "History of the Classification of the Human Blood," *Bull. Hist. Med.*, vol. 8 (1940), pp. 696–720, 785–805.

51 Otto Folin, "A System of Blood Analysis," *J. Bio-chem.*, vol. 38 (1919), p. 82.

52 Archibald Garrod, "Medicine from the Chemical Standpoint," *Br. Med. J.*, vol. 2 (1914), p. 233. See also D. D. Van Slyke, "Ivar Christian Bang," *Scand. J. Clin. Lab. Invest.*, vol. 31 (1958), pp. 18–23; Sir Almoth Wright, *Handbook of the Technique of the Teat and Capillary Glass Tube* (London: Constable, 1912).

53 Folin, "Blood Analysis," p. 82. See also the paper of Otto Folin and W. Denis, "Nitrogenous Waste Products in the Blood in Nephritis: Their Significance and the Methods for their Determination," *Boston Med. Surg. J.*, vol. 169 (1913), pp. 467–8. For an analysis of the state of blood testing a decade later, see Reed Rockwood, "Chemical Tests of the Blood, Indications and Interpretations," *J.A.M.A.*, vol. 91 (1928), pp. 157–66.

54 Henry L. Elsner, "On the Practical Value of the Newer Methods of Examination in the Diseases of the Stomach," *N. Y. Med. J.*, vol. 57 (1893), p. 487. See also Julius Friedenwald and Samuel Morrison, "The History of the Development of the Stomach Tube with Some Notes on the Duodenal Tube," *Bull. Hist. Med.*, vol. 4 (1936), pp. 448–54.

55 J. M. Purser, "On the Modern Diagnosis of Diseases of the Stomach," *Dublin J. Med. Sci.*, vol. 90 (1890), pp. 469–72.

56 Ibid., pp. 462–9.

57 "The Physical Examination of the Stomach, and the Value of the Absence of Free Hydrochloric Acid as a Sign of Cancer," *Boston Med. Surg. J.*, vol. 118 (1888), p. 582.

58 Alexander Haig, "The Human Body as an Analytical Laboratory," *Br. Med. J.*, vol. 2 (1901), pp. 1078–81. See also Elsner, "Practical Value of Newer Methods," p. 487.

59 Edward L. Young, "Clinical Functional Tests, Methods: The Place of the Phenosulphonephthalein Test in Nephritis," *Boston Med. Surg. J.*, vol. 169 (1913), pp. 466–7; C. Achard, "The Diagnosis of Renal Insufficiency," *Boston Med. Surg. J.*, vol. 143 (1900), p. 239; Louis Heitzmann, "On Some Recent Advances in Urinology," *Boston Med. Surg. J.*, vol. 153 (1905), p. 695.

60 Richard C. Cabot, "The Limitations of Urinary Diagnosis," *Bull. Johns Hopkins Hosp.*, vol. 15 (1904), p. 176.

61 Henry Head, "Disease and Diagnosis," *Br. Med. J.*, vol. 1 (1919), pp. 365–6; Richard C. Cabot, "The Historical Development and Relative Value of Laboratory and Clinical Methods of Diagnosis," *Boston Med. Surg. J.*, vol. 157 (1907), p. 152.

62 William Welch, "The Evolution of Modern Scientific Laboratories," *Bull. Johns Hopkins Hosp.*, vol. 7 (1896), pp. 19–24.

63 Ibid., p. 23; Raymond Wallace, "Laboratory Diagnosis – Its Relation to the General Practitioner," *Interstate Med. J.*, vol. 10 (1903), p. 148; "The William Pepper Laboratory of Clinical Medicine," *Boston Med. Surg. J.*, vol. 133 (1895), pp. 603–4.

64 Stuart M'Donald, "Clinical Pathology," *Scottish Med. Surg. J.*, vol. 10 (1902), pp. 226–7; Theodore C. Janeway, "Some Sources of Error in Laboratory Clinical Diagnosis," *Med. News.*, vol. 78 (1901), p. 700; Victor A. Robertson, "Laboratory Aids to Diagnosis for the General Practitioner," *Med. News*, vol. 84 (1904), p. 259.

65 C. N. B. Camac, "Hospital and Ward Clinical Laboratories," *J.A.M.A.*, vol. 35 (1900), pp. 219–27; James B. Herrick, "The Relation of the Clinical Laboratory to the Practitioner of Medicine," *Boston Med. Surg. J.*, vol. 156 (1907), pp. 763–8.

66 William Osler, discussion of M. H. Fussell's, "Blood Examination: Its Value to the General Practitioner," *J.A.M.A.*, vol. 35 (1900), p. 230.

67 Mark W. Richardson, "On the Bacteriological Examination of the Stools in Typhoid Fever, and its Value in Diagnosis," *Boston Med. Surg. J.*, vol. 137 (1897), p. 433.

68 "The Early Diagnosis of Diphtheria and the Physician's Duty when Confronted with Cases of Doubtful Character, Presenting Symptoms of Diphtheria," *J.A.M.A.*, vol. 25 (1895), p. 118.

69 J. C. Culbertson, "Diphtheria: Its Specific Diagnosis," *J.A.M.A.*, vol. 21 (1893), p. 699.

70 Theobold Smith, "Public Health Laboratories," *Boston Med. Surg. J.*, vol. 143 (1900), pp. 491–3.

71 Frederick Gay and J. G. Fitzgerald, "The Serum Diagnosis of Syphilis," *Boston Med. Surg. J.*, vol. 160 (1909), pp. 157–61; Roger I. Lee and Wyman Whittemore, "The Wassermann Reaction in Syphilis and Other Diseases," *Boston Med. Surg. J.*, vol. 160 (1909), pp. 410–12; A. C. Kimberlin, "The Psychologic Value of a Correct Diagnosis," *J. Indiana State Med. Assoc.*, vol. 5 (1912), p. 271; W. P. Lucas, "The Wassermann Reaction in its Application to Medicine," *Boston Med. Surg. J.*, vol. 169 (1913), pp. 116–20.

72 "Urinary Examination," *Med. Surg. Rep.*, vol. 48 (1883), p. 701. See also J. H. Musser, *A Practical Treatise in Medical Diagnosis* (Philadelphia: Lea Brothers, 1894), p. 21.

73 Lucius A. Fritze, "The Laboratory Service of Divisional Laboratories," *J. Iowa*

State Med. Soc., vol. 9 (1919), pp. 378–82; Helen Clapesattle, *The Doctors Mayo* (Minneapolis: University of Minnesota Press, 1941), pp. 573–4.

CHAPTER 7. MEDICAL SPECIALISM AND THE
CENTRALIZATION OF MEDICAL CARE

1 S. Weir Mitchell, *The Early History of Instrumental Precision in Medicine* (New Haven: Tuttle, Morehouse & Taylor, 1892), p. 3.
2 John S. Billings, "Our Medical Literature,"*Lancet*, vol. 2 (1881), p. 267. For an excellent account of the history of specialization from ancient times to the twentieth century, consult George Rosen, *The Specialization of Medicine, with Particular Reference to Ophthalmology* (New York: Froben Press, 1944). Rosemary Stevens has written a valuable account of medical specialization in the United States in *American Medicine and the Public Interest* (New Haven: Yale University Press, 1971).
3 J. Russell Reynolds, "Specialism in Medicine," *Lancet*, vol. 2 (1881), pp. 655–8.
4 Felix Semon, "The Relations of Laryngology, Rhinology, and Otology with Other Arts and Sciences,"*Br. Med. J.*, vol. 2 (1904), p. 713; Everett A. Bates, "Some Perplexities in Modern Medicine," *Boston Med. Surg. J.*, vol. 172 (1915), p. 846.
5 Maurice Leven, *The Incomes of Physicians* (Chicago: University of Chicago Press, 1932), pp. 25–7; Stevens, *American Medicine and the Public Interest*, p. 421.
6 A. T. Cabot, "Science in Medicine," *Boston Med. Surg. J.*, vol. 137 (1897) pp. 481–2.
7 J. M. Da Costa, *Modern Medicine* (Philadelphia: J. B. Lippincott, 1872), pp. 18–19. See also "Proctologists,"*J.A.M.A.*, vol. 32 (1899), p. 1066; Oliver Wendell Holmes, "Medical Highways and By–ways," *Boston Med. Surg. J.*, vol. 106 (1882), p. 507.
8 Frederick C. Shattuck, "Specialism in Medicine," *J.A.M.A.*, vol. 35 (1900), pp. 723–6.
9 In Great Britain during the twentieth century, the generalist maintained his status more successfully than in the United States, because in Britain general practice was considered a special field with well-delineated professional and administrative tasks: "On the one side are all the hospital specialties, from general medicine and surgery to radiotherapy, with a monopoly of the hospitals; on the other, and professionally distinct, is the general practitioner, who as the doctor of first contact has a monopoly of patients"; Rosemary Stevens, *Medical Practice in Modern England: The Impact of Specialization and State Medicine* (New Haven: Yale University Press, 1966), p. 356. Despite this circumstance specialism has grown in Great Britain, although at a slower pace than in the United States. In 1929 about one British practitioner in five was a specialist; by the mid-1960s the number of specialists and generalists was about equal (ibid., p. 355).
10 "The Real Reason for the Passing of the General Practitioner," *Boston Med. Surg. J.*, vol. 136 (1897), p. 142. See also Wilmot Herringham, "The Consultant,"*Br. Med. J.*, vol. 2 (1920), p. 37; James B. Herrick, "The Practitioner of the Future,"*J.A.M.A.*, vol. 103 (1934), p. 881; Shattuck, "Specialism in Medicine," pp. 724–5.

11 James L. Toll, discussion of D. Y. Keith's, "The Value of the X-Ray in Diagnosis," *Ky. Med. J.*, vol. 16 (1918), p. 164. See also Gilman Osgood, "The Country Doctor's Relations with the Metropolitan Institutions and Specialists," *Boston Med. Surg. J.*, vol. 159 (1908), pp. 291–7; John L. Hildreth, "The General Practitioner and the Specialist," *Boston Med. Surg. J.*, vol. 155 (1906), pp. 79–83.

12 J. R. Cowan, "The Value of Laboratory Methods to the Country Practitioner," *Boston Med. Surg. J.*, vol. 154 (1906), p. 258.

13 Leven, *Incomes of Physicians*, p. 120.

14 Ibid., p. 118.

15 Ibid., pp. 27–8.

16 Vernon R. Jones, "The County and Community Diagnostic Laboratory," *Ky. Med. J.*, vol. 20 (1922), p. 837.

17 Charles F. Painter, "Educational Requirements for Twentieth Century Practice: Who Should Determine Them and How They May Best Be Achieved," *Boston Med. Surg. J.*, vol. 194 (1962), p. 1059. See also for an interesting survey of rural medicine, William Allen Pusey, "Medical Education and Medical Service. . . ," *J.A.M.A.*, vol. 86 (1926), pp. 1501–8.

18 W. J. Breeding, "The Question of an Adequate Supply of Rural Physicians in Tennessee. . . ," *J. Tenn. State Med. Assoc.*, vol. 19 (1926), p. 148.

19 Ralph W. Tuttle, "The Other Side of Country Practice," *N. Engl. J. Med.*, vol. 199 (1928), p. 874. See also Painter, "Educational Requirements for Twentieth Century Practice," pp. 1058–60.

20 "The Relation of the Expert in Internal Medicine to the General Practitioner," *Boston Med. Surg. J.*, vol. 184 (1921), p. 497. See also E. C. Davis, "A Plea for More Thorough Examinations Before Operations Are Performed," *J. Med. Assoc. Ga.*, vol. 10 (1921), p. 655.

21 Herringham, "The Consultant," p. 37.

22 Paul A. White, "The Diagnostic Net-Surgical Viewpoint," *J. Iowa State Med. Soc.*, vol. 16 (1926), p. 159.

23 Helen Clapesattle, *The Doctors Mayo* (Minnesota: University of Minnesota Press, 1941), p. 530. See also "Report of the General Executive Committee, 1915," cited in Frederic A. Washburn, *The Massachusetts General Hospital: Its Development, 1900–1935* (Boston: Houghton Mifflin, 1939), p. 259.

24 Lewellys Barker, "Group Diagnosis and Group Therapy," *Wis. Med. J.*, vol. 19 (1920), p. 332. See also James B. Herrick, "Modern Diagnosis," *J.A.M.A.*, vol. 92 (1929), pp. 518–22; Nathaniel W. Faxon, "The Country Doctor and the Hospital," *Boston Med. Surg. J.*, vol. 177 (1917), pp. 167–71; J. J. Weber, "An Interesting Development of the Growing Tendency Towards Group Diagnosis . . . ," *Mod. Hosp.*, vol. 13 (1919), p. 178.

25 Lavina L. Dock and Isabel M. Stewart, *A Short History of Nursing* (New York: Putman, 1925), p. 95.

26 John Aikin, *Thoughts on Hospitals* (London: Printed for Joseph Johnson, 1771), pp. 9–10.

27 Florence Nightingale, *Notes on Nursing: What It Is, and What It Is Not* (London: Harrison, 1860); Florence Nightingale, *Notes on Hospitals*, 3rd ed. (London: Longman, Green, Longman, Roberts, and Green, 1863).

28 Harvey Cushing, *Realignments in Greater Medicine: Their Effect upon Surgery and the Influence of Surgery upon Them* (London: Oxford University Press, 1914),

p. 25. See also Bates, "Some Perplexities in Modern Medicine," p. 848.

29 C. Rufus Rorem, *Capital Investment in Hospitals* (Washington: Committee on the Costs of Medical Care, 1930), p. 9; *Health Resources Statistics: Health Manpower and Health Facilities, 1975* (Washington: U.S. Department of Health, Education, and Welfare, 1976), pp. 339, 342.

30 Raymond Pearl, "Modern Methods in Handling Hospital Statistics," *Bull. Johns Hopkins Hosp.*, vol. 32 (1921), p. 186. See also Richard C. Cabot, "On the Relation between Laboratory Work and Clinical Work," *Boston Med. Surg. J.*, vol. 164 (1911), pp. 833–4.

31 *Committee on the Costs of Medical Care, Final Report* (Chicago: University of Chicago Press, 1932), pp. 26–30, 58–66.

32 See Clapesattle, *The Doctors Mayo*, for a complete history of the Mayo Clinic's origins.

33 I. S. Falk, C. Rufus Rorem, and Martha D. Ring, *The Costs of Medical Care* (Chicago: University of Chicago Press, 1933), pp. 388–9.

34 *Committee on the Costs of Medical Care*, pp. 39–41, 76–9; Warren T. Vaughan, "Group Medicine: A Critical Survey," *South. Med. J.*, vol. 16 (1923), pp. 727–8.

35 C. Rufus Rorem, *Private Group Clinics* (Washington: Committee on the Costs of Medical Care, 1931), p. 93.

36 Ibid., p. 109.

37 Ibid., p. 104.

38 James Hunter, "The Economic Aspect of the Modern Diagnostic Survey," *J. Med. Soc. N. J.*, vol. 17 (1920), pp. 341–2.

39 Washburn, *The Massachusetts General Hospital*, pp. 259–62.

40 V. L. Schrager, "Roentgen Diagnosis in Relation to Clinical Teamwork," *J. Roentgenol.*, vol. 2 (1919), pp. 58–9. See also Leon Solomon, "Modern Day Diagnosis – Clinical and Laboratory Diagnostic Methods as Practiced by the Staff of the Solomon Clinic," *Ky. Med. J.*, vol. 18 (1920), pp. 15–20; *Committee on the Costs of Medical Care*, pp. 66–8, 81–2, 133–5, 169.

41 Barker, "Group Diagnosis and Group Therapy," p. 336.

42 Herrick, "Modern Diagnosis," p. 519.

43 Rorem, *Private Group Clinics*, pp. 86–8.

44 *Committee on the Costs of Medical Care*, pp. 65, 85; Leven, *Incomes of Physicians*, p. 7; James R. Cantwell, ed., *Profile of Medical Practice* (Chicago: American Medical Association, 1976) pp. 78–9.

45 Louis J. Goodman, "The Growth of Group Practice," in Henry R. Mason, ed., *Reference Data on Socioeconomic Issues of Health* (Chicago: American Medical Association, 1976), pp. 8–12.

46 Michael J. Halberstam, "Liberal Thought, Radical Theory and Medical Practice," *N. Engl. J. Med.*, vol. 284 (1971), p. 1181.

47 *Health Resources Statistics*, p. 444.

CHAPTER 8. THE SHORTCOMINGS OF TECHNOLOGY IN MEDICAL DECISION MAKING

1 Cecil Kent Austin, "Medical Impressions of America," *Boston Med. Surg. J.*, vol. 166 (1912), p. 801.

2 Sydney R. Miller, "Contemporary Fads and Fallacies, Therapeutic and Diagnostic, which Reflect Dangerous Professional Credulity," *Pa. Med. J.*, vol. 35 (1932), pp. 348–9. See also Ralph G. Stillman, "The Significance of Laboratory Tests and Methods," *N. Y. State J. Med.*, vol. 35 (1935), pp. 757–9; Alfred Stengel, "Importance of Accurate Medical Histories and Careful Physical Examinations," *Pa. Med. J.*, vol. 37 (1934), p. 812.

3 Tinsley R. Harrison, "The Value and Limitation of Laboratory Tests in Clinical Medicine," *J. Med. Assoc. Ala.*, vol. 13 (1944), p. 382.

4 Walter J. McNerney and Study Staff, *Hospital and Medical Economics: A Study of Population, Services, Costs, Methods of Payment, and Controls*, vol. 1 (Chicago: Hospital Research and Educational Trust, 1962), pp. 607–8, 615–17.

5 For the statistics on Yale-New Haven Hospital, consult David Seligson, "Clinical Laboratory Automation," *J. Chronic Dis.*, vol. 19 (1966), p. 509. A similar increase in laboratory testing was noted at the Massachusetts General Hospital, Boston, where in fiscal year 1958–59, 183,650 laboratory tests were performed; in 1963–64, 333,248; and in 1968–69, 611,660 (personal communication from Dr. William Beck, Director of Clinical Laboratories).

6 "Laboratory Posture," *N. Engl. J. Med.*, vol. 268 (1963), p. 1196. See also H. M. Marvin, "The Therapeutic Trial," *Conn. State Med. J.*, vol. 18 (1954), p. 850; Ellis Kellert, "Laboratory Tests vs. Stethoscopes," *Am. Pract. Dig. Treat.*, vol. 4 (1953), pp. 460–3.

7 Roy N. Barnett, et al., "Multiphasic Screening by Laboratory Tests – An Overview of the Problem," *Am. J. Clin. Pathol.*, vol. 54 (1970), p. 486; R. S. Murley, "The Use and Misuse of Laboratory Services in Surgical Practice," *Proc. Royal Soc. Med.*, vol. 58 (1965), p. 504; D. M. Young, et al., "The Advent of Chemical Screening Techniques," *Can. Med. Assoc. J.*, vol. 98 (1968), p. 868.

8 U.S. Congress, Senate, Committee on Human Resources, *Clinical Laboratory Improvement Act of 1977, Report to Accompany S. 705*, 95th Cong., 1st sess., 1977, S. Rept. 90-360, p. 4.

9 In Beverly, England, the volume of laboratory testing in hospitals has doubled every seven years since 1920 (H. F. Barnard, "Growth of Medical Laboratory Work during 1920–2000," *Br. Med. J.*, vol. 1 (1976), pp. 383–4). Another survey found that from 1958 to 1965, many hospital laboratories throughout England had doubled their work while, in the same period, the number of patients treated at these hospitals rose by only one quarter ("Is our Pathology Really Necessary?" *Lancet*, vol. 2 (1966), pp. 46–7). However, a study of the demand for laboratory services in England and Wales from 1959 to 1972, both within and outside of hospitals, showed demand rising about 7 percent a year, a smaller rate of increase than in the two hospital laboratory use studies (J. S. A. Ashley, "Demand for Laboratory Services," *Br. Med. Bull.*, vol. 30 (1974), pp. 234–6). At the Edinburgh Royal Infirmary, the test load had doubled every five years from 1921 to 1966 ("Data Processing in Clinical Pathology," *J. Clin. Path.*, vol. 21 (1968), p. 234). In Canada, laboratory testing was growing at a rapid rate also (Irwin H. Hilliard, "The Threat of the Modern Laboratory to the Art and Science of Medicine," *Can. Med. Assoc. J.*, vol. 85 (1961), p. 483).

10 L. T. Skeggs, Jr., "An Automatic Method for Colorimetric Analysis," *Am. J. Clin. Path.*, vol. 28 (1957), pp. 311–22. The abstract of this article first appeared in *Clin. Chem.*, vol. 2 (1956), p. 241. For an examination of the auto-

matic analyzer's reception see, Andrés Ferrari and Ralph Overman, "Medical Technology," *Ann. N. Y. Acad. Sci.*, vol. 166 (1969), pp. 1027–30.

11 Robert M. Schmidt, "Control of Diagnostic Hematology Products," in S. M. Lewis and J. F. Coster, eds., *Quality Control in Hematology* (London: Academic Press, 1975), pp. 174, 182; Tate M. Minckler, "Laboratory Automation: Perspectives," *Med. Instrum.*, vol. 8 (1974), p. 296; Richard H. Dixon and John Laszlo, "Utilization of Clinical Chemistry Services by Medical House Staff," *Arch. Intern. Med.*, vol. 134 (1974), p. 1066.

12 S. Cochrane Shankes, "Fifty Years of Radiology," *Br. Med. J.*, vol. 1 (1950), p. 46; James F. Brailsford, "Factors which Influence the Value of a Radiological Investigation," *Lancet*, vol. 1 (1952), p. 679.

13 McNerney, *Hospital and Medical Economics*, p. 615.

14 Brailsford, "Value of a Radiological Investigation," pp. 679–80. See also John L. McClenahan, "Wasted X-Rays," *Radiol.*, vol. 96 (1970), pp. 453–6.

15 I. E. Kirsh, "Routine Roentgenographic Examinations," *J.A.M.A.*, vol. 213 (1970), p. 300.

16 Russell S. Bell and John W. Loop, "The Utility and Futility of Radiographic Skull Examination for Trauma," *N. Engl. J. Med.*, vol. 284 (1971), pp. 236–9.

17 Institute of Medicine, *Computed Tomographic Scanning* (Washington: National Academy of Sciences, 1977); Michel M. Ter-Pogossian, "The Challenge of Computed Tomography," *Am. J. Roentgenol.*, vol. 127 (1976), p. 1; Patrick F. Sheedy et al., "Computed Tomography of the Body: Initial Clinical Trial with the EMI Prototype," ibid., p. 48; Hillier L. Baker, Jr., "Computed Tomography and Neuroradiology: A Fortunate Primary Union," ibid., p. 101; Kenneth R. Davis et al., "Some Limitations of Computed Tomography in the Diagnosis of Neurological Diseases," ibid., p. 121; Lee E. Cloe, "Health Planning for Computed Tomography: Perspectives and Problems," ibid., pp. 188–9.

18 U.S. Congress, *Clinical Laboratory Improvement Act of 1977, Report*, p. 4.

19 Paul F. Griner and Benjamin Liptzin, "Use of the Laboratory in a Teaching Hospital: Implications for Patient Care, Education, and Hospital Costs," *Ann. Intern. Med.*, vol. 75 (1971), pp. 157–63; Dixon and Laszlo, "Utilization of Clinical Chemistry Services," pp. 1064–7; Christopher C. Kowin, Richard H. Pierce, and John Stanley, "Admissions Screening: Clinical Benefits," *Ann. Intern. Med.*, vol. 83 (1975), pp. 197–203.

20 David E. Rogers, "On Technologic Restraint," *Arch. Intern. Med.*, vol. 135 (1975), p. 1395.

21 Miller, "Contemporary Fads and Fallacies," p. 349.

22 Marcus Backer, "The Trend Away from Clinical Medicine," *Conn. State Med. J.*, vol. 21 (1957), p. 99.

23 "Routine Laboratory Tests," *N. Engl. J. Med.*, vol. 275 (1966), p. 56. See also "Laboratory Posture," *N. Engl. J. Med.*, vol. 268 (1963), p. 1196.

24 James B. Herrick, "The Relation of the Clinical Laboratory to the Practitioner of Medicine," *Boston Med. Surg. J.*, vol. 156 (1907), p. 763. See also Francis W. Peabody, "The Physician and the Laboratory," *Boston Med. Surg. J.*, vol. 187 (1922), pp. 327–8; Lewis A. Conner, "Relation of Laboratory Aids to the Practice of Medicine and Surgery," *J.A.M.A.*, vol. 81 (1923), pp. 871–3.

25 Richard D. Loewenberg, "On the Psychology of Some Diagnostic Errors," *J.*

Insur. Med., vol. 6 (1951), p. 33. See also Bertram H. Roberts and Nea M. Norton, "The Prevalence of Psychiatric Illness in a Medical Out–Patient Clinic," *N. Engl. J. Med.*, vol. 246 (1952), p. 86.

26 Lucien Achard, "The Place of the Modern Medical Laboratory in the Diagnosis of Disease," *Med. Rec.*, vol. 101 (1922), p. 419. See also W. W. Herrick, "The Clinician and Research," *Minn. Med.*, vol. 3 (1920), p. 49; William S. Thayer, "On the Diagnostic Importance of Physical Examination," *Mil. Surg.*, vol. 65 (1929), p. 512.

27 Patrick C. J. Ward, et al., "Systematic Instruction in Interpretive Aspects of Laboratory Medicine," *J. Med. Educ.*, vol. 51 (1976), pp. 648–9; James K. Shipper et al., "Medical Students' Unfamiliarity with the Cost of Diagnostic Tests," ibid., vol. 50 (1975), pp. 683–4; Griner and Liptzin, "Use of the Laboratory," p. 162. A U.S. Senate committee studying the application and cost of laboratory tests, cited lack of adequate courses on this subject as a cause of unnecessary laboratory use (U.S. Congress, *Clinical Laboratory Improvement Act of 1977, Report*, p. 21).

28 C. Macfie Campbell, "Psychiatry and the Practice of Medicine," *Boston Med. Surg. J.*, vol. 190 (1924), p. 1058; James Mackenzie, *The Future of Medicine* (London: Oxford University Press, 1919), p. 179.

29 R. Macnair Wilson, *The Beloved Physician: Sir James Mackenzie* (London: John Murray, 1926), pp. 245–6.

30 George P. Robb and Israel Steinberg, "Visualization of the Chambers of the Heart, the Pulmonary Circulation, and the Great Blood Vessels in Man: A Practical Method," *Am. J. Roentgenol. Radium Ther.*, vol. 41 (1939), pp. 1–2.

31 Harvey W. Van Allen, "The Limitations of the Roentgen Method of Diagnosis," *N. Engl. J. Med.*, vol. 215 (1936), p. 483; W. Burton Wood, "Pulmonary Tuberculosis in General Practice," *Lancet*, vol. 2 (1930), p. 726.

32 Walter C. Alvarez, *Nervousness, Indigestion, and Pain* (New York: Paul B. Hoeber, 1943), p. 111.

33 Walter C. Alvarez, "Diagnostic Time Savers for Overworked Physicians," *J.A.M.A.*, vol. 122 (1943), p. 933. See also Raymond W. Brust, "History and Physical Signs Versus Expensive Diagnostic Aids," *Med. Rec.*, vol. 148 (1938), p. 437; W. R. Houston, "Diagnosis: Purpose and Scope," *Int. Clin.*, vol. 1 (1937), pp. 239–40.

34 William Seaman Bainbridge, "Clinical and Laboratory Diagnoses," *Med. J. Rec.*, vol. 136 (1932), p. 269.

35 Louis K. Diamond and F. Stanley Porter, "The Inadequacies of Routine Bleeding and Clotting Times," *N. Engl. J. Med.*, vol. 259 (1958), p. 1025.

36 "Statement of the American College of Surgeons and the American Academy of Orthopaedic Surgeons before the Secretary's (HEW) Commission on Medical Malpractice," *Bull. Am. Coll. Surg.*, vol. 57, No. 5 (1972), fig. 5, p. 14. See also Nathan Hersey, "The Defensive Practice of Medicine," *Milbank Mem. Fund Q.*, vol. 50 (1972), pp. 69–97.

37 "Why Most MDs Practice 'Defensive Medicine,' " *Amer. Med. News*, March 28, 1977, p. 3, supplement.

38 Marjorie Smith Mueller and Paula A. Piro, "Private Health Insurance in 1974: A Review of Coverage, Enrollment, and Financial Experience," *Soc. Secur. Bull.*, vol. 39, no. 3 (1976), p. 9. Some indication that increased laboratory use is related to elimination of laboratory charges to patients is found in Donald K.

Freeborn et al., "Determinants of Medical Care Utilization: Physicians' Use of Laboratory Services," *Am. J. Pub. Health*, vol. 62 (1972), p. 851.

39 A. H. Douthwaite, "Pitfalls in Medicine," *Br. Med. J.*, vol. 2 (1956), p. 899; Hilliard, "Threat of Modern Laboratory," p. 484; "Routine Tests," *N. Engl. J. Med.*, vol. 275 (1966), p. 56.

40 D. N. Baron, "The Laboratory and the Clinician," *Radiogr.*, vol. 19 (1953), p. 12; "Misdiagnosis," *Lancet*, vol. 1 (1953), p. 1034; William Dock, "The Place of the Gadget in the History and the Practice of Medicine," *Stanford Med. Bull.*, vol. 13 (1955), p. 142.

41 David P. Barr, "Hazards of Modern Diagnosis and Therapy – The Price We Pay," *J.A.M.A.*, vol. 159 (1955), p. 1456.

42 James B. Herrick, "The Clinician of the Future," *J.A.M.A.*, vol. 86 (1926), p. 4. See also for comments on the physicians' deference to the laboratory, Reed Rockwood, "Chemical Tests of the Blood; Indications and Interpretations," *J.A.M.A.*, vol. 91 (1928), pp. 157–8; M. P. Overholser, "On Laboratory Diagnosis," *N. Y. Med. J.*, vol. 79 (1904), pp. 631–2; Archibald Garrod, "The Laboratory and the Ward," *Contributions to Medical Biological Research Dedicated to Sir William Osler. . .* , vol. 1 (New York: Paul B. Hoeber, 1919), p. 63; Richard C. Cabot, "The Ideal of Accuracy in Clinical Work: Its Importance, Its Limitations," *Boston Med. Surg. J.*, vol. 151 (1904), pp. 557–60.

43 C. F. Hoover, "The Reputed Conflict Between the Laboratories and Clinical Medicine," *Science*, vol. 71 (1930), p. 492.

44 Ibid., p. 496.

45 Franklin W. White, "Remarks on Diagnosis and Treatment of Disease of the Stomach," *Boston Med. Surg. J.*, vol. 170 (1914), p. 827. See also C. Thurstan Holland, "Radiology in Clinical Medicine and Surgery," *Br. Med. J.*, vol. 1 (1917), p. 288; James Brailsford, "Reflections on the Teaching of Radiology," *Br. J. Radiol.*, vol. 18 (1945), p. 252.

46 Desmond O'Neill, ed., *Modern Trends in Psychosomatic Medicine* (London: Butterworth, 1955), p. 3. See also for other comments on the doctor's waning self–reliance: Emmet L. Holt, "Medical Tendencies and Medical Ideals," *J.A.M.A.*, vol. 48 (1907), p. 845; A. C. Kimberlin, "The Psychologic Value of a Correct Diagnosis," *J. Indiana State Med. Assoc.*, vol. 5 (1912), p. 271; Harvey Cushing, "The Physician and the Surgeon," *Boston Med. Surg. J.*, vol. 187 (1922), p. 627.

47 Jasper Halpenny, "On Clinical and Laboratory Methods of Diagnosis," *Can. Med. Assoc. J.*, vol. 14 (1924), p. 672. See also Urban Maes, "A Plea for Clinical Diagnosis in Present Day Medicine," *New Orleans Med. Surg. J.*, vol. 101 (1948–49), p. 363.

48 Elisabeth Kübler–Ross, *On Death and Dying* (New York: Macmillan, 1970), p. 9.

49 Alvan R. Feinstein, "What Kind of Basic Science for Clinical Medicine?" *N. Engl. J. Med.*, vol. 283 (1970), p. 848; "Routine Tests – the Physician's Responsibility," *N. Engl. J. Med.*, vol. 274 (1966), p. 222.

50 "Medicine and Medical Schools in America," *Br. Med. J.*, vol. 2 (1907), p. 1846.

51 Georges Baril, "The Correlation of Laboratory Findings with the Clinical Aspects of Disease," *Can. Med. Assoc. J.*, vol. 24 (1931), pp. 532–3; J. C. Waddell, "Present Day Diagnosis," *Nebr. State Med. J.*, vol. 14 (1929), pp. 349–50;

Arthur A. Eisenberg, "Errors in Surgical Diagnosis, Avoidable and Unavoidable. . . ," *Bull. Am. Coll. Surg.*, vol. 9 (1925), p. 55.

52 Theodore Tieken, "A Plea for Better Understanding of Physical Diagnosis," *J.A.M.A.*, vol. 76 (1921), p. 1736. See also Leon K. Balduaf, "The Laboratory in Diagnosis," *Ky. Med. J.*, vol. 20 (1922), p. 357.

53 John Adam, "Medical Diagnosis and Modern Discoveries," *Br. Med. J.*, vol. 1 (1902), p. 501.

54 Walter C. Alvarez, "The Art of Medicine," *Minn. Med.*, vol. 14 (1931), p. 228.

55 C. E. Watson, "Physical Diagnosis," *W. Va. Med. J.*, vol. 16 (1921), p. 194; Waddell, "Present Day Diagnosis," pp. 349–50.

56 James B. Herrick, "The Importance of the History and Physical Examination in Diagnosis," *J. Indiana State Med. Assoc.*, vol. 24 (1931), p. 71.

57 James J. Waring, "The Vicissitudes of Auscultation," *Am. Rev. Tuberc.*, vol. 34 (1936), p. 6. See also James B. Herrick, "In Defense of the Stethoscope," *Ann. Intern. Med.*, vol. 4 (1930), p. 113; R. A. Young, "The Stethoscope: Past and Present," *Lancet*, vol. 2 (1930), p. 883; "Physical Signs: Are they Worthwhile?" (South–west London Medical Society Meeting), *Lancet*, vol. 1 (1937), p. 1464.

58 Instruments Collection, Francis A. Countway Library of Medicine, Boston, Massachusetts.

59 "Stethoscope Versus X-Rays," *Br. Med. J.*, vol. 2 (1945), p. 856. See also F. M. Pottenger, "Why is Physical Examination of the Chest Being Neglected?" *Trans. Am. Ther. Soc.*, vol. 46 (1946), p. 88; Izod Bennett, "Discussion on the Stethoscope Versus X-Rays," *Proc. R. Soc. Med.*, vol. 39 (1946), pp. 355–7.

60 R. C. Hutchinson, "Stethoscope Versus X-Rays," *Br. Med. J.*, vol. 1 (1946), p. 31.

61 Samuel A. Levine, "A Plea for the Stethoscope," *Rocky Mt. Med. J.*, vol. 49 (1952), pp. 1029–33.

62 Urban Maes, "The Lost Art of Clinical Diagnosis," *Am. J. Surg.*, vol. 82 (1951), p. 107.

63 Stanley Wiener and Morton Nathanson, "Physical Examination: Frequently Observed Errors," *J.A.M.A.*, vol. 236 (1976), pp. 852–5.

64 George L. Engel, "Are Medical Schools Neglecting Clinical Skills?" *J.A.M.A.*, vol. 236 (1976), pp. 861–3.

65 John M. Scudder, *Specific Diagnosis: A Study of Disease* (Cincinnati: Wilstach, Baldwin and Co., 1874), p. 29. See also Somerville Scott Alison, *The Physical Examination of the Chest in Pulmonary Consumption* . . . (London: John Churchill, 1861), p. 169.

66 Russell H. Oppenheimer, "Significance of Symptoms in Medical Teaching," *South. Med. J.*, vol. 23 (1930), p. 856.

67 C. Ward Crampton, "Synthetic Diagnosis," *Med. Clin. North Am.*, vol. 14 (1930), p. 449.

68 Paul D. White, "Errors in the Interpretation of Cardiovascular Symptoms and Signs," *Ann. Intern. Med.*, vol. 9 (1936), p. 1703. For other discussions of the history's neglect, see Parley Nelson, "History Taking," *Northwest Med.*, vol. 27 (1928), p. 245; Oliver Thomas Osborne, "The Evaluation of Symptoms," *Med. J. Rec.*, vol. 138 (1933), p. 334; Richard F. Herndon, "The Value of Symptoms," *Ill. Med. J.*, vol. 66 (1934), p. 388; Ralph H. Major, "Diagnosing Disease without Instruments of Precision," *J. Kans. Med. Soc.*, vol. 40 (1939), pp. 408–12; Stengel, "Importance of Accurate Medical Histories," p. 812; George

Blumer, "History Taking," *Conn. State Med. J.*, vol. 13 (1949), p. 449; Tinsley R. Harrison, "Two Views of Present Trends in the Teaching of Internal Medicine," *Ann. Intern. Med.*, vol. 73 (1970), p. 476; and J. R. Hampton et al., "Relative Contributions of History–taking, Physical Examination, and Laboratory Investigation to Diagnosis and Management of Medical Outpatients," *Br. Med. J.*, vol. 1 (1975), pp. 486–9.

69 Sir Almoth E. Wright, "Vaccine Therapy: Its Administration, Value and Limitations," *Proc. Royal Soc. Med.*, vol. 3, part 1 (1910), pp. 5–10.

70 Leslie Zieve, "Misinterpretation and Abuse of Laboratory Tests by Clinicians," *Ann. N.Y. Acad. Sci.*, vol. 134 (1966), pp. 563–72; A. F. Brown, "Pitfalls in the Interpretation of Laboratory Observations," *J. Int. Coll. Surg.*, vol. 34 (1960), p. 683; John Laszlo, "Automated 'Chemistries,' " *Arch. Intern. Med.*, vol. 133 (1974), pp. 1068–9; "The Clinical Laboratory and Training for Internal Medicine," *Am. J. Med.*, vol. 8 (1950), p. 690.

71 George W. Pickering, "Disorders of Contemporary Society and Their Impact on Medicine," *Ann. Intern. Med.*, vol. 43 (1955), p. 925. See also Alvarez, *Nervousness, Indigestion and Pain*, p. 113.

CHAPTER 9. SELECTION AND EVALUATION OF EVIDENCE IN MEDICINE

1 James Mackenzie, *The Future of Medicine* (London: Oxford University Press, 1919), pp. 61–5. See also R. Macnair Wilson, *The Beloved Physician: Sir James Mackenzie* (London: John Murray, 1926), pp. 93–103.

2 A. Chauffard, "Medical Prognosis: Its Methods, Its Evolution, Its Limitations," *Br. Med. J.*, vol. 2 (1913), pp. 287–8. See also Dyce Duckworth, "The Prognosis of Disease," *Br. Med. J.*, vol. 2 (1896), pp. 251–8; P. H. Pye–Smith, "Observations on Prognosis," *Guy's Hosp. Rep.*, vol. 49 (1888), pp. 59–86; "The Art of Prognosis," *Boston Med. Surg. J.*, vol. 157 (1907), p. 677.

3 John C. Hemmeter, "Science and Art in Medicine: Their Influence on the Development of Medical Thinking," *J.A.M.A.*, vol. 46 (1906), pp. 243–8; "The Present Decline of Art in Medicine," *Lancet*, vol. 2 (1905), pp. 1555–6; Emmet L. Holt, "Medical Tendencies and Medical Ideals," *J.A.M.A.*, vol. 48 (1907), p. 846; Frederick C. Shattuck, "The Science and Art of Medicine in Some of Their Aspects," *Boston Med. Surg. J.*, vol. 157 (1907), p. 63.

4 Sigmund Freud, "Recommendations for Physicians on the Psychoanalytic Method of Treatment" (1912), in Philip Reiff, ed., *Sigmund Freud: Therapy and Technique* (New York: Macmillan, 1963), p. 122. A principal disciple of Freud and transmitter of his theories in the United States was James J. Putnam; see his "The Present Status of Psychoanalysis," *Boston Med. Surg. J.*, vol. 170 (1914), pp. 897–903.

5 Lewellys F. Barker, "Some Experience with the Simpler Methods of Psychotherapy and Re-Education," *Am. J. Med. Sci.*, vol. 132 (1906), pp. 500–3; Richard C. Cabot, "Mind Cure: Its Service to the Community," *Detroit Med. J.*, vol. 7 (1907), pp. 277–8.

6 Richard C. Cabot, "Suggestions for the Reorganization of Hospital Out–Patient Departments, with Special Reference to the Improvement of Treatment," *Maryland Med. J.*, vol. 50 (1907), pp. 88–9. For an excellent historical account

of medical social work in America, consult the book written by Cabot's principal associate in establishing the discipline at the Massachusetts General Hospital – Ida M. Cannon, *On the Social Frontier of Medicine: Pioneering in Medical Social Service* (Cambridge: Harvard University Press, 1952). See also Richard C. Cabot, *Social Service and the Art of Healing* (New York: Moffat, Yard and Co., 1909).

7 Celia Burns Stendler, "New Ideas for Old: How Freudianism Was Received in the United States from 1900 to 1925," *J. Ed. Psychol.*, vol. 38 (1947), pp. 193–206.

8 Lawrence K. Lunt, "Attitudes in Relation to Illness," *N. Engl. J. Med.*, vol. 219 (1938), p. 560; Ernest Jones, "The Unconscious Mind and Medical Practice," *Br. Med. J.*, vol. 1 (1938), p. 1355; W. R. Houston, "The Doctor Himself as a Therapeutic Agent," *Ann. Intern. Med.*, vol. 11 (1938), p. 1420; Louis Hamman, "The Relationship of Psychiatry to Internal Medicine," *Ment. Hyg.*, vol. 23 (1939), p. 181.

9 William C. Menninger, "Psychiatric Experience in the War: 1941–1946," *Am. J. Psychiatr.*, vol. 103 (1946–47), p. 578.

10 Karl Menninger, "Changing Concepts of Disease," *Ann. Intern. Med.*, vol. 29 (1948), pp. 318–25; David Barr, "The Responsibilities of the Internist," *Ann. Intern. Med.*, vol. 27 (1947), pp. 199–201; Bernard B. Raginsky, "Psychosomatic Medicine: Its History, Development and Teaching," *Am. J. Med.*, vol. 5 (1948), pp. 866–8.

11 Carl Binger, "What Can We Learn from a Medical History," *Am. J. Med.*, vol. 6 (1949), pp. 751–5; Florence Powdermaker, "The Techniques of the Initial Interview and Methods of Teaching Them," *Am. J. Psychiatr.*, vol. 104 (1948), pp. 642–6; Clark W. Heath, "An Interview Method for Obtaining Personal Histories," *N. Engl. J. Med.*, vol. 234 (1946), pp. 251–7; Stanley Wiener and Morton Nathanson, "Physical Examination: Frequently Observed Errors," *J.A.M.A.*, vol. 236 (1976), p. 853.

12 Stewart Wolf, et al., "Instruction in History Taking," *J. Med. Educ.*, vol. 27 (1952), pp. 244–7; Ainslie Meares, "Communication with the Patient," *Lancet*, vol. 1 (1960), pp. 663–7. An early application of the videotape to record and study nonverbal communication between medical students and patients occurred in 1968 at the Harvard Medical School, in a course entitled "Seminar in Clinical Interviewing," (Medicine 703.3) *Elective Catalogue, 1968–69*.

13 Theodore Reik, *Listening with the Third Ear* (New York: Farrar, Straus & Giroux, 1954), pp. 131–56.

14 Erik Erikson, "The Nature of Clinical Evidence," *Daedalus*, vol. 87 (Fall, 1958), p. 67. See also Eric Berne, "The Nature of Intuition," *Psychiatr. Q.*, vol. 23 (1949), pp. 203–25. For a noteworthy analysis of the medical interview see Michael Balint, *The Doctor, His Patient and the Illness* (London: Pitman Paperbacks, 1968).

15 Mackenzie, *Future of Medicine*, pp. 94–5. See also James Mackenzie, *Symptoms and their Interpretation* (London: Shaw and Sons, 1920), pp. 20–9.

16 William H. Broadbent, "The Croonian Lectures on the Pulse," *Br. Med. J.*, vol. 1 (1887), p. 657; Edouard Seguin, *Medical Thermometry and Human Temperature* (New York: William Wood, 1876), pp. 252–3; Harvey Cushing, "On Routine Determinations of Arterial Tension in the Operating Room and Clinic," *Boston Med. Surg. J.*, vol. 148 (1903), p. 252; James E. Talley, "The Elec-

trocardiograph as a Clinical Instrument," *Am. J. Med. Sci.*, vol. 147 (1914), p. 698.

17 Abraham Flexner, *Medical Education in the United States and Canada* (Boston: Merrymount Press, 1910), pp. 91–2; James B. Herrick, "The Relationship of the Clinical Laboratory to the Practitioner of Medicine," *Boston Med. Surg. J.*, vol. 156 (1907), p. 766; Richard C. Cabot, "The Historical Development and Relative Value of Laboratory and Clinical Methods of Diagnosis," *Boston Med. Surg. J.*, vol. 157 (1907), pp. 150–3; F. B. Eaton, "The Relative Value of Clinical Medical and Surgical Knowledge to That of the Laboratory," *J.A.M.A.*, vol. 48 (1907), pp. 2176–7; James B. Herrick, "Modern Diagnosis," *J.A.M.A.*, vol. 92 (1929), p. 520.

18 "Errors in Observation," *Br. Med. J.*, vol. 1 (1905), pp. 547–8; Byrom Bramwell, "Mistakes," *Lancet*, vol. 2 (1911), pp. 281–5; Richard C. Cabot, "Diagnostic Pitfalls Identified During A Study of Three Thousand Autopsies," *J.A.M.A.*, vol. 59 (1912), pp. 2295–8; Adolphe Abrahams, "Common Errors in Diagnosis," *Practitioner* (London), vol. 44 (1915), pp. 380–95.

19 J. Mitchell Bruce, "Inattention and Inexactness in Ordinary Diagnosis," *Clin. J.*, vol. 17 (1900–01), pp. 17–22; Theodore C. Janeway, "Some Sources of Error in Laboratory Clinical Diagnosis," *Med. News*, vol. 78 (1901), pp. 700–6; Richard C. Cabot, "The Relation of Bacteriology to Medicine," *Boston Med. Surg. J.*, vol. 142 (1900), p. 482; Richard C. Cabot, "Clinical Examination of the Urine," *J.A.M.A.*, vol. 44 (1905), pp. 837–42, 943–50; William P. Boardman, "Interpretation of the Wassermann Reaction," *Boston Med. Surg. J.*, vol. 183 (1920), pp. 538–9.

20 Robert A. Kilduffe, " 'Diagnostic' or 'Clinical' Laboratories and their Standardization," *J. Med. Soc. N. J.*, vol. 24 (1927), p. 525. See also Charles P. Emerson, "The Accuracy of Certain Clinical Methods," *Bull. Johns Hopkins Hosp.*, vol. 14 (1903), pp. 9–18; J. C. Ohlmacher, "The Relation of the Laboratory to Clinical Medicine in the Light of Present–Day Medical Advancement," *J.-Lancet*, vol. 42 (1922), pp. 460–3.

21 E. H. R. Altounyan, "The Visual Diagnosis of Disease," *Lancet*, vol. 2 (1928), pp. 684–5; Albert S. Welch, "The Relation of the Clinician to the Laboratory," *J. Kansas Med. Soc.*, vol. 26 (1926), pp. 85–7; Bowman Corning Crowell, "The Mutual Relations Existing Between the Clinic and the Laboratory," *J. Lab. Clin. Med.*, vol. 11 (1925), pp. 37–43; Frederick H. Lamb, "Symposium on Surgical Diagnosis: Laboratory Procedures," *J. Iowa State Med. Soc.*, vol. 11 (1921), p. 245.

22 D. L. Harris, "The Danger of Laboratory Diagnosis," *St. Louis Med. Rev.*, vol. 58 (1909), pp. 117–20.

23 Francis H. Slack, "An Investigation of the Reliability of Laboratory Tests and a Discussion of Techniques of Laboratories in and Near Boston," *Boston Med. Surg. J.*, vol. 187 (1922), pp. 441–6; 474–9, 540–3.

24 A.M.A. Council on Medical Education and Hospitals, "Clinical Laboratory Service in the United States," *N. Engl. J. Med.*, vol. 198 (1928), pp. 110–11.

25 "Accurate Blood Tests for Syphilis," *J.A.M.A.*, vol. 115 (1940), p. 386. See also "Efficiency of State and Local Laboratories in the Performance of Serodiagnostic Tests for Syphilis," *Am. J. Public Health*, vol. 27 (1937), pp. 15–23.

26 J. G. Snavely and Walter R. C. Golden, "A Survey of the Accuracy of Certain Chemical Determinations," *Conn. State Med. J.*, vol. 13 (1949), p. 193.

27 William P. Belk and F. William Sunderman, "A Survey of the Accuracy of Chemical Analyses in Clinical Laboratories," *Am. J. Clin. Pathol.*, vol. 17 (1947), pp. 855–6.
28 Henry Bauer, "The National Laboratory Crisis," *Hosp. Pract.*, vol. 2, no. 2, (1967), p. 67.
29 Bradley E. Copeland, "Reliability of Medical Laboratories," *N. Engl. J. Med.*, vol. 276 (1967), pp. 873–4. See also "Evaluation of Laboratory Tests," *N. Engl. J. Med.*, vol. 278 (1968), p. 221; William Kaufmann and Raymond Vanderline, "Medical Laboratory Evaluation," *N. Engl. J. Med.*, vol. 277 (1967), p. 1024; J. H. Flokstra, A. B. Varley, and J. A. Hagans, "Reproducibility and Accuracy of Clinical Laboratory Determinations," *Am. J. Med. Sci.*, vol. 251 (1966), pp. 646–55.
30 Laurence P. Skendzel and Rudolf J. Meulling, Jr., "Report on Small Hospital Laboratories; 1966 Survey of the College of American Pathologists," *N. Engl. J. Med.*, vol. 277 (1967), pp. 180–5.
31 U.S. Congress, Senate, Committee on Human Resources, *Clinical Laboratory Improvement Act of 1977, Report to Accompany S. 705*, 95th Cong., 1st sess., 1977, S. Rept. 90–360, pp. 3, 6.
32 Ibid., pp. 4–6. See also U.S. Congress, Senate, Subcommittee on Health and Scientific Research of the Committee on Human Resources, *Clinical Laboratory Improvement Act of 1977, Hearings on S. 705*, 95th Cong., 1st sess., 29 and 30 March 1977, pp. 141–2, 499, 512–13, 526, 545, 553, 581–5; Barbara Culliton, "Clinical Labs: Bills Aimed at Correcting 'Massive' Problems," *Science*, vol. 192 (1976), pp. 531–3.
33 *Laboratory Improvement Act of 1977, Hearings*, p. 451.
34 Center for Disease Control, "Summary of Selected CDC Data on Performance by Participant Clinical Laboratories: 1969–1975," (Atlanta: U.S. Department of Health, Education, and Welfare, 1976).
35 Dr. Donald R. Bruska, *Laboratory Improvement Act of 1977, Hearings*, p. 214. See also John A. Koepke, "Inter-Laboratory Trials: The Quality Control Survey Programme of the College of American Pathologists," in S. M. Lewis and J. F. Coster, eds., *Quality Control in Hematology* (London: Academic Press, 1975), p. 55; R. M. Schmidt, "Control of Diagnostic Hematology Products," in ibid., pp. 182–4; Ralph R. Grams, "Clinical Laboratories: Influence of Increased Productivity and New Laboratory Instruments on Health Care," *South. Med. J.*, vol. 69 (1976), pp. 1397–8.
36 John Laszlo, "Automated 'Chemistries:' A Multiphasic Misadventure," *Arch. Intern. Med.*, vol. 133 (1974), p. 1068. See also George Z. Williams, "Effects of Automation on Laboratory Diagnosis," *Calif. Med.*, vol. 108 (1968), p. 44.
37 J. H. Musser, "The Internist and Radiology," *Radiol.*, vol. 11 (1923), p. 252. See also Ester M. Sunderlöf, "X-Ray Diagnosis and Therapy," *Boston Med. Surg. J.*, vol. 182 (1920), pp. 393–6; George Dock, "X Ray Work from the Viewpoint of an Internist," *Am. J. Radiol.*, vol. 8 (1921), pp. 321–7; Russell D. Carman, "Limitations of Roentgenologic Diagnosis," *N. Y. State J. Med.*, vol. 22 (1922), p. 303; Frank S. Bissell, "Cooperative Diagnosis," *Minn. Med.*, vol. 11 (1928), pp. 792–4.
38 Evarts A. Graham, "Some Functional Tests and Their Significance," *N. Engl. J. Med.* vol. 199 (1928), p. 2. See also Hugh J. Means, "The Uses and Limitations of the X-Ray," *Ohio State Med., J.*, vol. 19 (1923), pp. 792–5; Leopold

Jaches, "Roentgen–Ray Diagnosis,"*J.A.M.A.*, vol. 90 (1928), p. 614; W. Edward Chamberlain, "Radiology as a Medical Specialty," *J.A.M.A.*, vol. 92 (1929), pp. 1033–5.

39 Carl C. Birkelo, et al., "Tuberculosis Case Findings. . . ,"*J.A.M.A.*, vol. 133 (1947), pp. 354–65. For an immediate reaction to the Birkelo study see, "The 'Personal Equation' in the Interpretation of Chest Roentgenogram,"*J.A.M.A.*, vol. 133 (1947), p. 399.

40 L. Henry Garland, "On the Scientific Evaluation of Diagnostic Procedures," *Radiol.*, vol. 52 (1949), p. 312. See also, "Evaluating Roentgenographic Techniques," *Public Health Rep.*, vol. 62 (1947), pp. 1431–2; and Jacob Yerushalmy, "Statistical Problems in Assessing Methods of Medical Diagnosis, with Special Reference to X-Ray Techniques," ibid., pp. 1432–56.

41 E. Groth–Petersen, A. Løvgreen, and J. Thillermann, "On the Reliability of the Reading of Photofluorograms and the Value of Dual Reading," *Acta Tuberc. Scand.*, vol. 26 (1952), pp. 13–37.

42 Henry B. Zwerling, et al., "The Clinical Importance of Lesions Undetected in a Mass Radiographic Survey of the Chest," *Am. Rev. Tuberc.*, vol. 64 (1951), pp. 249–55.

43 A. L. Cochrane and L. Henry Garland, "Observer Error in the Interpretation of Chest Films: An International Investigation," *Lancet*, vol. 2 (1952), pp. 505–9; L. Henry Garland," The Problem of Observer Error,"*Bull. N. Y. Acad. Med.*, vol. 36 (1960), p. 583; William J. Tuddenham, "Problems of Perception in Chest Roentgenology: Facts and Fallacies," *Radiol. Clin. North Am.*, vol. 1 (1963), pp. 277–89.

44 L. G. Davies, "Observer Variation in Reports on Electrocardiograms," *Br. Heart J.*, vol. 20 (1958), pp. 153–61.

45 Robert A. Bruce and Stephen R. Yarnall, "Computer–aided Diagnosis of Cardiovascular Disorders," *J. Chronic Dis.*, vol. 19 (1966), p. 478.

46 *Physical Defects – the Pathway to Correction* (New York: American Child Health Association, 1930), pp. 80–96.

47 C. M. Fletcher, "The Clinical Diagnosis of Pulmonary Emphysema – An Experimental Study,"*Proc. R. Soc. Med.*, vol. 45 (1952), p. 579.

48 J. Scott Butterworth and Edmund H. Reppert, "Auscultatory Acumen in the General Medical Population,"*J.A.M.A.*, vol. 174 (1960), pp. 32–4.

49 A. L. Cochrane, P. J. Chapman, and P. D. Oldham, "Observers Error in Taking Medical Histories,"*Lancet*, vol. 1 (1951), pp. 1007–9.

50 See for example F. William Sunderman, Jr., "Current Concepts of 'Normal Values,' 'Reference Values,' and 'Discrimination Values' in Clinical Chemistry," *Clin. Chem.*, vol. 21 (1975), p. 1873.

51 Thomas J. Scheff, "Decision Rules, Types of Error, and their Consequences in Medical Diagnosis,"*Behav. Sci.*, vol. 8 (1963), pp. 97–107; David E. Rogers, "On Technologic Restraint," *Arch. Intern. Med.*, vol. 135 (1975), p. 1397.

52 Richard Asher, "Clinical Sense: The Use of the Five Senses,"*Br. Med. J.*, vol. 1 (1960), p. 985.

53 R. E. Colman, "Clinical Records, the Laboratory, and the General Practitioner," *Northwest Med.*, vol. 20 (1921), p. 255.

54 L. Henry Garland, "Studies on the Accuracy of Diagnostic Procedures," *Am. J. Roentgenol.*, vol. 82 (1959), pp. 32–5; Peter Stradling and R. N. Johnson, "Reducing Observer Error in a 70–MM. Chest Radiography Service for Gen-

eral Practitioners," *Lancet*, vol. 1 (1955), pp. 1247–50; "Repetition – Often the Price of Accuracy," *J. Indiana Med. Assoc.*, vol. 55 (1962), p. 54.

55 M. L. J. Abercrombie, "The Observer and His Errors," *J. Psychosom. Res.*, vol. 8 (1964–65), pp. 169–75.

56 Garland, "Scientific Evaluation of Diagnostic Procedures," pp. 312–27; I. D. P. Wootton, E. J. King, and J. Maclean Smith, "The Quantitative Approach to Hospital Biochemistry. . . ," *Br. Med. Bull.*, vol. 7 (1951), pp. 307–11.

57 Alvan R. Feinstein, *Clinical Judgment* (Baltimore: Williams & Wilkins, 1967), pp. 4–8, 29, 285–6, 324–34.

58 Lorrin M. Koran, "The Reliability of Clinical Methods, Data and Judgments," *N. Engl. J. Med.*, vol. 293 (1975), p. 700.

59 Garland, "Studies on the Accuracy of Diagnostic Procedures," p. 36.

60 "Observer Error," *Lancet*, vol. 1 (1954), p. 88; C. M. Fletcher, "Observer Error," ibid., p. 212; Davies, "Observer Variation in Reports on Electrocardiograms," p. 159.

CHAPTER 10. TELECOMMUNICATION, AUTOMATION, AND MEDICAL PRACTICE

1 R. T. H. Laennec, *A Treatise on Diseases of the Chest*, trans. John Forbes, 1st ed. (London: T. and G. Underwood, 1821), pp. xix, xxiii, 288; John Bell, "Some general remarks on the use of the Stethoscope, as an aid in forming correct diagnosis of Diseases of the Lungs. . . ," *N.Y. Med. Physical J.*, vol. 3 (1824), pp. 271–3; Lester S. King, "Auscultation in England, 1821–1837," *Bull. Hist. Med.*, vol. 33 (1959), pp. 447–50.

2 Frederic J. Farre, "Clinical Observation," *Lancet*, vol. 2 (1857), p. 409. See also P. M. Latham, "Lectures on Subjects Connected with Clinical Medicine," *Lond. Med. Gaz*, vol. 17 (1835–36), p. 280; Sir William Withey Gull, "Some Guiding Thoughts to the Study of Medicine," in *A Collection of the Published Writings of. . .*, ed. Theodore Dyke Acland (London: New Sydenham Society, 1896), p. 11.

3 James Clark, *Medical Notes on Climate, Diseases, Hospitals, and Medical Schools in France, Italy, and Switzerland. . .*(London: T. and G. Underwood, 1820), pp. 127–8.

4 Eduoard Seguin, *Medical Thermometry and Human Temperature* (New York: William Wood, 1876), pp. 360–1.

5 "The Telephone," *Br. Med. J.*, vol. 2 (1878), p. 43.

6 "The Telephone as a Medium of Consultation and Medical Diagnosis," *Br. Med. J.*, vol. 2 (1879), p. 897.

7 John L. Hildreth, "The General Practitioner and the Specialist," *Boston Med. Surg. J.*, vol. 155 (1906), p. 79. This problem persisted all during the twentieth century, as shown in John Lister, "The Doctor and his Telephone," *N. Engl. J. Med.*, vol. 252 (1955), p. 909.

8 "Consultations by Telegraph," *Lancet*, vol. 1 (1887), p. 230. See also "The Telephone," *J.A.M.A.*, vol. 11 (1888), p. 791.

9 "Some Recent Instruments of Precision," *Med. Surg. Rep.*, vol. 41 (1879), p. 236. See also John G. McKendrick, "Notes on the Microphone and Telephone in Auscultation," *Br. Med. J.*, vol. 1 (1878), p. 856.

10 C. J. Blake, "The Telephone and Microphone in Auscultation," *Boston Med. Surg. J.*, vol. 103 (1880), pp. 486–7.

11 "The Microphone in Diagnosis," *Lancet*, vol. 1 (1878), p. 766; Edward Joseph Eve, "The Microphone as Diagnosticator of the Entire Physical Organism," *Atlanta Med. Surg. J.*, vol. 2 (1885–86), pp. 129–31.

12 Julius Hérisson, *The Sphygmometer, An Instrument which Renders the Action of the Arteries Apparent to the Eye. . .*, trans. E. S. Blundell (London: Longman, Rees, Orme, Brown, Green, and Longman, 1835), p. 14.

13 Somerville Scott Alison, *The Physical Examination of the Chest in Pulmonary Consumption. . .*(London: John Churchill, 1861), pp. 346–7. See also "Sphygmography by Telegraph," *Br. Med. J.*, vol. 2 (1869), pp. 355–6.

14 Seguin, *Medical Thermometry*, pp. 360–1.

15 W. Einthoven, "Le Télécardiogramme,"*Arch. Int. Physiol.*, vol. 4 (1906–07), p. 139 (trans. by S. J. R.).

16 Walter B. James and Horatio B. Williams, "The String Galvanometer and the Electrocardiogram in Health," *Am. J. Med. Sci.*, vol. 140 (1910), p. 413.

17 "A Telephonic Stethoscope," *Sci. Am.*, vol. 102 (1910), pp. 496, 509.

18 J. Gershon-Cohen, et al., "Telediagnosis: Three Years of Experience with Diagnosis by Telephone–Transmitted Roentgenograms,"*J.A.M.A.*, vol. 148 (1952), pp. 731–2.

19 E. Grey Dimond and Fred Berry, "Transmission of Electrocardiograms over Standard Telephone Lines,"*J. Lab. Clin. Med.*, vol. 40 (1952), pp. 792–3.

20 George W. Jackson, C. F. Taylor, and J. L. Morgan, "The Telephone Electrocardiograph: The Practical Application of an Ingenious Device," *J. Kans. Med. Soc.*, vol. 57 (1956), pp. 4–6.

21 Harold M. Schmeck, Jr., "House Call by Computer," *New York Times*, July 9, 1967, Section 4, p. 6E.

22 Kenneth T. Bird, Milton Henry Clifford, and Thomas F. Dwyer, *Teleconsultation: A New Health Information Exchange System, The 03 Annual Report* (Boston: Massachusetts General Hospital, 1971). See also Kenneth T. Bird, "Cardiopulmonary Frontiers: Quality Health Care via Interactive Television," *Chest*, vol. 61 (1972), pp. 204–5; John Noble Wilford, "Distant Diagnosis Over TV Is Demonstrated Publically," *New York Times*, July 9, 1968, p. 78.

23 B. Drummond Ayres, Jr., "Big City Help for Rural Doctor," *New York Times*, April 7, 1971, p. 24. See also Scott I. Allen and Michael Otten, "The Telephone as a Computer Input–Output Terminal for Medical Information," *J.A.M.A.*, vol. 208 (1969), pp. 673–9.

24 Office of Charles and Ray Eames, *A Computer Perspective* (Cambridge: Harvard University Press, 1973), p. 7.

25 Gerry Feigen, "Triple Bromides," *Bull. San Franc. Med. Soc.*, vol. 29, no. 6 (1956), p. 10.

26 Lee B. Lusted, "Computers in Medicine – A Personal Perspective,"*J. Chronic Diseases*, vol. 19 (1966), p. 367.

27 "Resolution Adopted by Conference," *IRE Trans. Med. Electron.*, vol. 7 (1960), p. 316.

28 François Paycha, "Diagnosis, Therapeutics, Prognosis, and Computers," *IRE Trans. Med. Electr.*, vol. 7 (1960), pp. 288–9.

29 Ibid.

30 Stephen E. Goldfinger, "The Problem–Oriented Medical Record: A Critique from a Believer," *N. Engl. J. Med.*, vol. 288 (1973), p. 607.
31 T. S. Eimerl, R. J. C. Pearson, and the Merseyside and North Wales Faculty of the College of General Practitioners, "Working–time in General Practice: How General Practitioners Use Their Time," *Br. Med. J.*, vol. 2 (1966), p. 1551; John Fry and J. B. Dillane, "Too Much Work?" *Lancet*, vol. 2 (1964), p. 633; Henry E. Payson, Eugene C. Gaenslen, and Fred L. Stargardter, "Time Study of an Internship on a University Medical Service," *N. Engl. J. Med.*, vol. 264 (1961), p. 441.
32 Martin Lipkin, et al., "Digital Computer as an Aid to Differential Diagnosis," *Arch. Intern. Med.*, vol. 108 (1961), pp. 56–72; Paycha, "Diagnosis, Therapeutics, Prognosis, and Computers," p. 289.
33 Thomas K. Chambers, "Drill for Auscultation," *Lancet*, vol. 1 (1861), p. 334.
34 Allon Peebles, *A Survey of Medical Facilities of Shelby County, Indiana* (Washington: Committee on the Costs of Medical Care, 1929), p. 35.
35 Osler Peterson, et al., "An Analytic Study of North Carolina General Practice, 1952–1954," *J. Med. Educ.*, vol. 31, Supplement (1956), pp. 46–7.
36 Ibid., p. 24.
37 Helen Clapesattle, *The Doctors Mayo* (Minneapolis: University of Minnesota Press, 1941), p. 385.
38 "Hospital Standardization Series: General Hospitals of 100 or More Beds," *Bull. Am. Coll. Surg.*, vol. 4, no. 4 (1920), p. 5.
39 *Massachusetts General Hospital Acts, Resolves, By-Laws and Rules and Regulations* (Boston: James Loring Press, 1837), Chapter 5, Article 7.
40 James Jackson, Letter of Resignation to the Hospital Board of Trustees, September 30, 1837, Archives of the Massachusetts General Hospital.
42 Byam Hollings, "Record Keeping at the Massachusetts General Hospital," *Mod. Hosp.*, vol. 2 (1914), pp. 94–5. See also Grace Whiting Meyers, "Care of Hospital Records According to the Method of the Massachusetts General Hospital, Boston, Mass.," *Int. Hosp. Rec.*, vol. 15 (1911), pp. 18–19.
42 The comments about the contents of the Massachusetts General Hospital records that follow are based on the author's examination of them.
43 *Massachusetts General Hospital East Clinical Records*, vol. 381 (1885), p. 229. As early as 1861, there is a suggestion in the medical literaature that doctors draw rough outlines of the chest on their clinical records to denote the location of lesions (Chambers, "Drill for Auscultation," pp. 333–4).
44 "Standard of Efficiency: First Hospital Survey of the College," *Bull. Am. Coll. Surg.*, vol. 3, no. 3 (1918), pp. 1–4; Eugene S. Kilgore, "Clinical Records in Relation to Teaching and Research – A Plan to Promote Conservation and Utilization of Material," *Boston Med. Surg. J.*, vol. 173 (1915), p. 767; E. A. Codman, "The Value of Case Records in Hospitals," *Mod. Hosp.*, vol. 9 (1917), pp. 426–8.
45 Raymond Pearl, "Modern Methods in Handling Hospital Statistics," *Bull. Johns Hopkins Hosp.*, vol. 32 (1921), p. 187. See also Halbert L. Dunn and Reed Rockwood, "A Record System Suitable for Both Clinical and Statistical Medicine," *Arch. Intern. Med.*, vol. 41 (1928), pp. 499–501; J. Lerman and J. H. Means, "The Use of Record Forms and Mechanical Methods of Analysis in the Study of Clinical Data," *N. Engl. J. Med.*, vol. 208 (1933), pp. 1135–43.
46 Pearl, "Modern Methods in Handling Hospital Statistics," pp. 187–8.

47 George Blumer, "History Taking," *Conn. State Med. J.*, vol. 13 (1949), pp. 450–1.
48 Clapesattle, *The Doctors Mayo*, pp. 522–3.
49 H. Auchincloss, "The Unit History System," *Med. Surg. Rep. Presbyt. Hosp. N.Y.*, vol. 10 (1918), pp. 30–73.
50 Dorothy L. Kurtz, *Unit Medical Records In Hospital and Clinic* (New York: Columbia University Press, 1943), p. 5. For an examination of a new concept for structuring the medical record according to the problems of the patient, see Lawrence L. Weed, "Medical Records that Guide and Teach," *N. Engl. J. Med.*, vol. 278 (1968), pp. 593–9, 652–7.
51 F. A. Nash, "The Mechanical Conservation of Experience, Especially in Medicine," *IRE Trans. Med. Electr.*, vol. 7 (1960), p. 240. See also "Devices for Diagnosis," *Ann. Intern. Med.*, vol 55 (1961), pp. 702–3.
52 F. A. Nash, "Diagnostic Reasoning and the Logoscope," *Lancet*, vol. 2 (1960), p. 1443.
53 Martin Lipkin and James D. Hardy, "Mechanical Correlation of Data in Differential Diagnosis of Hematological Diseases," *J.A.M.A.*, vol. 166 (1958), pp. 113–25.
54 R. Ebald and R. Lane, "Digital Computers and Medical Logic," *IRE Trans. Med. Electr.*, vol. 7 (1960), pp. 286–8; Keeve Brodman, "Diagnostic Decisions by Machine," *IRE Trans. Med. Electr.*, vol. 7 (1960), pp. 216–19; R. Gross, "From Intuition to Computation: Development and problems of medical diagnosis," *Methods Inf. Med.*, vol. 5 (1966), pp. 35–9; Katherine O. Elsom, et al., "Physicians' Use of Objective Data in Clinical Diagnoses," *J.A.M.A.*, vol. 201 (1967), pp. 519–26.
55 Robert S. Ledley, "Using Electronic Computers in Medical Diagnosis," *IRE Trans. Med. Electr.*, vol. 7 (1960), p. 279.
56 "Implications of Computer Technology on the Future Development of Clinical Medicine," *Gastroenterolog.* vol. 50 (1966), p. 450; G. Octo Barnett, "Computers in Patient Care," *N. Engl. J. Med.*, vol. 279 (1968), p. 1322.
57 Jordan J. Baruch, "Doctor-Machine Symbiosis," *IRE Trans. Med. Electr.*, vol. 7 (1960), pp. 290–3; Theodore D. Sterling, James Nickson, and Seymour V. Pollack, "Is Medical Diagnosis a General Computer Problem?" *J.A.M.A.*, vol. 198 (1966), pp. 281–6.
58 Lee B. Lusted, "Diagnostic Video Data Processing," *IRE Trans. Med. Electr.*, vol. 7 (1960), p. 293.
59 "Radiology Clinical Science Most Susceptible to Computerization," *Hosp. Trib.*, vol. 6 (February 16, 1972), pp. 1, 18. See also Gwilym S. Lodwick, Theodore E. Keats, and John P. Dorst, "The Coding of Roentgen Images for Computer Analysis as Applied to Lung Cancer," *Radiol.*, vol. 81 (1963), pp. 185–200.
60 Arthur L. Klatsky, et al., "Auscultation of the Adult Heart by Machine," *N. Engl. J. Med.*, vol. 279 (1968), p. 230. See also Charles E. Kossmann, "Electrocardiographic Analysis by Computer," *J.A.M.A.*, vol. 191 (1965), pp. 922–4.
61 K. Brodman, et al., "The Cornell Medical Index: An Adjunct to Medical Interview," *J.A.M.A.*, vol. 140 (1949), pp. 530–4.
62 Warner V. Slack, et al., "A Computer-Based Medical-History System," *N. Engl. J. Med.*, vol. 274 (1966), p. 197.

63 "On the History and Physical Examination of the Patient," *Med. Times*, vol. 89 (1962), pp. 1112–15; John G. Mayne, William Weksel, Paul N. Sholtz, "Towards Automating the Medical History," *Mayo Clin. Proc.*, vol. 43 (1968), p. 1; Donald W. Simborg, Arthur E. Rikli, and Paul Hall, "Experimentation in Medical History–Taking," *J.A.M.A.*, vol. 210 (1969), pp. 1443–5; Richard Stillman, et al., "An On Line Computer System for Initial Psychiatric Inventory," *Am. J. Psychiatr.*, vol. 125, supplement (1969), pp. 8–11.

64 Allen G. Brailey, Jr., "Anti–Amnesis–by–Computer," *N. Engl. J. Med.*, vol. 280 (1969), p. 1186; J. A. V. Bates, "Preparation of Clinical Data for Computers, *Br. Med. Bull.*, vol. 24 (1968), pp. 199–205; Alvan R. Feinstein, *Clinical Judgment* (Baltimore: Williams & Wilkins, 1967), p. 299; Howard P. Lewis, "Reflections from Our Mirrors," *Ann. Intern. Med.*, vol. 53 (1960), p. 1205.

65 Isaac W. Brewer, "The Physical Condition of American Men of Military Age," *N.Y. Med. J.*, vol. 107 (1918), pp. 216–17; C. E. Yount, "The American Youth as Mirrored by the World War: Some Timely Lessons," *Southwest. Med.*, vol. 4 (1920), p. 18.

66 James A. Tobey, "The Health Examination Movement," *The Nation's Health*, vol. 5 (1923), p. 611.

67 Ibid., p. 648.

68 Haven Emerson, "The Protection of Health through Periodic Medical Examinations," *J. Mich. Med. Soc.*, vol. 21 (1922), p. 399.

69 "Precautionary X–Rays," *Boston Med. Surg. J.*, vol. 167 (1912), pp. 560–1.

70 C. Kelly Canelo, et al., "A Multiphasic Screening Survey in San Jose," *Calif. Med.*, vol. 71 (1949), pp. 409–13; A. L. Chapman, "The Concept of Multiphasic Screening," *Public Health Rep.*, vol. 64 (1949), pp. 1311–14; Lester Breslow, "Multiphasic Screening Examinations – An Extension of the Mass Screening Technique," *Am. J. Public Health*, vol. 40 (1950), pp. 274–8.

71 Morris F. Collin, "Automated Multiphasic Screening and Diagnosis," *Am. J. Public Health*, vol. 54 (1964), pp. 741–3; Morris F. Collin, "Value of Multiphasic Health Checkups," *N. Engl. J. Med.*, vol. 280 (1969), pp. 1072–3; Sidney Garfield, "The Delivery of Medical Care," *Sci. Am.*, vol. 222 (1970), pp. 15–23.

72 Sir James F. Goodhart, "The Passing of Morbid Anatomy," *Lancet*, vol. 2 (1912), p. 1130.

73 Sir Henry Dale, "Some Epochs in Medical Research," *Lancet*, vol. 2 (1935), p. 931.

74 Karl T. Compton, "Possibilities in Biological Engineering," *Ann. Intern. Med.*, vol. 12 (1938), p. 870.

75 Hans Berger's first publication of his work on the electroencephalogram is "Ueber das Elektroenkephalogramm des Menschen," *Arch. Psychiatr. Nervenkr.*, vol. 87 (1929), pp. 527–70. The early diagnostic uses of this are well discussed in W. Grey Walter, "The Technique and Application of Electro–encephalography," *J. Neurol. Psychiatr.*, vol. 1 (1938), pp. 359–85; Frederick A. Gibbs, "Diagnostic and Prognostic Value of the Electroencephalogram," *J.A.M.A.*, vol. 118 (1942), pp. 216–19; Frederick A. Gibbs, "Electroencephalography," *Am. J. Psychiatr.*, vol. 101 (1944–45), pp. 530–3.

76 Sidney Licht, *Electrodiagnosis and Electromyography* (Baltimore: Elizabeth Licht, 1956), pp. 15–18.

77 George Hevesy, "The Absorption and Translocation of Lead by Plants: A

Contribution to the Application of the Method of Radioactive Indicators in the Investigation of the Change of Substance in Plants," *Biochem. J.*, vol. 17 (1923), pp. 439–45. Hevesy has written on the history of the subject in "Some Historical Remarks on the Application of Radioactive Indicators," *Cardiol.*, vol. 21 (1952), pp. 226–32. An excellent review article of early medical uses of radioactive isotopes is John Ross, "Artificial Radioactive Isotopes in Biology and Medicine," *N. Engl. J. Med.*, vol. 226 (1942), pp. 854–60. An informative post–World War II editorial is "Atom Bomb and Medical Research," *N. Engl. J. Med.*, vol. 235 (1946), pp. 342–3. A valuable book about later developments is John H. Lawrence, Bernard Manowitz, and Benjamin S. Loeb, *Radioisotopes and Radiation* (New York: McGraw-Hill, 1964).

78 Lee Lusted, "Medical Electronics," *N. Engl. J. Med.*, vol. 252 (1955), pp. 580–1; Kurt S. Lion, "Technology and Medicine," *Arch. Phys. Med.*, vol. 27 (1946), pp. 279–84.

79 Ralph W. Alman and Joseph F. Fazekas, "Apparatus for Continuous Blood Pressure Observation," *N. Engl. J. Med.*, vol. 248 (1953), pp. 105–7.

80 George Radcliffe, "The Necessity of Physiological Monitoring in the General Hospital," *Trans. N. Y. Acad. Sci.*, vol. 23 (1960–61), p. 52. See also George Godber, "Measurement and Mechanization in Medicine," *Lancet*, vol. 2 (1964), p. 1193; David D. Rutstein and Murray Eden, *Engineering and Living Systems: Interfaces and Opportunities* (Cambridge: M.I.T. Press, 1970), pp. 99–102.

81 Philip A. Smith, "Some Problems and Approaches to Automation of Medical Diagnosis," *Behav. Sci.*, vol. 6 (1961), pp. 88–9; John S. Hanson and Burton S. Tabakin, "Electrocardiographic Telemetry in Skiers," *N. Engl. J. Med.*, vol. 271 (1964), pp. 181–5; Charles C. Norland and Herbert J. Semler, "Angina Pectoris and Arrhythmias Documented by Cardiac Telemetry," *J.A.M.A.*, vol. 190 (1964), pp. 115–18.

82 G. Douglas Talbott, "Computers in Cardiology – A Look Towards the Future," *Ohio State Med. J.*, vol. 62 (1966), pp. 897–8; Robert A. Bruce and Stephen Yarnall, "Computer–Aided Diagnosis of Cardiovascular Disorders," *J. Chronic Diseases*, vol. 19 (1966), pp. 479–81; Thomas C. Gibson, et al., "Telecardiography and the Use of Simple Computers," *N. Engl. J. Med.*, vol. 267 (1962), pp. 1218–24.

83 Bernard S. Bloom and Osler L. Peterson, "End Results, Cost and Productivity of Coronary Care Units," *N. Engl. J. Med.*, vol. 288 (1973), pp. 72–8; Thomas P. Hackett, N. H. Cassem, and Howard A. Wishnie, "The Coronary Care Unit: An Appraisal of its Psychologic Hazards," *N. Engl. J. Med.*, vol. 279 (1968), p. 1368; F. Patrick McKegney, "The Intensive Care Syndrome. . .," *Conn. Med.*, vol. 30 (1966), pp. 633–6; "Monitoring Fever," *Biomed. Eng.*, vol. 4 (1969), p. 259; J. M. Rawls, "Patient Monitoring: A Clinician's Point of View," *Biomed. Eng.*, vol. 4 (1969), pp. 264–7.

84 Rosemary Stevens, *American Medicine and The Public Interest* (New Haven: Yale University Press, 1971), p. 420.

85 Fry and Dillane, "Too Much Work?" pp. 632–4; Mardoqueo I. Salomon, "Medical Assistants or Quasi–Physicians," *N. Engl. J. Med.*, vol. 277 (1967), p. 1373; Garfield, "The Delivery of Medical Care," p. 20; Frederick J. Moore, "The Need for New Technologies to Offset the Shortage of Physicians," *Arch. Intern. Med.*, vol. 125 (1970), p. 355; Eugene A. Stead, "Conserving Costly Talents – Providing Physicians' New Assistants," *J.A.M.A.*, vol. 198 (1966),

pp. 1108–9; William B. Schwartz, "Medicine and the Computer," *N. Engl. J. Med.*, vol. 283 (1970), p. 1258.

86 See for expressions of this belief Leonard A. Walker, "Frontiers of Medicine II. Electronic Computers in Medicine," *Northwest Med.*, vol. 59 (1960), p. 658; Gross, "From Intuition to Computation," p. 38; Bernard V. Dryer, "Thinking Men and Thinking Machines in Medicine," *J. Med. Educ.*, vol. 38 (1963), p. 88; Garfield, "The Delivery of Medical Care," p. 23; Schwartz, "Medicine and the Computer," p. 1258.

87 Richard M. Bailey, "Economies of Scale in Outpatient Medical Practice," *Group Pract.*, vol. 17 (1968), pp. 24–33.

88 Lee B. Lusted, "Computer Programming of Diagnostic Tests," *IRE Trans. Med. Electr.*, vol. 7 (1960), p. 255. See also Sir George Godber, "Measurement and Mechanisation in Medicine," *Lancet*, vol. 2 (1964), p. 1193.

89 John H. Houck, "We Need to Restore these Pioneer Efforts," *Am. J. Psychiatr.*, vol. 125, supplement (1969), p. 33; James V. Maloney and Gilbert Bradham, "Computers in Medicine," *Annu. Rev. Med.*, vol. 16 (1965), pp. 249–50. A major effort to bridge the barriers between engineers and physical scientists and physicians occurred in 1971 when Harvard Medical School and the Massachusetts Institute of Technology began a cooperative program to jointly train medical students during the first two years of the medical curriculum.

90 "Medical Manners," *Br. Med. J.*, vol. 2 (1963), p. 128. See also Bernard S. Linn, "Statistics, Computers, and Clinical Judgment," *Lancet*, vol. 2 (1969), p. 48; Carl Binger, *The Two Faces of Medicine* (New York: Norton, 1967), p. 19; George W. Pickering, "Manners Makyth Man: A Plea for the Importance of Character in Medicine," *Br. Med. J.*, vol. 2 (1963), p. 133.

91 Feinstein, *Clinical Judgment*, p. 379. See also H. P. Rome, "Human Factors and Technical Difficulties in the Application of Computers to Medicine," in Nathan S. Kline and Eugene Laska, eds., *Computers and Electronic Devices in Psychiatry* (New York: Grune and Stratton, 1968), pp. 41–2; Maloney and Bradham, "Computers in Medicine," p. 249.

92 "Machine–Made Diagnoses," *Br. Med. J.*, vol. 1 (1895), p. 36.

93 "Computers and Medicine," *Ann. Intern. Med.*, vol. 70 (1969), p. 653. See also "Computers in Medicine," *Can. Med. Assoc., J.*, vol. 100 (1969), p. 393.

94 "Dialogue of Tomorrow," *Lancet*, vol. 1 (1960), p. 1022.

95 Alvan G. Foraker, "The End of an Era," *N. Engl. J. Med.*, vol. 272 (1965), p. 37.

96 "Medical Judgment – The Master Computer," *N. Y. State J. Med.*, vol. 68 (1968), pp. 739–40.

97 Jerrold S. Maxmen, *The Post–Physician Era: Medicine in the Twenty-First Century* (New York: Wiley, 1976), pp. 7, 282.

98 Albert H. Schwictenberg, "What about the Future?" *J.A.M.A.*, vol. 191 (1965), p. 928.

99 Feinstein, *Clinical Judgment*, pp. 369–70.

Bibliography

This bibliography is divided into sections according to subject matter. I have not included all of the material examined in preparing this book. In making the necessary choice among publications, I have tried to cite those that provide a broad background, as well as some of the most important sources already given in the notes.

GENERAL REFERENCES

Derry, T. K., and Williams, Trevor I. *A Short History of Technology*. Oxford: Oxford University Press, 1961.
Ellul, Jacques. *The Technological Society*. New York: Knopf, 1967.
Garrison, Fielding H. *An Introduction to the History of Medicine*. 4th ed., 1929. Reprint, Philadelphia: Saunders, 1966.
Kranzberg, Melvin, and Pursell, Carroll W., Jr. *Technology in Western Civilization*. 2 vols. New York: Oxford University Press, 1967.
McLuhan, Marshall. *Understanding Media: The Extensions of Man*. New York: McGraw–Hill, 1965.
Morton, Leslie T. *Garrison and Morton's Medical Bibliography*. 2nd ed. New York: Argosy, 1965.
O'Malley, C. D., ed. *The History of Medical Education*. Berkeley: University of California Press, 1970.
Singer, Charles, and Underwood, E. Ashworth. *A Short History of Medicine*. Oxford: Oxford University Press, 1962.
Skinner, Henry Alan. *The Origin of Medical Terms*. Baltimore: Williams & Wilkins, 1961.

COMPUTER AND AUTOMATED DIAGNOSIS

Amlinger, P. R. "Biotelemetry and Computer Analysis of Electrocardiograms." *Methods of Information in Medicine*, vol. 8 (1969), pp. 120–7.
Barnett, G. Octo. "Computers in Patient Care." *New England Journal of Medicine*, vol. 279 (1968), pp. 1321–7.
Boyle, J. A., and Anderson, J. A. "Computer Diagnosis: Clinical Aspects." *British Medical Bulletin*, vol. 24 (1968), pp. 224–9.
Brodman, Keeve, et al. "Interpretation of Symptoms with a Data–Processing Machine." *Archives of Internal Medicine*, vol. 103 (1959), pp. 776–82.
Bruce, Robert A., and Yarnall, Stephen R. "Computer–Aided Diagnosis of Cardiovascular Disorders." *Journal of Chronic Diseases*, vol. 19 (1966), pp. 473–84.
Caceres, C. A. "Will we lose our practice to a computer?" *Medical Instrumentation*, vol. 8 (1974), pp. 311–12.
Caceres, C. A., and Ayers, W. R. "Health Testing with Automated Techniques."

Bibliography

Bulletin of the New York Academy of Medicine, vol. 45 (1969), pp. 1277–87.

"Conference on Diagnostic Data Processing." *IRE Transactions on Medical Electronics*, vol. 7 (1960), pp. 232–317. [An important conference with many valuable papers presented.]

Cooper, James K., et al. "Role of a Digital Computer in a Diagnostic Center." *Journal of the American Medical Association*, vol. 193 (1965), pp. 911–15.

Gross, R. "From Intuition to Computation. Development and problems of medical diagnosis." *Methods of Information in Medicine*, vol. 5 (1966), pp. 35–9.

Ingram, Marylou, and Preston, Kendall, Jr. "Automatic Analysis of Blood Cells." *Scientific American*, vol. 223 (1970), pp. 72–82.

Johnson, David L., and Kobler, Arthur L. "The Man–Computer Relationship." *Science*, vol. 138 (1963), pp. 873–9.

Ledley, Robert S., and Lusted, Lee B. "Reasoning Foundations of Medical Diagnosis." *Science*, vol. 130 (1959), pp. 9–21.

Lodwick, Gwilym S., et al. "Computer–Aided Analysis of Radiographic Images." *Journal of Chronic Diseases*, vol. 19 (1966), pp. 485–96.

Lusted, Lee B. "Computer Techniques in Medical Diagnosis." In *Computers in Biomedical Research*, ed. Ralph W. Stacy and Bruce D. Waxman, vol. 1, pp. 319–38. New York: Academic Press, 1965.

Maxmen, Jerrold S. *The Post-Physician Era.* New York: Wiley, 1976.

Mayne, John G., Weksel, William, and Sholtz, Paul N. "Toward Automating the Medical History." *Mayo Clinic Proceedings*, vol. 43 (1968), pp. 1–25.

Payne, L. C. "The Basic Principles and Brief History of Computer Technology," *British Medical Bulletin*, vol. 24 (1968), pp. 189–93.

Rawles, J. M. "Patient Monitoring: A Clinician's Point of View." *Bio–Medical Engineering*, vol. 4 (1969), pp. 264–7.

Rome, H. P. "Microsociology of Automation: Medical Sector." *Methods of Information in Medicine*, vol. 5 (1966), pp. 161–7.

Scadding, J. G. "Diagnosis: The Clinician and the Computer." *Lancet*, vol. 2 (1967), pp. 877–82.

Schwartz, William B. "Medicine and the Computer: The Promise and Problems of Change." *New England Journal of Medicine*, vol. 283 (1970), pp. 1257–64.

Slack, Warner V., et al. "A Computer–Based Medical–History System." *New England Journal of Medicine*, vol. 274 (1966), pp. 194–8.

"A Computer–Based Physical Examination System." *Journal of the American Medical Association*, vol. 200 (1967), pp. 224–8.

Spencer, William A., et al. "The Impact of Electronics on Medicine." *Postgraduate Medicine*, vol. 36 (1964), pp. 291–6, 516–23.

Starkweather, J. A., Kamp, M., and Monto, A. "Psychiatric Interview Simulation by Computer." *Methods of Information in Medicine*, vol. 6 (1967), pp. 15–23.

Stern, R. B., Knill-Jones, R. P., and Williams, R. "Clinician Versus Computer in the Choice of 11 Different Diagnoses of Jaundice Based on Formalised Data." *Methods of Information in Medicine*, vol. 13 (1974), pp. 79–82.

CONCEPTS AND CLASSIFICATION OF DISEASE

Aitken, William. "On the Progress of Scientific Pathology." *British Medical Journal*, vol. 2 (1888), pp. 348–59.

Bichat, Xavier. *General Anatomy, applied to physiology and medicine.* Translated by George Hayward. Boston: Richardson and Lord, 1822.

Bruce, J. Mitchell. "The Dominance of Etiology in Modern Medicine." *British Medical Journal*, vol. 2 (1910), pp. 246–51.

Buchanan, Scott. *The Doctrine of Signatures: A Defense of Theory in Medicine.* London: Kegan, Paul, Trench, Trubner & Co., 1938.

Dewhurst, Kenneth. "Locke and Sydenham on the Teaching of Anatomy." *Medical History*, vol. 2 (1958), pp. 1–12.

Engel, George L. "A Unified Concept of Health and Disease." *Perspectives in Biology and Medicine*, vol. 3 (1960), pp. 459–85.

Faber, Knud. "Nosography in Modern Internal Medicine." *Annals of Medical History*, vol. 4 (1922), pp. 1–63.

Foster, Michael. "Relations of Physiology and Pathology. – The Professional Aspect of Physiology." *British Medical Journal*, vol. 2 (1880), pp. 285–9.

Foucault, Michel. *The Birth of the Clinic: An Archeology of Medical Perception.* Translated by A. M. Sheridan Smith. New York: Pantheon Books, 1973.

Gairdner, W. T. "The Progress of Pathology." *British Medical Journal*, vol. 2 (1874), pp. 515–17.

Gant, F. J. "What Has Pathological Anatomy Done for Medicine and Surgery?" *Lancet*, vol. 2 (1857), pp. 239–42, 262–5, 335–6, 359–60, 385–7, 411–13, 437–9, 463–5, 491–3.

Goodhart, James F. "The Passing of Morbid Anatomy." *Lancet*, vol. 2 (1912), pp. 1129–33.

Greenfield, W. S. "Pathology, Past and Present." *British Medical Journal*, vol. 2 (1881), pp. 695–8, 731–4.

Jackson, J. B. S. "Morbid Anatomy." *Medical Communications of the Massachusetts Medical Society*, vol. 8 (1854), pp. 201–32.

Jarcho, Saul. "Morgagni and Auenbrugger in the Retrospect of Two Hundred Years." *Bulletin of the History of Medicine*, vol. 35 (1961), pp. 489–96.

King, Lester S. "Boissier de Sauvages and 18th Century Nosology." *Bulletin of the History of Medicine*, vol. 40 (1966), pp. 43–51.

The Growth of Medical Thought. Chicago: University of Chicago Press, 1963.

Klemperer, Paul. "Pathologic Anatomy at the End of the Eighteenth Century." *Journal of Mt. Sinai Hospital*, vol. 24 (1957), pp. 589–603.

"The Pathology of Morgagni and Virchow." *Bulletin of the History of Medicine*, vol. 32 (1958), pp. 24–38.

Krumbhaar, E. B. *Pathology.* 1937. Reprint, New York: Macmillan (Hafner Press), 1962.

Lewis, Thomas. "The Relation of Physiology to Medicine." *British Medical Journal*, vol. 2 (1920), pp. 459–62.

Long, Esmond R. *A History of Pathology.* New York: Dover, 1965.

Lush, Brandon, ed. *Concepts of Medicine.* New York: Pergamon Press, 1961.

McMenemey, W. H. "Cellular Pathology, with Special Reference to the Influence of Virchow's Teachings on Medical Thought and Practice." In *Medicine and Science in the 1860s*, ed. F. N. L. Poynter, pp. 13–44. London: Wellcome Institute of the History of Medicine, 1968.

Menninger, Karl. "Changing Concepts of Disease." *Annals of Internal Medicine*, vol. 29 (1948), pp. 318–25.

Morgagni, J. B. *The Seats and Causes of Diseases Investigated by Anatomy.* Translated by Benjamin Alexander, with a Preface, Introduction and a new translation of five letters by Paul Klemperer. 1769. Facsimile, New York: Macmillan (Hafner Press), 1960.

Pagel, Walter. *Paracelsus: An Introduction to Philosophical Medicine in the Era of the Renaissance.* Basel: S. Karger, 1958.

Rather, L. J. "Towards a Philosophical Study of the Idea of Disease." In *The Historical Development of Physiological Thought,* ed. Chandler McC. Brooks and Paul F. Cranefield, pp. 351–73. New York: Macmillan (Hafner Press), 1959.

Robson, A. W. Mayo. "The Position of Pathology with Regard to Clinical Diagnosis." *British Medical Journal,* vol. 1 (1906), pp. 601–5.

Seguin, C. Alberto. "The Concept of Disease." *Psychosomatic Medicine,* vol. 8 (1946), pp. 252–7.

Shryock, Richard Harrison. "The Interplay of Social and Internal Factors in the History of Modern Medicine." *Scientific Monthly,* vols. 76–7 (1953), pp. 221–30.

Snapper, I. *Meditations on Medicine and Medical Education: Past and Present.* New York: Grune and Stratton, 1956.

Sydenham, Thomas. *Medical Observations concerning the History and the Cure of Acute Diseases. The Works of Thomas Sydenham, M.D.* 2 vols. Translated from the Latin by R. G. Latham. London: Sydenham Society, 1848–50.

Temkin, Owsei. "The Role of Surgery in the Rise of Modern Medical Thought." *Bulletin of the History of Medicine,* vol. 25 (1951), pp. 248–59.

Vallee, Bert L., and Wacker, Warren E. C. "Medical Biology: A Perspective." *Journal of the American Medical Association,* vol. 184 (1963), pp. 485–9.

Virchow, Rudolf. *Cellular Pathology as based upon Physiological and Pathological Histology.* Translated from the 2nd edition of the original by Frank Chance. London: John Churchill, 1860.

"The Influence of Morgagni on Anatomical Thought." Translated by Madame L. Wolffsohn. *Lancet,* vol. 1 (1894), pp. 843–6.

"The Position of Pathology among the Biological Studies." *British Medical Journal,* vol. 1 (1893), pp. 561–5.

Williams, Thomas. "On the Pathology of Cells." *Guy's Hospital Reports,* vol. 1 (1843), pp. 423–61.

Wolfe, David E. "Sydenham and Locke on the Limits of Anatomy." *Bulletin of the History of Medicine,* vol. 35 (1961), pp. 193–220.

DIAGNOSIS AND THE PRACTICE OF MEDICINE

Adam, John. "Medical Diagnosis and Modern Discoveries." *British Medical Journal,* vol. 1 (1902), pp. 499–502.

Aitken, William. *The Science and Practice of Medicine,* 2 vols. 5th ed. London: Griffin, 1868.

Alvarez, Walter C. "The Neglected Art of Diagnosis by Eye and Ear." *Geriatrics,* vol. 12 (1957), pp. 542–8.

Asher, Richard. "Clinical Sense: The Use of the Five Senses." *British Medical Journal,* vol. 1 (1960), pp. 985–93.

Balint, Michael. *The Doctor, His Patient and the Illness.* 2nd ed. London: Pitman, 1964.

Barker, Lewellys F. "The Development of the Science of Diagnosis." *Journal of the South Carolina Medical Association*, vol. 12 (1917), pp. 278–84.

Barr, David P. "Hazards of Modern Diagnosis and Therapy – The Price We Pay." *Journal of the American Medical Association*, vol. 159 (1955), pp. 1452–6.

"The Responsibilities of the Internist." *Annals of Internal Medicine*, vol. 27 (1947), pp. 195–201.

Bates, Everett A. "Some Perplexities in Modern Medicine." *Boston Medical and Surgical Journal*, vol. 172 (1915), pp. 843–51.

Berne, Eric. "The Nature of Intuition." *Psychiatric Quarterly*, vol. 23 (1949), pp. 203–26.

Blumer, George. "On the Importance of Observation and Induction in Diagnosis." *Rhode Island Medical Journal*, vol. 18 (1935), pp. 20–7.

"Some Discursive Remarks on Bedside Diagnosis." *Yale Journal of Biology and Medicine*, vol. 6 (1933–34), pp. 571–81.

Brown, Lawrason. *The Story of Clinical Pulmonary Tuberculosis*. Baltimore: Williams & Wilkins, 1941.

Brunton, T. Lauder. "The Method of Zadig in Medicine." *Lancet*, vol. 1 (1892), pp. 3–7.

Cabot, Richard C. "The Ideal of Accuracy in Clinical Work: Its Importance, Its Limitations." *Boston Medical and Surgical Journal*, vol. 151 (1904), pp. 557–60.

Social Service and the Art of Healing. New York: Moffat, Yard and Company, 1909.

Campbell, C. Macfie. "Psychiatry and the Practice of Medicine." *Boston Medical and Surgical Journal*, vol. 190 (1924), pp. 1053–61.

Christian, Henry A., ed. *The Oxford Medicine by Various Authors*, vol. 1, part 1. New York: Oxford University Press, 1949.

Clendinning, John. "Clinical Lectures on the Examination of the Sick . . ." *London Medical Gazette*, vol. 1 (1839–40), pp. 711–18.

Crombie, D. L. "Diagnostic Process." *Journal of the College of General Practitioners*, vol. 6 (1963), pp. 579–89.

Crookshank, F. G. "The Theory of Diagnosis." *Lancet*, vol. 2 (1926), pp. 939–42, 995–9.

Cushing, Harvey. "The Physician and the Surgeon." *Boston Medical and Surgical Journal*, vol. 187 (1922), pp. 623–30.

Draper, George. "Disease: A Psychosomatic Reaction." *Journal of the American Medical Association*, vol. 90 (1928), pp. 1281–5.

Dudley, H. A. F. "The Clinical Task." *Lancet*, vol. 2 (1970), pp. 1352–4.

Elliotson, John. *The Principles and Practice of Medicine; Founded on the Most Extensive Experience in Public Hospitals and Private Practice; and Developed in a Course of Lectures, Delivered at University College, London*. London: Joseph Butler, 1839.

Elsom, Katharine O., et al. "Physicians' Use of Objective Data in Clinical Diagnoses." *Journal of the American Medical Association*, vol. 201 (1967), pp. 519–26.

Engle, Ralph L., Jr., and Davis, B. J. "Medical Diagnosis: Present, Past, and Future." *Archives of Internal Medicine*, vol. 112 (1963), pp. 512–43.

Erikson, Erik H. "The Nature of Clinical Evidence." *Daedalus*, vol. 87 (Fall 1958), pp. 65–87.

Feinstein, Alvan R. *Clinical Judgment*. Baltimore: Williams and Wilkins, 1967.

Fidler, Antony. *Whither Medicine: From Dogma to Science?* London: Thomas Nelson, 1946.

Bibliography

Foster, Balthazar. *Method and Medicine. An Essay.* London: John Churchill and Sons, 1870.

Galdston, Iago. "Diagnosis in Historical Perspective." *Bulletin of the History of Medicine,* vol. 9 (1941), pp. 367–84.

Hall, Marshall. *An Essay on the Symptoms and History of Diseases; considered chiefly in their relation to diagnosis.* London: Longman, Hurst, Rees, Orme, and Brown, 1822.

"On Diagnosis." *Edinburgh Medical and Surgical Journal,* vol. 14 (1818), pp. 236–42.

Hemmeter, John C. "Science and Art in Medicine. Their Influence on the Development of Medical Thinking." *Journal of the American Medical Association,* vol. 46 (1906), pp. 243–8.

Herrick, James B. "Some Features of Present Day Diagnosis." *Journal of the American Medical Association,* vol. 111 (1938), pp. 981–90.

Holt, L. Emmett. "Medical Tendencies and Medical Ideals." *Journal of the American Medical Association,* vol. 48 (1907), pp. 845–9.

Horder, Lord, Thomas Jeeves. "Clinical Medicine: A Farewell Lecture." *Lancet,* vol. 1 (1936), pp. 179–82.

Houston, W. R. "Diagnosis: Purpose and Scope." *International Clinics,* vol. 1 (1937), pp. 232–49.

Jacquez, John A., ed. *The Diagnostic Process.* Ann Arbor: University of Michigan Press, 1963.

Keele, Kenneth D. *The Evolution of Clinical Methods in Medicine.* Springfield: Thomas, 1963.

Lain Entralgo, Pedro. *Doctor and Patient.* New York: McGraw-Hill, 1969.

Latham, P. M. *Lectures on subjects connected with clinical medicine.* London: Longman, Rees, Orme, Brown, Green, and Longman, 1836.

Laycock, Thomas. "The Physiognomical Diagnosis of Disease." *Medical Times and Gazette,* vol. 1 (1862), pp. 1–3, 51–4, 101–3, 151–4, 185, 205–8, 287–9, 341–4, 449–51, 551–4, 635–7.

Lehmann, Heinz E. "Empathy and Perspective or Consensus and Automation? Implications of the New Deal in Psychiatric Diagnosis." *Comprehensive Psychiatry,* vol. 8 (1967), pp. 265–76.

Lewin, Bertram D. "Counter–Transference in the Technique of Medical Practice." *Psychosomatic Medicine,* vol. 8 (1946), pp. 195–9.

Lindsay, James Alexander. "The Art of Observing." *Lancet,* vol. 2 (1889), pp. 1102–5.

Louis, P. Ch. A. *An Essay on Clinical Instruction.* London: S. Highley, 1834.

Mackenzie, James. *The Future of Medicine.* London: Oxford University Press, 1919.
Symptoms and Their Interpretations. London: Shaw & Sons, 1920.

Maes, Urban. "The Lost Art of Clinical Diagnosis." *American Journal of Surgery,* vol. 82 (1951), pp. 107–10.

Meador, Clifton K. "The Art and Science of Nondisease." *New England Journal of Medicine,* vol. 272 (1965), pp. 92–5.

Meehl, Paul E. "Wanted – A Good Cookbook." *American Psychologist,* vol. 11 (1956), pp. 263–72.

Menninger, Karl. *The Vital Balance: The Life Process in Mental Health and Illness.* New York: Viking Press, 1963.

Miller, Sydney R. "Contemporary Fads and Fallacies, Therapeutic and Diagnostic, which Reflect Dangerous Professional Credulity." *Pennsylvania Medical Journal*, vol. 35 (1932), pp. 347–54.

Musser, John H. *A Practical Treatise on Medical Diagnosis for Students and Physicians.* Philadelphia: Lea Bros. and Co., 1894.

Nash, F. A. "Diagnostic Reasoning and the Logoscope." *Lancet*, vol. 2 (1960), pp. 1442–6.

Newman, Charles. "Diagnostic Investigation before Laennec." *Medical History*, vol. 4 (1960), pp. 322–9.

The Evolution of Medical Education in the Nineteenth Century. London: Oxford University Press, 1957.

Oesterlen, Friedrich. *Medical Logic.* Translated and edited by George Whitley. London: Sydenham Society, 1855.

Pearl, Raymond. "Modern Methods in Handling Hospital Statistics." *Bulletin Johns Hopkins Hospital*, vol. 32 (1921), pp. 184–94.

Pickering, George. "Manners Makyth Man: A Plea for the Importance of Character in Medicine." *British Medical Journal*, vol. 2 (1963), pp. 133–5.

Poynter, F. N. L., and Bishop, W. J. *A Seventeenth Century Doctor and His Patients: John Symcotts, 1592?–1662.* Bedfordshire Historical Record Society, vol. 31. Luton, England: Bedfordshire Historical Record Society, 1951.

Pratt, Joseph H. "A Sketch of the Development of Medical Diagnosis." *Boston Medical and Surgical Journal*, vol. 193 (1925), pp. 200–10.

Putnam, James J. "Not the Disease Only, But Also the Man." *Boston Medical and Surgical Journal*, vol. 141 (1899), pp. 53–7.

Richardson, Maurice H. "On Certain Evil Tendencies in Medicine and Surgery." *Boston Medical and Surgical Journal*, vol. 159 (1908), pp. 711–16, 752–6, 791–5.

Riese, Walther. "The Structure of Galen's Diagnostic Reasoning." *Bulletin of the New York Academy of Medicine*, vol. 44 (1968), pp. 778–91.

Romano, John. "Requiem or Reveille: The Clinician's Choice." *Journal of Medical Education*, vol. 38 (1963), pp. 584–90.

Ryle, John A. "Clinical Sense and Clinical Science." *Lancet*, vol. 1 (1939), pp. 1083–7.

"The Study of Symptoms." *Lancet*, vol. 1 (1931), pp. 737–41.

Savory, William. "Symptoms in Perspective." *Lancet*, vol. 2 (1892), pp. 923–5.

Scudder, John M. *Specific Diagnosis: A Study of Disease with Special Reference to the Administration of Remedies.* Cincinnati: Wilstach, Baldwin and Co., 1874.

Shryock, Richard H. "The History of Quantification in Medical Science." *Isis*, vol. 52 (1961), pp. 215–37.

Siegel, Rudolph E. "Clinical Observation in Hippocrates: An Essay on the Evolution of the Diagnostic Art." *Journal of Mt. Sinai Hospital*, vol. 31 (1964), pp. 285–303.

"Statement of the American College of Surgeons and the American Academy of Orthopaedic Surgeons before the Secretary's (HEW) Commission on Medical Malpractice." *Bulletin of the American College of Surgeons*, vol. 57, no. 5 (1972), pp. 10–15.

Stokes, John H. *Modern Clinical Syphilology: Diagnosis – Treatment – Case Studies.* Philadelphia: W. B. Saunders, 1927.

"The Art of Detecting Diseases." *London Medical Repository and Review*, vol. 24 (1825), pp. 1–20, 313–31.

Bibliography

"The Limits of Exact Knowledge in Medicine." *British Medical Journal*, vol. 1 (1886), pp. 120–1.

Todd, John W. "The Superior Clinical Acumen of the Old Physicians: A Myth." *Lancet*, vol. 1 (1953), pp. 482–4.

Underwood, E. Ashworth. "The History of the Quantitative Approach in Medicine." *British Medical Bulletin*, vol. 7 (1951), pp. 265–74.

Weed, Lawrence L. "Medical Records that Guide and Teach." *New England Journal of Medicine*, vol. 278 (1968), pp. 593–9, 652–7.

Wilson, R. Macnair. *The Beloved Physician: Sir James Mackenzie*. New York: Macmillan, 1926.

ELECTROCARDIOGRAPHY

Barker, Lewellys F. "Electrocardiography and Phonocardiography. A Collective Review." *Bulletin Johns Hopkins Hospital*, vol. 21 (1910), pp. 358–89.

Burch, George E. "Development in Clinical Electrocardiography since Einthoven." *American Heart Journal*, vol. 61 (1961), pp. 324–46.

Einthoven, Wilhelm [or Willem]. "The Different Forms of the Human Electrocardiogram and Their Signification." *Lancet*, vol. 1 (1912), pp. 853–61.

"Le Télécardiogramme." *Archives Internationales de Physiologie*, vol. 4 (1906–07), pp. 132–64 and graph.

Herrick, James B. "Thrombosis of the Coronary Arteries." *Journal of the American Medical Association*, vol. 72 (1919), pp. 387–90.

James, Walter B., and Williams, Horatio B. "The String Galvanometer and the Electrocardiogram in Health." *American Journal of Medical Sciences*, vol. 140 (1910), pp. 408–21, 644–69.

Lewis, Thomas. *The Mechanism and Graphic Registration of the Heart Beat*. 3rd ed. London: Shaw & Sons, 1925.

The Mechanism of the Heart Beat. London: Shaw & Sons, 1911.

Marvin, H. M. "The Use and Abuse of the Electrocardiogram in Medical Practice." *New England Journal of Medicine*, vol. 226 (1942), pp. 213–17.

Smith, S. Calvin. "The Clinical Value of Electrocardiography." *Pennsylvania Medical Journal*, vol. 21 (1917), pp. 10–18.

Talley, James E. "The Electrocardiograph as a Clinical Instrument." *American Journal of Medical Sciences*, vol. 147 (1914), pp. 692–8.

Waller, Augustus D. "A Demonstration on Man of Electromotive Changes Accompanying the Heart's Beat." *Journal of Physiology*, vol. 8 (1887), pp. 229–34.

"The Electromotive Properties of the Human Heart." *British Medical Journal*, vol. 2 (1888), pp. 751–4.

Wiggers, Carl J. "Some Significant Advances in Cardiac Physiology during the Nineteenth Century." *Bulletin of the History of Medicine*, vol. 34 (1960), pp. 1–15.

HEALTH EXAMINATION AND SCREENING FOR DISEASE

Boucot, Katharine R., et al. "Chest X-Ray Surveys in General Hospitals, A Critical Review." *Annals of Internal Medicine*, vol. 31 (1949), pp. 889–98.

Brailsford, James F. "Mass Radiography." *Post–Graduate Medical Journal*, vol. 20 (1944), pp. 135–42.
Breslow, Lester. "Multiphasic Screening Examinations – An Extension of the Mass Screening Technique." *American Journal of Public Health*, vol. 40 (1950), pp. 274–8.
"Periodic Health Examinations and Multiple Screening." *American Journal of Public Health*, vol. 49 (1959), pp. 1148–56.
Buck, Robert W. "The Physical Examination of Groups." *New England Journal of Medicine*, vol. 221 (1939), pp. 883–7.
Canelo, C. Kelly, et al. "A Multiphasic Screening Survey in San José." *California Medicine*, vol. 71 (1949), pp. 409–13.
"Chest X-Ray Screening Recommendations for TB–RD Associations." *National Tuberculosis and Respiratory Disease Association Bulletin*, vol. 57, no. 9 (1971), pp. 3–5.
Collen, Morris F. "Multiphasic Screening as a Diagnostic Method in Preventive Medicine." *Methods of Information in Medicine*, vol. 4 (1965), pp. 71–4.
Collen, Morris F., and Linden, Corinne. "Screening in a Group Practice Prepaid Medical Care Plan As Applied to Periodic Health Examinations." *Journal of Chronic Diseases*, vol. 2 (1955), pp. 400–8.
Dodson, John M. "The Periodic Physical Examination of the Apparently Healthy – Its Development and Present Status." *International Journal of Medicine and Surgery*, vol. 44 (1931), pp. 197–203.
Downing, Andrew F. "The Physical Examination as a Civil Service Instrument." *Boston Medical and Surgical Journal*, vol. 179 (1918), pp. 181–93.
Emerson, Haven. "The Protection of Health through Periodic Medical Examinations." *Journal of the Michigan State Medical Society*, vol. 21 (1922), pp. 399–403.
"Ethical and Social Issues in Screening for Genetic Disease." *New England Journal of Medicine*, vol. 286 (1972), pp. 1129–32.
Ferrer, H. P. *Screening for Health: Theory and Practice*. London: Butterworth, 1968.
Fiske, Eugene L. "The Purposes of the Life Extension Institute." *Boston Medical and Surgical Journal*, vol. 192 (1925), pp. 136–9.
Fremont–Smith, Maurice. "Periodic Examination of Supposedly Well Persons." *New England Journal of Medicine*, vol. 248 (1953), pp. 170–3.
Goodenough, Florence L. *Mental Testing: Its History, Principles, and Applications.* New York: Rinehart and Co., 1949. Reprint, New York: Johnson Reprint, 1969.
Gould, George M. "A System of Personal Biologic Examinations: The Condition of Adequate Medical and Scientific Conduct of Life." *Journal of the American Medical Association*, vol. 35 (1900), pp. 134–8.
Lee, Roger I. "The Physical Examination of Apparently Healthy Individuals: Its Importance, Limitations and Opportunities." *Boston Medical and Surgical Journal*, vol. 188 (1923), pp. 929–37.
Lewis, William W. "Mobile X-Ray Units: A Critical Look." *National Tuberculosis and Respiratory Disease Association Bulletin*, vol. 57 (1971), pp. 4–10.
Perrott, George St. J. "Some Public Health Implications of Selective Service Rejections." *Bulletin of the New York Academy of Medicine*, vol. 23 (1947), pp. 420–35.
Sadusk, Joseph F., Jr., and Robbins, Lewis C. "Proposal for Health–Hazard Ap-

praisal in Comprehensive Health Care." *Journal of the American Medical Association*, vol. 203 (1968), pp. 1108–12.

Thorner, Robert M. "Whither Multiphasic Screening?" *New England Journal of Medicine*, vol. 280 (1969), pp. 1037–42.

Tobey, James A. "The Health Examination Movement." *The Nation's Health*, vol. 5 (1923), pp. 610–11, 648–9.

"A Layman's View of Health Examinations." *Boston Medical and Surgical Journal*, vol. 191 (1924), pp. 875–8.

White, B. V., and Geschickter, C. F. *Diagnosis in Daily Practice*. Philadelphia: Lippincott, 1947.

Yount, C. E. "The American Youth as Mirrored by the World War: Some Timely Lessons." *Southwestern Medicine*, vol. 4 (1920), pp. 13–19.

HEMATOLOGICAL DIAGNOSIS

Ancell, Henry. "The Physiology and Pathology of the Blood, and the Other Animal Fluids." *Lancet*, vol. 2 (1839), pp. 661–71.

Andral, G. *Pathological Hematology. An Essay on the Blood in Disease*. Philadelphia: Lea and Blanchard, 1844.

Baxter, E. Buchanan, and Willcocks, Frederick. "A Contribution to Clinical Haemometry." *Lancet*, vol. 1 (1880), pp. 361–2, 397–9, 439–41.

Cabot, Richard C. "The Diagnostic and Prognostic Importance of Leucocytosis." *Boston Medical and Surgical Journal*, vol. 130 (1894), pp. 277–82.

Coupland, Sidney. "Anaemia." *British Medical Journal*, vol. 1 (1881), pp. 419–21.

Craig, Charles I. *The Wassermann Test*. St. Louis: Mosby, 1918.

Daland, Judson. "A Volumetric Study of the Red and White Corpuscles of Human Blood in Health and Disease, by Aid of the Haematokrit." *University Medical Magazine*, vol. 4 (1891), pp. 85–102.

Dreyfus, Camille. *Some Milestones in the History of Hematology*. New York: Grune & Stratton, 1957.

Folin, Otto, and Wu, Hsien. "A System of Blood Analysis." *Journal of Biological Chemistry*, vol. 38 (1919), pp. 81–91.

Garrod, Alfred B. "Observations on Certain Pathological Conditions of the Blood and Urine in Gout, Rheumatism and Bright's Disease." *Medico–Chirurgical Transactions*, vol. 31 (1848), pp. 83–97.

Gowers, W. R. "On the Numeration of Blood–Corpuscles." *Lancet*, vol. 2 (1877), pp. 797–8.

Henry, Frederick P., and Nancrede, Chas. B. "Blood–Cell Counting: A Series of Observations with the Hématimètre of MM. Hayem and Nachet, and the Haemacytometer of Dr. Gowers." *Boston Medical and Surgical Journal*, vol. 100 (1879), pp. 489–99.

Hewes, Henry F. "Practical Blood Examination." *Boston Medical and Surgical Journal*, vol. 145 (1901), pp. 121–6.

Hewson, William. *The Works of William Hewson*. Edited by George Gulliver. London: Sydenham Society, 1846.

Hunt, Joseph W. "Observations on the Blood in Anaemia." *Lancet*, vol. 2 (1880), pp. 89–91.

Lanius, J. Maria. "The Opinion of the College of Physicians at Rome, concerning Dr. Vieusions's [sic] Analysis of Human Blood." In *Philosophical Transactions* and Collections to the End of the Year MDCC. Abridged and Disposed under General Heads. vol. 3, pp. 242–7. 5th ed. Adapted by John Lowthorp. London, 1749.

Magendie, François. *Lectures on the Blood; and the changes which it undergoes during disease.* Philadelphia: Haswell, Barrington, and Haswell, 1839.

Rees, George Owen. "Observations on the Blood, with Reference to its Peculiar Condition in the Morbus Brightii." *Guy's Hospital Reports*, vol. 1 (1843), pp. 317–30.

Rockwood, Reed. "Chemical Tests of the Blood: Indications and Interpretations." *Journal of the American Medical Association*, vol. 91 (1928), pp. 157–66.

Sabine, Jean Captain. "History of the Classification of Human Blood Corpuscles." *Bulletin of the History of Medicine*, vol. 8 (1940), pp. 696–720, 785–805.

Sailer, Joseph. "Diagnosis by Means of the Serum of the Blood: A Critical Study." *Proceedings of the Pathological Society of Philadelphia*, vol. 5 (1901–02), pp. 253–66.

Scudamore, Charles. *An Essay on the Blood.* London: Longman, Hurst, Rees, Orme, Brown and Green, 1824.

Southworth, Thomas S. "The Technique and Diagnostic Value of Ehrlich's Method of Staining the White Blood–Corpuscles." *New York Medical Journal*, vol. 57 (1893), pp. 2–7.

Tholozan, J. D. "On the present state of knowledge acquired in Haematology, and the Practical Consequences which thence result." *Edinburgh Medical and Surgical Journal*, vol. 80 (1853), pp. 359–409.

Verso, M. L. "The Evolution of Blood–Counting Techniques." *Medical History*, vol. 8 (1964), pp. 149–58.

Vieussens, Raymond. "The Constituent Parts of Human Blood." In *Philosophical Transactions and Collections to the End of the Year MDCC. Abridged and Disposed under General Heads.* vol. 3, pp. 235–42. 5th ed. Adapted by John Lowthorp. London, 1749.

Welch, William H. "Principles Underlying the Serum Diagnosis of Typhoid Fever and the Methods of Its Application." *Journal of the American Medical Association*, vol. 29 (1897), pp. 301–9.

LABORATORY AND CHEMICAL DIAGNOSIS

Arnold, Horace D. "The Relation of Laboratory Research to the General Practitioner of Medicine." *Boston Medical and Surgical Journal*, vol. 149 (1903), pp. 473–8.

Bainbridge, William Seaman. "Clinical and Laboratory Diagnoses." *Medical Journal and Record*, vol. 136 (1932), pp. 265–70.

Baril, Georges. "The Correlation of Laboratory Findings with the Clinical Aspects of Disease." *Canadian Medical Association Journal*, vol. 24 (1931), pp. 531–6.

Barnett, Roy N. et al. "Multiphasic Screening by Laboratory Tests – An Overview of the Problem." *American Journal of Clinical Pathology*, vol. 54 (1970), pp. 983–92.

Baron, D. N. "The Laboratory and the Clinician." *Radiography*, vol. 19 (1953), pp. 9–13.

Bauer, Henry. "The National Laboratory Crisis." *Hospital Practice*, vol. 2, no. 2 (1967), pp. 67–73.

Bibliography

Bulloch, William. *The History of Bacteriology.* London: Oxford University Press, 1938.

Cabot, Richard C. "The Historical Development and Relative Value of Laboratory and Clinical Methods of Diagnosis." *Boston Medical and Surgical Journal,* vol. 157 (1907), pp. 150–3.

"On the Relation between Laboratory Work and Clinical Work." *Boston Medical and Surgical Journal,* vol. 164 (1911), pp. 880–3.

"The Relation of Bacteriology to Medicine." *Boston Medical and Surgical Journal,* vol. 142 (1900), pp. 479–87.

The Serum Diagnosis of Disease. New York: William Wood and Co., 1899.

Camac, C. N. B. "Hospital and Ward Clinical Laboratories." *Journal of the American Medical Association,* vol. 35 (1900), pp. 219–27.

Conn, H. W. "Bacteriology in Our Medical Schools." *Science,* vol. 11 (1888), pp. 123–6.

Culliton, Barbara J. "Clinical Labs: Bills Aimed at Correcting 'Massive' Problems." *Science,* vol. 192 (1976), pp. 531–3.

"Data Processing in Clinical Pathology." *Journal of Clinical Pathology,* vol. 21 (1968), pp. 231–5, 296–301.

Davis, Audrey B. "Rudolf Schindler's Role in the Development of Gastroscopy." *Bulletin of the History of Medicine,* vol. 46 (1972), pp. 150–70.

Dixon, Richard H., and Laszlo, John. "Utilization of Clinical Chemistry Services by Medical House Staff." *Archives of Internal Medicine,* vol. 134 (1974), pp. 1064–7.

Elsner, Henry L. "On the Value to the Physician of Modern Methods of Diagnosis." *Boston Medical and Surgical Journal,* vol. 146 (1902), pp. 101–8.

Ford, William W. *Bacteriology.* 1939. Reprint, New York: Macmillan (Hafner Press), 1964.

Foster, W. D. *A Short History of Clinical Pathology.* Edinburgh: Livingstone, 1961.

Gage, Stephen DeM., and Earle, Edith. "Diagnostic Chemistry as a Routine Function of a State Laboratory." *American Journal of Public Health,* vol. 12 (1922), pp. 665–9.

Garrod, Alfred B. "The Chemistry of Pathology and Therapeutics." *Lancet,* vol. 1 (1848), pp. 353–5, 381–3.

Garrod, Archibald E. "The Laboratory and the Ward." In *Contributions to Medical and Biological Research, Dedicated to Sir William Osler, Bart., M.D., F.R.S., in Honour of his Seventieth Birthday, July 12, 1919,* by his Pupils and Co-workers, vol. 1, pp. 59–69. New York: Paul B. Hoeber, 1919.

"Medicine from the Chemical Standpoint." *British Medical Journal,* vol. 2 (1914), pp. 228–34.

Gay, Frederick P., and Fitzgerald, J. G. "The Serum Diagnosis of Syphilis." *Boston Medical and Surgical Journal,* vol. 160 (1909), pp. 157–61.

Griner, Paul F. and Liptzin, Benjamin. "Use of the Laboratory in a Teaching Hospital: Implications for Patient Care, Education, and Hospital Costs." *Annals of Internal Medicine,* vol. 75 (1971), pp. 157–63.

Ham, Thomas Hale. "Laboratory Data in Clinical Medicine: Units of Measure, Costs, and Quantitative Significance of Results." *New England Journal of Medicine,* vol. 241 (1949), pp. 488–96.

Harris, D. L. "The Danger of Laboratory Diagnosis, with Especial Reference to the Use of the City Bacteriological Laboratory by the Medical Profession." *St. Louis Medical Review*, vol. 58 (1909), pp. 117–20.

Harrison, Tinsley R. "The Value and Limitation of Laboratory Tests in Clinical Medicine." *Journal of the Medical Association of the State of Alabama*, vol. 13 (1944), pp. 381–4.

Herrick, James B. "The Relation of the Clinical Laboratory to the Practitioner of Medicine." *Boston Medical and Surgical Journal*, vol. 156 (1907), pp. 763–8.

Hoover, C. F. "The Reputed Conflict between the Laboratories and Clinical Medicine." *Science*, vol. 71 (1930), pp. 491–7.

Iglehart, John K. "Health Report/Congress and HEW Focus on Multi–Billion Dollar Clinical Labs." *National Journal Reports*, vol. 6 (1974), pp. 153–16.

Jaksch, Rudolf von. *Clinical Diagnosis: the bacteriological, chemical and microscopical evidence of disease.* 2nd ed. Translated by James Cagney. London: Charles Griffin, 1890.

Jones, Vernon R. "The County and Community Diagnostic Laboratory." *Kentucky Medical Journal*, vol. 20 (1922), pp. 836–41.

Jordan, Arthur. "The Development of Chemical Pathology." *Journal of Clinical Pathology*, vol. 18 (1965), pp. 274–6.

Kaplan, Stanley M. "Laboratory Procedures as an Emotional Stress." *Journal of the American Medical Association*, vol. 161 (1956), pp. 677–81.

Kellert, Ellis. "Laboratory Tests vs. Stethoscopes." *American Practitioner and Digest of Treatment*, vol. 4 (1953), pp. 459–63.

Koch, R. *On the Bacteriological Diagnosis of Cholera. . .* Translated by George Duncan. Edinburgh: David Douglas, 1894.

"On the Investigation of Pathogenic Organisms" and "The Etiology of Tuberculosis." In *Recent Essays by Various Authors on Bacteria in Relation to Disease*, ed. W. Watson Cheyne, pp. 1–66, 67–264. London: New Sydenham Society, 1886.

Levinson, A. "History of Cerebrospinal Fluid." *American Journal of Syphilis*, vol. 2 (1918), pp. 267–75.

M'Donald, Stuart. "Clinical Pathology." *Scottish Medical and Surgical Journal*, vol. 10 (1902), pp. 226–36.

"Physiological Chemistry and Its Relation to Medical Practice." *Boston Medical and Surgical Journal*, vol. 138 (1898), pp. 332–5.

Purser, J. M. "On the Modern Diagnosis of Diseases of the Stomach." *Dublin Journal of Medical Science*, vol. 90 (1890), pp. 449–87.

Rollo, John. *Cases of the Diabetes Mellitus . . .* 2nd ed. London: C. Dilly, 1798.

"Routine Laboratory Tests," *New England Journal of Medicine*, vol. 275 (1966), p. 56.

Salter, William T. "Fundamental Misconceptions Involving Clinical Pathology." *New England Journal of Medicine*, vol. 222 (1940), pp. 143–8.

Skeggs, Leonard T., Jr. "An Automatic Method for Colorimetric Analysis." *American Journal of Clinical Pathology*, vol. 28 (1957), pp. 311–22.

Smith, Theobald. "Public Health Laboratories." *Boston Medical and Surgical Journal*, vol. 143 (1900), pp. 491–3.

Stengel, Alfred. "Chemical and Biological Methods in Diagnosis." *Transactions of the Congress of American Physicians and Surgeons*, vol. 7 (1907), pp. 17–47.

Stillman, Ralph G. "The Significance of Laboratory Tests and Methods." *New York State Journal of Medicine*, vol. 35 (1935), pp. 757–66.

Van Slyke, Donald D. "A Method for the Determination of Carbon Dioxide and

Carbonates in Solution." *Journal of Biological Chemistry*, vol. 30 (1917), pp. 347–68.

Vecchio, Thomas J. "Predictive Value of a Single Diagnostic Test in Unselected Populations." *New England Journal of Medicine*, vol. 274 (1966), pp. 1171–3.

Welch, William H. "The Evolution of Modern Scientific Laboratories." *Bulletin Johns Hopkins Hospital*, vol. 7 (1896), pp. 19–24.

Williams, George Z. "Effects of Automation on Laboratory Diagnosis." *California Medicine*, vol. 108 (1968), pp. 43–5.

Wright, Almoth E. *Handbook of the Technique of the Teat and Capillary Glass Tube*. London: Constable, 1912.

Wyeth, John M. "The Value of Clinical Microscopy, Bacteriology and Chemistry in Surgical Practice." *Boston Medical and Surgical Journal*, vol. 144 (1901), pp. 541–7.

LARYNGOSCOPY

Bryan, Joseph Hammond. "The History of Laryngology and Rhinology and the Influence of America in the Development of This Specialty." *Annals of Medical History*, vol. 5 (1933), pp. 151–70.

Cutter, Ephraim. "On the Laryngoscope and Rhinoscope." *Boston Medical and Surgical Journal*, vol. 69 (1863), pp. 389–98.

Czermak, J. N. *On the Laryngoscope and Its Employment in Physiology and Medicine*. Translated by George D. Gibb. London: New Sydenham Society, 1861.

Johnson, George. "On Some Practical Gains Which Have Resulted from the Use of the Laryngoscope." *British Medical Journal*, vol. 1 (1874), pp. 675–8.

"The Laryngoscope and its Applications [book review]." *British and Foreign Medico–Chirurgical Review*, vol. 30 (1862), pp. 340–50.

Mackenzie, Morell. *The Use of the Laryngoscope in Diseases of the Throat, with an Appendix on Rhinoscopy*. Philadelphia: Lindsay and Blakiston, 1865.

Milligan, William. "The Rise and Progress of Laryngology: Its Relation to General Medicine and Its Position in the Medical Curriculum." *British Medical Journal*, vol. 1 (1922), pp. 547–53.

Ruppaner, Antoine. "The Practice of Laryngoscopy and Rhinoscopy." *New York Medical Journal*, vol. 6 (1867), pp. 1–25, 126–47.

Semeleder, Friederich. *Rhinoscopy and Laryngoscopy; Their Value in Practical Medicine*. Translated by Edward T. Caswell. New York: William Wood, 1866.

Semon, Felix. "The Relations of Laryngology, Rhinology, and Otology with Other Arts and Sciences." *British Medical Journal*, vol. 2 (1904), pp. 713–19.

Stevenson, R. Scott, and Guthrie, Douglas. *A History of Oto–Laryngology*. Edinburgh: E. & S. Livingstone, 1949.

Watson, Eben. "Laryngoscopy and Its Revelations." *Lancet*, vols. 1 and 2 (1865), pp. 588–91, and 5–8.

MICROSCOPY IN DIAGNOSIS

Baker, Henry. *The Microscope Made Easy*. . .London: Printed for R. Dodsley, M. Cooper, and J. Coff, 1744.

Beale, Lionel. *The Microscope, in Its Application to Practical Medicine*. 2nd ed. London; John Churchill, 1858.

Bell, Thomas. "Observations on the Use of the Microscope, in Investigations Connected with Anatomy, Physiology, and Pathology." *Transactions of the Medical Society of London*, vol. 1 (1846), pp. 1–24.

Bradbury, S. *The Evolution of the Microscope*. Oxford: Pergamon Press, 1967.

Carpenter, William Benjamin. *The Microscope and Its Revelations*. London: John Churchill, 1856.

Clay, Reginald S., and Court, Thomas H. *The History of the Microscope*. London: Charles Griffin, 1932.

Conn, H. J. *The History of Staining*. New York: W. F. Humphrey Press, 1933.

Dobbell, Clifford. *Antony van Leeuwenhoek and his 'Little Animals.'* New York: Russell & Russell, 1958.

Donaldson, Francis. "The Practical Application of the Microscope to the Diagnosis of Cancer." *American Journal of the Medical Sciences*, vol. 25 (1853), pp. 43–68.

"History and Applications of the Microscope [book review]." *Edinburgh Medical and Surgical Journal*, vol. 73 (1850), pp. 161–86.

Hooke, Robert. *Micrographia: or some Physiological Descriptions of Minute Bodies Made by Magnifying Glasses with Observations and Inquiries Thereupon*. London: Jo. Martyn & Ja. Allestry, 1665.

Hughes, Arthur. *A History of Cytology*. London: Abelard–Schuman, 1959.

Lister, Joseph Jackson. "On some properties in achromatic–object glasses applicable to the improvement of the microscope." *Philosophical Transactions of the Royal Society of London*, vol. 120 (1830), pp. 187–200.

Medicus [pseud.]. "Does a minute knowledge of Anatomy contribute greatly to the Discrimination and Cure of Diseases?" *Edinburgh Medical and Surgical Journal*, vol. 5 (1809), pp. 66–72.

Paddock, Frank K. "Use of the Microscope as a Means of Diagnosis." *Boston Medical and Surgical Journal*, vol. 74 (1866), pp. 95–9.

Quekett, John. *A Practical Treatise on the Use of the Microscope*. London: Hippolyte Baillière, 1848.

Rooseboom, M. "The History of the Microscope." *Proceedings Royal Microscopical Society*, vol. 2 (1967), pp. 266–93.

Sims, J. Marion. "Illustrations of the Value of the Microscope in the Treatment of the Sterile Condition." *British Medical Journal*, vol. 2 (1868), pp. 465–6, 492–4.

Singer, Charles. "Notes on the Early History of Microscopy." *Proceedings of the Royal Society of Medicine*, vol. 7 (1913), pp. 247–79.

Tyson, James. "Some Reasons Why the Microscope Should Be Used by Every Physician." *Medical and Surgical Reporter*, vol. 39 (1878), pp. 45–8.

OBSERVER VARIATION AND ERROR

Abrahams, Adolphe. "Errors in Diagnosis." *Lancet*, vol. 2 (1932), pp. 661–4.

Addison, Thomas. "On the Difficulties and Fallacies Attending Physical Diagnosis in Diseases of the Chest." *Guy's Hospital Reports*, vol. 4 (1846), pp. 1–36.

Belk, William P., and Sunderman, F. William. "A Survey of the Accuracy of Chemical Analyses in Clinical Laboratories." *American Journal of Clinical Pathology*, vol. 17 (1947), pp. 853–61.

Birkelo, Carl C., et al. "Tuberculosis Case Finding: A Comparison of the Effectiveness of Various Roentgenographic and Photofluorographic Methods." *Journal of the American Medical Association*, vol. 133 (1947), pp. 359–66.

Bibliography

Boyle, Charles Murray. "Difference between Patients' and Doctors' Interpretation of Some Common Medical Terms." *British Medical Journal*, vol. 2 (1970), pp. 286–9.

Brailsford, James F. "Factors Which Influence the Value of a Radiological Investigation." *Lancet*, vol. 1 (1952), pp. 679–83.

Bramwell, Byrom. "Mistakes." *Lancet*, vol. 2 (1911), pp. 281–5.

Butterworth, J. Scott, and Reppert, Edmund H. "Auscultatory Acumen in the General Medical Population." *Journal of the American Medical Association*, vol. 174 (1960), pp. 32–4.

Cabot, Richard C. "Diagnostic Pitfalls Identified during a Study of Three Thousand Autopsies." *Journal of the American Medical Association*, vol. 59 (1912), pp. 2295–8.

Cochrane, A. L., Chapman, P. J., and Oldham, P. D. "Observers' Errors in Taking Medical Histories." *Lancet*, vol. 1 (1951), pp. 1007–9.

Comroe, Julius H., and Botelho, Stella. "The Unreliability of Cyanosis in the Recognition of Arterial Anoxemia." *American Journal of the Medical Sciences*, vol. 214 (1947), pp. 1–6.

Davies, L. G. "Observer Variation in Reports on Electrocardiograms." *British Heart Journal*, vol. 20 (1958), pp. 153–61.

Derryberry, Mayhew. "Reliability of Medical Judgments on Malnutrition." *Public Health Reports*, vol. 53 (1938), pp. 263–8.

Emerson, Charles P. "The Accuracy of Certain Clinical Methods." *Bulletin Johns Hopkins Hospital*, vol. 14 (1903), pp. 9–18.

Fletcher, C. M. "The Clinical Diagnosis of Pulmonary Emphysema – An Experimental Study." *Proceedings of the Royal Society of Medicine*, vol. 45 (1952), pp. 577–84.

Garland, L. Henry. "The Problem of Observer Error." *Bulletin of the New York Academy of Medicine*, vol. 36 (1960), pp. 570–84.

"On the Scientific Evaluation of Diagnostic Procedures." *Radiology*, vol. 52 (1949), pp. 309–27.

Groth–Petersen, E., Løvgreen, A., and Thillemann, J. "On the Reliability of the Reading of Photofluorograms and the Value of Dual Reading." *Acta Tuberculosia Scandinavica*, vol. 26 (1952), pp. 13–37.

Horvath, William J. "The Effect of Physician Bias in Medical Diagnosis." *Behavioral Science*, vol. 9 (1968), pp. 334–40.

Johnson, M. L. "Observer Error: Its Bearing on Teaching." *Lancet*, vol. 2 (1955), pp. 422–4.

Koran, Lorrin M. "The Reliability of Clinical Methods, Data and Judgments." *New England Journal of Medicine*, vol. 293 (1975), pp. 642–6, 695–701.

Kreitman, N. "The Reliability of Psychiatric Diagnosis." *Journal of Mental Science*, vol. 107 (1961), pp. 876–86.

MacDonnell, Robert L. "Propositions on the 'Fallacies of Physical Diagnosis in Diseases of the Chest.' By Thomas Addison." *British American Journal of Medical and Physical Science*, vol. 3 (1847), pp. 1–7.

Ritchie, Charles. "On Diagnosis." *Edinburgh Medical and Surgical Journal*, vol. 16 (1820), pp. 53–62.

Scheff, Thomas J. "Decision Rules, Types of Error, and Their Consequences in Medical Diagnosis." *Behavioral Science*, vol. 8 (1963), pp. 97–107.

Skendzel, Laurence P., and Muelling, Rudolph J., Jr. "Report on Small Hospital

Laboratories: 1966 Survey of the College of American Pathologists." *New England Journal of Medicine*, vol. 277 (1967), pp. 180–5.

Slack, Francis H. "An Investigation of the Reliability of Laboratory Tests and a Discussion of Technique of Laboratories in and Near Boston." *Boston Medical and Surgical Journal*, vol. 187 (1922), pp. 441–6, 474–9, 540–3.

Swartout, H. O. "Ante Mortem and Post Mortem Diagnoses." *New England Journal of Medicine*, vol. 211 (1934), pp. 539–42.

Tonks, David B. "A Study of the Accuracy and Precision of Clinical Chemistry Determinations in 170 Canadian Laboratories." *Clinical Chemistry*, vol. 9 (1963), pp. 217–33.

Tuddenham, William J. "Problems of Perception in Chest Roentgenology: Facts and Fallacies." *Radiologic Clinics of North America*, vol. 1 (1963), pp. 277–89.

Wooton, I. D. P., King, E. J., and Smith, J. Maclean. "The Quantitative Approach to Hospital Biochemistry: Normal Values and the Use of Biochemical Determinations for Diagnosis and Prognosis." *British Medical Bulletin*, vol. 7 (1951), pp. 307–11.

Zieve, Leslie. "Misinterpretation and Abuse of Laboratory Tests by Clinicians." *Annals of the New York Academy of Sciences*, vol. 134 (1966), pp. 563–72.

OPHTHALMOLOGY

Allbutt, Thomas Clifford. *On the use of the ophthalmoscope in diseases of the nervous system and of the kidneys; also in certain other general disorders.* London: Macmillan, 1871.

Arrington, George E. *A History of Ophthalmology.* New York: MD Publications, 1959.

Dix, John H. "On the Ophthalmoscope – Its Uses and Methods of Application." *Boston Medical and Surgical Journal*, vol. 54 (1856), pp. 409–20, 429–31.

Ewing, A. E. "Test Objects for the Illiterate." *Journal of Ophthalmology*, vol. 3 (1920), pp. 5–22.

Helmholtz, H. von. *Description of an Ophthalmoscope for the Investigation of the Living Eye.* Translated by Thomas Hall Shastid. Chicago: Cleveland Press, 1916.

Jackson, Edward, et al. "Report on the Value of Objective Tests for the Determination of Ametropia, Opthalmoscopy, Ophthalmometry, Skiascopy." *Journal of the American Medical Association*, vol. 23 (1894), pp. 337–9.

Keyes, Thomas E. "Contributions Leading to the Invention of the Ophthalmoscope." *Proceedings of the Staff Meetings of the Mayo Clinic*, vol. 26 (1951), pp. 209–16.

Koenigsberger, Leo. *Hermann von Helmholtz.* Translated by Frances A. Welby. Oxford: Clarendon Press, 1906.

Pallen, Montrose A. "Vision, and Some of Its Anomalies, as Revealed by the Ophthalmoscope." *Transactions of the American Medical Association*, vol. 11 (1858), pp. 859–934 and illustrations.

Robertson, Argyll. "The Progress of Ophthalmology: a Sketch." *Edinburgh Medical Journal*, vol. 8 (1862), pp. 40–50.

Rucker, C. Wilbur. *A History of the Ophthalmoscope.* Rochester, N.Y.: Whiting Printers, 1971.

Shakespeare, Edward O. "Description of a New Ophthalmoscope and Ophthalmometer, devised for Clinical Use and for Physiological and Therapeutic In-

295

vestigations upon Man and Animals." *American Journal of the Medical Sciences*, vol. 71 (1876), pp. 45–61.

Snellen, H. *Test–Types for the Determination of the Acuteness of Vision*. Utrecht: P. W. Van de Weijier, 1862.

Thau, William. "Purkyně: A Pioneer in Ophthalmology." *Archives of Ophthalmology*, n.s. vol. 27 (1942), pp. 299–316.

Vernon, Bowater J. "Hints to Beginners on the Use of the Ophthalmoscope." *Students' Journal and Hospital Gazette*, vol. 2 (1874), pp. 133–4.

Williams, E. "The Ophthalmoscope; The Principles on Which It Is Based – The Manner of Its Application – and Its Practical Advantages; with a Report of Some Cases." *Medical Times and Gazette*, vol. 9 (1854), pp. 7–9, 30–2.

Zander, Adolf. *The Ophthalmoscope: Its Varieties and Its Use*. Translated by Robert Brudenell Carter. London: Robert Hardwicke, 1864.

PATIENT'S HISTORY

Blumer, George. "History Taking." *Connecticut State Medical Journal*, vol. 13 (1949), pp. 449–53.

Brodman, Keeve, et al. "The Cornell Medical Index: An Adjunct to Medical Interview." *Journal of the American Medical Association*, vol. 140 (1949), pp. 530–4.

Galton, Francis. *Life History Album*. 2nd ed. London: Macmillan, 1902.

Hampton, J. R., et al. "Relative Contributions of History-taking, Physical Examination, and Laboratory Investigation to Diagnosis and Management of Medical Outpatients." *British Medical Journal*, vol. 2 (1975), pp. 486–9.

Herrick, James B. "The Importance of the History and Physical Examination in Diagnosis." *Journal of the Indiana State Medical Association*, vol. 24 (1931), pp. 69–72.

Marcondes, Durval. "New Aspects of the Clinical Interview: Countertransference Difficulties." *Psychosomatic Medicine*, vol. 22 (1960), pp. 211–17.

Meares, Ainslie. "Communication with the Patient." *Lancet*, vol. 1 (1960), pp. 663–7.

Powdermaker, Florence. "The Techniques of the Initial Interview and Methods of Teaching Them." *American Journal of Psychiatry*, vol. 104 (1948), pp. 642–6.

Richardson, Maurice H. "On the Significance of Clinical Histories before and after Operative Demonstration of the Real Lesion." *Boston Medical and Surgical Journal*, vol. 158 (1908), pp. 469–73, 513–20.

Riese, W. "The Structure of the Clinical History." *Bulletin of the History of Medicine*, vol. 16 (1944), pp. 437–49.

Riesman, David. "Some Observations on Interviewing in a State Mental Hospital." *Bulletin of the Menninger Clinic*, vol. 23 (1959), pp. 7–19.

Stengel, Alfred. "Importance of Accurate Medical Histories and Careful Physical Examinations." *Pennsylvania Medical Journal*, vol. 37 (1934), pp. 811–14.

Whitehorn, John C. "Guide to Interviewing and Clinical Personality Study." *Archives of Neurology and Psychiatry*, vol. 52 (1944), pp. 197–216.

Wolf, Stewart, et al. "Instruction in Medical History Taking." *Journal of Medical Education*, vol. 27 (1952), pp. 244–52.

PHYSICAL DIAGNOSIS

Alison, Somerville Scott. *The Physical Examination of the Chest in Pulmonary Consumption.* . . . London: John Churchill, 1861.

Auenbrugger, Leopold. *Nouvelle méthode pour reconnaître les maladies internes de la poitrine.* Edited by J. N. Corvisart. Paris: Migneret, 1808.

"On Percussion of the Chest." Translated by John Forbes. Introduction by Henry E. Sigerist. *Bulletin of the History of Medicine*, vol. 4 (1936), pp. 373–403.

Inventum novum ex percussione thoracis humani ut signo abstrusos interni pectoris morbos detegendi Vindobonae: J. T. Trattner, 1761.

Balfour, George W. "On the Evolution of Cardiac Diagnosis from Harvey's Days Till Now." *Edinburgh Medical Journal*, vol. 32 (1887), pp. 1065–81.

Barth, J.-B.-P., and Roger, Henri. *A Practical Treatise on Auscultation.* Translated by Patrick Newbigging. Lexington, Kentucky: Scrugham & Dunlop, 1847.

Bell, John. "Some general remarks on the use of the Stethoscope, as an aid in forming a correct diagnosis of Diseases of the Lungs, together with some observations on the symptom called by M. Laennec, Pectoriloquy." *New–York Medical and Physical Journal*, vol. 3 (1824), pp. 269–81.

Bennet, Henry. "Remarks on the Comparative Value of Auscultation Practised With and Without the Stethoscope." *Lancet*, vol. 1 (1843–44), pp. 461–6.

Blake, C. J. "The Telephone and Microphone in Auscultation." *Boston Medical and Surgical Journal*, vol. 103 (1880), pp. 486–7.

Bowditch, Henry I. *The Young Stethoscopist, or the Student's Aid to Auscultation.* 1846. Reprint, New York and London: Macmillan (Hafner Press), 1964.

Buck, Robert W. "Physical Diagnosis Prior to Auenbrugger." *New England Journal of Medicine*, vol. 209 (1933), pp. 239–41.

Cammann, D. M. "An Historical Sketch of the Stethoscope." *New York Medical Journal*, vol. 43 (1886), pp. 465–6.

Clark, James. *Medical Notes on Climate, Diseases, Hospitals, and Medical Schools in France, Italy, and Switzerland* . . . London: T. G. Underwood, 1820.

Comins, Nicholas P. "New Stethoscope." *London Medical Gazette*, vol. 4 (1829), pp. 427–30.

Corvisart, J.–N. *An Essay on the Organic Diseases and Lesions of the Heart and Great Vessels.* Translated by Jacob Gates. 1812. Reprint, New York: Macmillan (Hafner Press), 1962.

Coues, William Pearce. "Laennec, the Man – 1781–1826." *Boston Medical and Surgical Journal*, vol. 195 (1926), pp. 208–11.

Dickinson, W. Howship. *The Tongue as an Indication in Disease.* London: Longmans, Green, 1888.

Flint, Austin. "On the Clinical Study of the Heart Sounds." *Journal of the American Medical Association*, vol. 3 (1884), pp. 85–91.

Physical Exploration of the lungs by means of auscultation and percussion. Philadelphia: Lea, Son and Co., 1882.

Forbes, John. *Original Cases with dissections and observations illustrating the use of the stethoscope and percussion in the diagnosis of diseases of the chest* . . . London: T. and G. Underwood, 1824.

Gairdner, W. T. "A Short Account of Cardiac Murmurs." *Edinburgh Medical Journal*, vol. 7 (1861–62), pp. 438–53.

297

Bibliography

Gerhard, W. W. *On the Diagnosis of Diseases of the Chest.* Philadelphia: Key & Biddle, 1836.

Grant, Klein, ed. *Memoir of the late James Hope, M.D., by Mrs. Hope; To Which Are Added Remarks on Classical Education, by Dr. Hope; and Letters from a Senior to a Junior Physician, by Dr. Burder.* 4th ed. London: J. Hatchard and Son, 1848.

Graves, Robert J. *Clinical Lectures delivered during the sessions of 1834–5 and 1836–7.* Philadelphia: Adam Waldie, 1838.

Graves, Robert J., and Stokes, W. "Dr. Clutterbuck versus the Stethoscope. Dr. Hope on Auscultation in Valvular Disease." *Dublin Journal of Medical Science,* vol. 14 (1838), pp. 178–80.

Guttmann, Paul. *A Handbook of Physical Diagnosis, comprising the Throat, Thorax, and Abdomen.* Translated from the 3rd German edition by Alex. Napier. New York: William Wood, 1880.

Herrick, James B. "In Defense of the Stethoscope." *Annals of Internal Medicine,* vol. 4 (1930–31), pp. 113–16.

Memories of Eighty Years. Chicago: University of Chicago Press, 1949.

"A Note Concerning the Long Neglect of Auenbrugger's 'Inventum Novum.' " *Archives of Internal Medicine,* vol. 71 (1943), pp. 741–8.

A Short History of Cardiology. Springfield: Thomas, 1942.

Holmes, Oliver Wendell. "Dissertation on the Question, How far are the external means of exploring the condition of the internal organs to be considered useful and important in medical practice?" *Library of Practical Medicine,* vol. 7 (1836). [One of three Boylston Prize Dissertations for 1836 on this subject; the other two were by Luther Bell and Robert W. Haxall.]

"The Stethoscope Song: A Professional Ballad," in *Poems,* pp. 272–7. Boston: Ticknor, Reed & Fields, 1850.

Hope, J. "Reply to Drs. Graves' and Stokes' Remarks on Dr. Hope, in Reference to Auscultation." *London Medical Gazette,* vol. 1 (1838–39), pp. 126–30.

A Treatise on the Diseases of the Heart and Great Vessels. Philadelphia: Haswell & Johnson, 1842.

Hudson, Alfred. "Laennec: His Labours, and Their Influence in Medicine." *British Medical Journal,* vol. 2 (1879), pp. 204–9.

Hudson, E. Darwin. *A Manual of the Physical Diagnosis of Thoracic Diseases.* New York: William Wood, 1887.

Hughes, H. M. *A Clinical Introduction to the Practice of Auscultation, and Other Modes of Physical Diagnosis: Intended to Simplify the Study of the Diseases of the Lungs and Heart.* Philadelphia: Lea and Blanchard, 1846.

Hutchinson, John. "On the Capacity of the Lungs and on the Respiratory Functions, with a View of Establishing a Precise and Easy Method of Detecting Disease by the Spirometer." *Medico–Chirurgical Transactions,* vol. 29 (1846), pp. 137–252.

Jackson, James. *Memoir of James Jackson, Jr.* Boston: I. R. Butts, 1835.

Jacobus, Arthur M. "Physical Examination a Requirement for a Correct Diagnosis and the Honest Treatment of the Sick." *Medical Record,* vol. 81 (1912), pp. 651–6.

Jarcho, Saul. "Auenbrugger, Laennec, and John Keats: Some Notes on the Early History of Percussion and Auscultation." *Medical History,* vol. 5 (1961), pp. 167–72.

"Observations on the History of Physical Diagnosis: Hippocrates, Auenbrugger, Laennec." *Journal of International College of Surgeons*, vol. 31 (1959), pp. 717–25.

Kennedy, Evory. *Observations on Obstetric Auscultation with an analysis of the evidences of pregnancy* . . . New York: Langley, 1843.

Kervan, Roger. *Laennec: His Life and Times*. Translated by D. C. Abrahams–Curiel. New York: Pergamon Press, 1960.

King, Lester S. "Auscultation in England, 1821–1837," *Bulletin of History of Medicine*, vol. 33 (1959), pp. 446–53.

Laennec, R. T. H. *A Treatise on the Diseases of the Chest*. Translation by John Forbes of the 1st French edition. London: T. and G. Underwood, 1821. (Reprinted by Macmillan (Hafner Press), New York, 1962.)

   A Treatise on the Diseases of the Chest, and on Mediate Auscultation. Translation by John Forbes of the 2nd French edition. London: T. and G. Underwood, 1827.

   A Treatise on the Diseases of the Chest, and on Mediate Auscultation. Translation by John Forbes of the 3rd French edition; with additional notes by Professor Gabriel Andral. New York: Samuel S. and William Wood, 1838.

Levine, Samuel A. "A Plea for the Stethoscope." *Rocky Mountain Medical Journal*, vol. 49 (1952), pp. 1029–34.

Longcope, Warfield T. "A Note on Laennec's Invention of the Stethoscope." *American Review of Tuberculosis*, vol. 19 (1929), pp. 1–8.

Major, Ralph H. "Physical Diagnosis in Antiquity." *Journal of the Kansas Medical Society*, vol. 63 (1962), pp. 497–9.

Malet, Henry. "The Physical Differences between Binaural and Uniaural Stethoscopes." *British Medical Journal*, vol. 2 (1882), pp. 774–5.

Mattson, M. "The Curability of Consumption, Considered in Reference to a New Method of Ascertaining the Healthy or Diseased Condition of the Lungs." *Boston Medical and Surgical Journal*, vol. 43 (1851), pp. 429–35, 449–57.

Morris, Stephen. "The Advent and Development of the Binaural Stethoscope." *Practitioner*, vol. 199 (1968), pp. 674–80.

Morrison, Hyman. "Laennec's Clinico–Pathological Studies." *Boston Medical and Surgical Journal*, vol. 195 (1926), pp. 211–13.

Newman, Charles. "Physical Signs in the London Hospitals: A Chapter in the History of the Introduction of Physical Examination." *Medical History*, vol. 2 (1958), pp. 195–201.

Otis, Edward O. "Some Methods of Chest Examination Supplementary to Auscultation and Percussion." *Boston Medical and Surgical Journal*, vol. 132 (1895), pp. 355–9.

Peyraud, G. "A History of the Improvements which Practical Medicine Has Derived from Auscultation." Translated by Charles A. Pope. *Western Journal of Medicine and Surgery*, vol. 6 (1842), pp. 1–58, 80–142.

Piorry, P. A. *De la percussion médiate et des signes obtenus à l'aide de ce nouveau moyen d'exploration, dans les maladies des organs thoraciques et abdominaux*. Paris: J.–S. Chaudé et J.–B. Ballière, 1828.

Pottenger, F. M. "An Historical Review of the Physical Examination of the Chest." *Annals of Internal Medicine*, vol. 30 (1949), pp. 766–77.

Pratt, Joseph H. "The Development of Physical Diagnosis." *New England Journal of Medicine*, vol. 213 (1935), pp. 639–44.

Ransome, Arthur. *On Stethometry*. London: Macmillan, 1876.

Bibliography

Risse, Guenter B. "Pierre A. Piorry (1794–1879), the French 'Master of Percussion.' " *Chest*, vol. 60 (1971), pp. 484–8.

Salter, Hyde. "Lectures on Dyspnoea." *Lancet*, vol. 2 (1865), pp. 111–13, 141–4, 225–9, 253–6, 281–3, 475–8.

Scudamore, Charles. *Observations on M. Laennec's Method of Forming a Diagnosis of the Diseases of the Chest by Means of the Stethoscope, and of Percussion; and upon Some Points of the French Practice of Medicine.* London: Longman, Rees, Orme, Brown, and Green, 1826.

Segall, Harold N. "A Simple Method for Graphic Description of Cardiac Auscultatory Signs." *American Heart Journal*, vol. 8 (1932–33), pp. 533–6.

Shattuck, Frederick C. *Auscultation and Percussion*. Detroit: George S. Davis, 1890.

Sheldon, Paul B., and Doe, Janet. "The Development of the Stethoscope: An Exhibition Showing the Work of Laennec and His Successors." *Bulletin of the New York Academy of Medicine*, vol. 11 (1935), pp. 608–26.

Skoda, Joseph. *A Treatise on Auscultation and Percussion*. Translated from the 4th ed. by W. Markham. London: Highley and Son, 1853.

Spittal, Robert. *A Treatise on Auscultation, Illustrated by Cases and Dissections.* Edinburgh: R. Grant & Sons, 1830.

"Stethoscope versus X Rays." [Debate at Royal Society of Medicine and letters to the Editor in response.] *British Medical Journal*, vol. 2 (1945), pp. 856–7; and vol. 1 (1946), pp. 31, 103, 182–3, 254–5, 292–3, 329, 410, 504, 628, 737.

Stokes, William. *An Introduction to the Use of the Stethoscope; with Its Application to the Diagnosis in Diseases of the Thoracic Viscera; Including the Pathology of these Various Affections.* Edinburgh: Maclachlan and Stewart, 1825.

Thayer, William S. "On the Diagnostic Importance of Physical Examination." *Military Surgeon*, vol. 65 (1929), pp. 497–514.

"To the Stethoscope." *Blackwood's Edinburgh Magazine*, vol. 61 (1847), pp. 361–7.

Viets, Henry R. "Some Editions of Laennec's Work on Mediate Auscultation." *Boston Medical and Surgical Journal*, vol. 195 (1926), pp. 213–17.

Waring, James J. "The Vicissitudes of Auscultation." *American Journal of Tuberculosis*, vol. 34 (1936), pp. 1–9.

Williams, Charles J. B. "On the Acoustic Principles and Construction of Stethoscopes and Ear–Trumpets." *Lancet*, vol. 2 (1873), pp. 664–6.

Memoirs of Life and Work. London: Smith, Elder, 1884.

A Rational Exposition of the Physical Signs of the Diseases of the Lungs and Pleura . . . Philadelphia: Carey and Lea, 1830.

Williams, C. Theodore. "Laënnec and the Evolution of the Stethoscope." *British Medical Journal*, vol. 2 (1907), pp. 6–8.

Wilson, A. B. Kinnier, Fothergill, L., and Taylor, Selwyn. "Some Applications of a New Electronic Stethoscope." *Lancet*, vol. 2 (1956), pp. 1027–8.

Young, R. A. "The Stethoscope: Past and Present." *Lancet*, vol. 2 (1930), pp. 883–8.

THE PULSE: ITS QUALITATIVE AND QUANTITATIVE EVALUATION

Bedford, D. Evan. "The Ancient Art of Feeling the Pulse." *British Heart Journal*, vol. 13 (1951), pp. 423–37.

"Blood Pressure Observations in Surgical Cases." Report of the Committee on Research for the Division of Surgery, Harvard Medical School, January, 1904. *Boston Medical and Surgical Journal*, vol. 150 (1904), pp. 255–72.

Bordeu, Théophile de. *Inquiries Concerning the Varieties of the Pulse and the Particular Crisis Each More Especially Indicates*. London: Printed for T. Lewis and G. Kearsly, 1764.

Bramwell, Byrom. *Student's Guide to the Examination of the Pulse, and Use of the Sphygmograph*. 2nd ed. Edinburgh: Maclachlan and Stewart, 1883.

Broadbent, W. H. *The Pulse*. London: Cassell, 1890.

Burdon-Sanderson, J. "The Characters of the Arterial Pulse, in Their Relation to the Mode and Duration of the Contraction of the Heart in Health and Disease." *British Medical Journal*, vol. 2 (1867), pp. 19–22, 39–40, 57–8.

Handbook of the Sphygmograph. London: Robert Hardwicke, 1867.

Currens, J. H., Brownell, G. L., and Aronow, S. "An Automatic Blood–Pressure–Recording Machine." *New England Journal of Medicine*, vol. 256 (1957), pp. 780–4.

Cushing, Harvey. "On Routine Determinations of Arterial Tension in Operating Room and Clinic." *Boston Medical and Surgical Journal*, vol. 148 (1903), pp. 250–6.

Falconer, W. *Observations Respecting the Pulse; Intended to Point Out with Greater Certainty, the Indications Which it Signifies; Especially in Feverish Complaints*. London: Printed for T. Cadell, Jr. and W. Davies, 1796.

Floyer, John. *The Physician's Pulse-Watch; or, an Essay to Explain the Old Art of Feeling the Pulse, and to Improve it by the help of a Pulse-Watch*. London: Printed for Sam. Smith and Benj. Walford, 1707.

Hérisson, Julius. *The Sphygmometer, an Instrument Which Renders the Action of the Arteries Apparent to the Eye. The Utility of This Instrument in the Study of Disease. Researches on the Affections of the Heart, and on the Proper Means of Discriminating Them Considered*. Translated by E. S. Blundell. London: Longman, Rees, Orme, Brown, Green, and Longman, 1835.

Holden, Edgar. *The Sphygmograph: Its Physiological and Pathological Indications*. Philadelphia: Lindsay & Blakiston, 1874.

Hope, James. "On the Pulse." *London Medical Gazette*, vol. 30 (1841–42), pp. 310–16.

Janeway, Theodore C. *The Clinical Study of the Blood–Pressure*. New York: D. Appleton, 1907.

Keyt, Alonzo T. *Sphygmography and Cardiography, Physiological and Clinical*. Edited by Asa B. Isham and M. H. Keyt. New York and London: Putnam, The Knickerbocker Press, 1887.

Lewis, William Hall, Jr. "The Evolution of Clinical Sphygmomanometry." *Bulletin of the New York Academy of Medicine*, vol. 17 (1941), pp. 871–81.

Lindsay, Lilian. "Sir John Floyer (1649–1734)." *Proceedings Royal Society of Medicine*, vol. 44 (1951), pp. 43–8.

Mackenzie, James. *The Study of the Pulse and the Movements of the Heart*. New York: Macmillan, 1902.

Mahomed, F. A. "Some of the Clinical Aspects of Chronic Bright's Disease." *Guy's Hospital Reports*, vol. 24 (1879), pp. 363–440.

Major, Ralph H. "The History of Taking the Blood Pressure." *Annals of Medical History*, vol. 2 (1930), pp. 47–55.

Bibliography

Marey, Etienne-Jules. "The Graphic Method in the Experimental Sciences, and on its Special Application to Medicine." *British Medical Journal*, vol. 1 (1876), pp. 1–3, 65–6.

Segall, Harold N. "Dr. N. C. Korotkoff: Discoverer of the Auscultatory Method for Measuring Arterial Pressure." *Annals of Internal Medicine*, vol. 63 (1965), pp. 147–9.

Townsend, Gary L. "Sir John Floyer (1649–1734) and His Study of Pulse and Respiration." *Journal of the History of Medicine*, vol. 22 (1967), pp. 286–316.

RADIOLOGY

Bell, Russell S., and Loop, John W. "The Utility and Futility of Radiographic Skull Examination for Trauma." *New England Journal of Medicine*, vol. 284 (1971), pp. 236–9.

Benatt, A. J. "Cardiac Catheterisation: A Historical Note." *Lancet*, vol. 1 (1949), pp. 746–7.

Blatz, Hanson. "Common Causes of Excessive Patient Exposure in Diagnostic Radiology." *New England Journal of Medicine*, vol. 271 (1964), pp. 1184–8.

Brailsford, James F. "Reflections on the Teaching of Radiology." *British Journal of Radiology*, vol. 18 (1945), pp. 249–57.

Brecher, Ruth, and Brecher, Edward. *The Rays: A History of Radiology in the United States and Canada*. Baltimore: Williams & Wilkins, 1969.

Cannon, Walter B. "The Movements of the Stomach Studied by Means of the Röntgen Rays." *American Journal of Physiology*, vol. 1 (1898), pp. 359–82.

Chamberlain, W. Edward. "Radiology as a Medical Specialty: Its Development, with Especial Reference to the Relations between Hospitals and Radiologists." *Journal of the American Medical Association*, vol. 92 (1929), pp. 1033–5.

Desjardins, Arthur U. "The Status of Radiology in America." *Journal of the American Medical Association*, vol. 92 (1929), pp. 1035–9.

Dock, George. "X-Ray Work from the Viewpoint of an Internist." *American Journal of Roentgenology*, vol. 8 (1921), pp. 321–7.

Donaldson, Samuel W. "Medical Facts That Can or Cannot Be Proved by Roentgen–Ray; Historical Review and Present Possibilities." *Annals of Internal Medicine*, vol. 18 (1943), pp. 535–40.

Edsall, David L. "The Attitude of the Clinician in Regard to Exposing Patients to the X-Ray." *Journal of the American Medical Association*, vol. 47 (1906), pp. 1425–9.

Gershon–Cohen, J., and Cooley, A. G. "Roentgenographic Facsimile: A Rapid Accurate Method for Reproducing Roentgenograms at a Distance via Wire or Radio Transmission." *American Journal of Roentgenology*, vol. 61 (1949), pp. 557–9.

Glasser, Otto. "W. C. Roentgen and the Discovery of the Roentgen Rays." *American Journal of Roentgenology and Radium Therapy*, vol. 25 (1931), pp. 437–50.

Dr. W. C. Röntgen. 2nd rev. ed. Springfield: Thomas, 1958.

Horder, Lord, Thomas. "The Influence of Radiology upon Our Conceptions of Disease." *British Medical Journal*, vol. 2 (1924), pp. 89–94.

Leonard, Charles Lester. "Recent Progress in the Roentgen-Ray Methods of Diagnosis." *Journal of the American Medical Association*, vol. 35 (1900), pp. 147–52.

Martin, Frederick C., and Fuchs, Arthur W. "The Historical Evolution of

Roentgen-Ray Plates and Films." *American Journal of Roentgenology and Radium Therapy*, vol. 26 (1931), pp. 540–8.

Reed, R. Harvey. "The X-Ray from a Medico–Legal Standpoint." *Journal of the American Medical Association*, vol. 30 (1898), pp. 1013–19.

"Report of the Committee of the American Surgical Association on the Medico–Legal Relations of the X-Rays." *American Journal of Medical Sciences*, vol. 120 (1900), pp. 7–35.

"The Responsibilities of the Medical Profession in the Use of X Rays and Other Ionising Radiation. Statement by the United Nations Scientific Committee on the Effects of Atomic Radiation." *Lancet*, vol. 1 (1957), pp. 467–8.

Richards, Dickinson W. "Right Heart Catheterization: Its Contributions to Physiology and Medicine." *Science*, vol. 125 (1957), pp. 1181–5.

Robb, George P., and Steinberg, Israel. "Visualization of the Chambers of the Heart, the Pulmonary Circulation, and the Great Blood Vessels in Man: A Practical Method." *American Journal of Roentgenology and Radium Therapy*, vol. 41 (1939), pp. 1–17.

Röntgen, W. C. "On a New Kind of Rays." *Nature*, vol. 53 (1896), pp. 274–6.

"Roentgen Rays." *Lancet*, vol. 2 (1896), pp. 1832–3.

Rowland, Sidney. "Report on the Application of the New Photography to Medicine and Surgery." *British Medical Journal*, vol. 1 (1896), pp. 361–2.

Safford, H. E. "The Present Status of the X-Ray in Diagnosis." *Physician and Surgeon*, vol. 20 (1898), pp. 538–44.

Shanks, S. Cochrane. "Fifty Years of Radiology." *British Medical Journal*, vol. 1 (1950), pp. 44–6.

Sosman, Merrill C. "Medicine as a Science: Roentgenology." *New England Journal of Medicine*, vol. 244 (1951), pp. 552–63.

Swinton, A. A. C. "Professor Röntgen's Discovery." *Nature*, vol. 53 (1896), pp. 276–7.

Williams, Francis H. "A Method for More Fully Determining the Outline of the Heart by Means of the Fluoroscope Together with Other Uses of This Instrument in Medicine." *Boston Medical and Surgical Journal*, vol. 135 (1896), pp. 335–7.

The Roentgen Rays . . . New York: Macmillan, 1901.

SOLO AND GROUP PRACTICE

Bailey, Richard M. "Economies of Scale in Outpatient Medical Practice." *Group Practice*, vol. 17, no. 7 (1968), pp. 24–33.

Barker, Lewellys F. "Group Diagnosis and Group Therapy." *Wisconsin Medical Journal*, vol. 19 (1920), pp. 329–37.

Billings, Frank. "The Trend of the Practice of Modern Medicine." *Journal of the American Medical Association*, vol. 78 (1922), pp. 1503–6.

Billings, John S. "Our Medical Literature." *Lancet*, vol. 2 (1881), pp. 265–70.

Collings, Joseph S. "General Practice in England Today: A Reconnaissance." *Lancet*, vol. 1 (1950), pp. 555–85.

Davis, Michael M., and Warner, Andrew R. *Dispensaries; Their Management and Development.* New York: Macmillan, 1918.

Eimerl, T. S., Pearson, R. J. C., and the Merseyside and North Wales Faculty of the College of General Practitioners. "Working–time in General Practice.

How General Practitioners Use Their Time." *British Medical Journal*, vol. 2 (1966), pp. 1549–54.

Faxon, Nathaniel W. "The Country Doctor and the Hospital." *Boston Medical and Surgical Journal*, vol. 177 (1917), pp. 167–71.

Fry, John, and Dillane, J. B. "Too Much Work? Proposals Based on a Review of Fifteen Years' Work in Practice." *Lancet*, vol. 2 (1964), pp. 632–4.

Garfield, Sidney R. "The Delivery of Medical Care." *Scientific American*, vol. 222 (1970), pp. 15–23.

Gutman, Jacob, "Group Diagnosis." *New York Medical Journal*, vol. 111 (1920), pp. 851–5.

Halberstam, Michael J. "Liberal Thought, Radical Theory and Medical Practice." *New England Journal of Medicine*, vol. 284 (1971), pp. 1180–5.

Herrick, James B. "Modern Diagnosis." *Journal of the American Medical Association*, vol. 92 (1929), pp. 518–22.

"The Practitioner of the Future." *Journal of the American Medical Association*, vol. 103 (1934), pp. 881–5.

Herringham, Wilmot. "The Consultant." *British Medical Journal*, vol. 2 (1920), pp. 36–40.

Hildreth, John L. "The General Practitioner and the Specialist." *Boston Medical and Surgical Journal*, vol. 155 (1906), pp. 79–83.

McGuire, Stuart. *The Profit and Loss Account of Modern Medicine and other papers.* Richmond, Virginia: Jenkins, 1915.

Morris, E. W. "The Hospitals." *British Medical Journal*, vol. 2 (1920), pp. 42–6.

Osler, William. "Remarks on Specialism." *Boston Medical and Surgical Journal*, vol. 126 (1892), pp. 457–9.

Peterson, Osler, et al. "An Analytic Study of North Carolina Medical Practice, 1952–1954."*Journal of Medical Education*, vol. 31, Supplement (1956), pp. 1–165.

Pettit, Rowsell, T. "The Diagnostic Hospital of a Small Community." *Modern Hospital*, vol. 17 (1921), pp. 195–9.

Proger, Samuel. "The Joseph H. Pratt Diagnostic Hospital." *New England Journal of Medicine*, vol. 220 (1939), pp. 771–9.

Reynolds, J. Russell. "Specialism in Medicine." *Lancet*, vol. 2 (1881), pp. 655–8.

Rosen, George. *The Specialization of Medicine, with Particular Reference to Ophthalmology.* New York: Froben Press, 1944.

Shattuck, Frederick C. "Specialism in Medicine." *Journal of the American Medical Association*, vol. 35 (1900), pp. 723–6.

Stevens, Rosemary. *American Medicine and the Public Interest.* New Haven: Yale University Press, 1971.

Tuttle, Ralph W. "The Other Side of Country Practice." *New England Journal of Medicine*, vol. 199 (1928), pp. 874–7.

Vaughan, Warren T. "Group Medicine: A Critical Survey."*Southern Medical Journal*, vol. 16 (1923), pp. 724–31.

TECHNOLOGY IN MEDICINE

Bradbury, John Buckley. "Modern Scientific Medicine." *British Medical Journal*, vol. 2 (1880), pp. 244–52.

Clendening, Logan. "The History of Certain Medical Instruments." *Annals of Internal Medicine*, vol. 4 (1930–31), pp. 176–89.

Compton, Karl T. "Possibilities in Biological Engineering." *Annals of Internal Medicine*, vol. 12 (1938), pp. 867–75.

Dock, William. "The Place of the Gadget in the History and the Practice of Medicine." *Stanford Medical Bulletin*, vol. 13 (1955), pp. 138–43.

Ferrari, Andrés, and Overman, Ralph. "Medical Technology." *Annals New York Academy of Sciences*, vol. 166 (1969), pp. 1027–30.

Godber, George. "Measurement and Mechanisation in Medicine." *Lancet*, vol. 2 (1964), pp. 1191–5.

Lion, Kurt S. "Technology and Medicine." *Archives of Physical Medicine*, vol. 27 (1946), pp. 279–84.

Lusted, Lee B. "Medical Electronics." *New England Journal of Medicine*, vol. 252 (1955), pp. 580–5.

Mitcham, Carl, and Mackey, Robert. "Bibliography of the Philosophy of Technology." *Technology and Culture*, vol. 14, no. 2, part II (1973), pp. S1–S205.

Mitchell, S. Weir. *The Early History of Instrumental Precision in Medicine*. New Haven: Tuttle, Morehouse & Taylor, 1892. This monograph has been printed, without appendix, as "The History of Instrumental Precision in Medicine," *Boston Medical and Surgical Journal*, vol. 125 (1891), pp. 309–16.

Moore, Frederick J. "The Need for New Technologies to Offset the Shortage of Physicians." *Archives of Internal Medicine*, vol. 125 (1970), pp. 351–5.

Rogers, David E. "On Technologic Restraint." *Archives of Internal Medicine*, vol. 135 (1975), pp. 1393–7.

Ross, Joseph F. "Artificial Radioactive Isotopes in Medicine and Biology." *New England Journal of Medicine*, vol. 226 (1942), pp. 854–60.

Rushmer, Robert F., and Huntsman, Lee L. "Biomedical Engineering." *Science*, vol. 167 (1970), pp. 840–4.

Rutstein, David D., and Eden, Murray. *Engineering and Living Systems*. Cambridge: M.I.T. Press, 1970.

Zinsser, Hans H. "Electronic Future of Medical Facilities." *Annals New York Academy of Sciences*, vol. 118 (1965), pp. 3–5.

"The Impact of New Technology on Medicine." *Transactions New York Academy of Sciences*, vol. 26 (1964), pp. 914–22.

THERMOMETRY

Bolton, Henry Carrington. *Evolution of the Thermometer 1592–1743*. Easton, Penn.: Chemical Publishing Co., 1900.

Boyle, Robert. *New Experiments and Observations Touching Cold*. London: Richard Davies, 1683.

Currie, James. *Medical Reports, on the Effects of Water, Cold and Warm, as a Remedy in Fever and Febrile Diseases*. Liverpool: Cadell and Davies, 1797.

Curtis, F. C. "Thermometry in Health and Disease." *New York Medical Journal*, vol. 16 (1872), pp. 618–27.

Engel, Hugo. "The Thermometer and Its Use in Medicine." *Medical and Surgical Reporter*, vol. 46 (1882), pp. 145–51.

Finlayson, James. "Use of the Clinical Thermometer." *British Medical Journal*, vol. 1 (1874), pp. 261–4.

Flint, Austin. "Remarks on the Use of the Thermometer in Diagnosis and Prognosis." *New York Medical Journal*, vol. 4 (1866–67), pp. 81–93.

Immisch, Moritz. "A Comparison between Mercurial and Avitreous Thermometers." *New York Medical Journal*, vol. 50 (1889), pp. 309–13.

McGuigan, Hugh A. "Medical Thermometry." *Annals of Medical History*, vol. 9 (1937), pp. 148–54.

Maclagan, T. J. "Thermometrical Observations." *Edinburgh Medical Journal*, vol. 13 (1868), pp. 601–25.

Martine, George. *Essays on the Construction and Graduation of Thermometers and on the Heating and Cooling of Bodies.* Edinburgh: Printed for William Creech, 1792.

Parkes, E. A. "On Pyrexia." *Medical Times and Gazette*, vol. 1 (1855), pp. 253–5, 279–80, 331–5, 535–7, 561–3.

Sawyer, James. "Clinical Thermometry." *Birmingham Medical Review*, vol. 4 (1875), pp. 109–17.

Seguin, E. *Medical Thermometry and Human Temperature.* New York: William Wood, 1876.

Woodhead, G. Sims, and Varrier–Jones, P. C. "Investigations on Clinical Thermometry: Continuous and Quasi–Continuous Temperature Records in Man and Animals in Health and Disease." *Lancet*, vol. 1 (1916), pp. 173–80.

Wunderlich, C. A. *On the Temperature in Diseases: A Manual of Medical Thermometry.* Translated by W. Bathhurst Woodman. London: New Sydenham Society, 1871.

URINARY DIAGNOSIS

Beale, Lionel S. *Kidney Diseases, Urinary Deposits, and Calculous Disorders; Their Nature and Treatment.* Philadelphia: Lindsay & Blakiston, 1869.

Berzelius, J. J. *The Kidneys and Urine.* Translated by N. H. Boye and F. Leaming. Philadelphia: Lea & Blanchard, 1843.

Bird, Golding. *Urinary Deposits: Their Diagnosis, Pathology, and Therapeutical Indications.* London: John Churchill, 1844.

Bremer, Ludwig. "The Meaning and Import of Casts in the Urine without Albumin, and the Inadequacy of the Ordinary Chemic Tests." *Journal of the American Medical Association*, vol. 25 (1895), pp. 575–7.

Brian, Tho. *The Pisse–Prophet or Certaine Pisse Pot Lectures.* London: 1637. Reprint (facsimile), Riker Laboratories, 1968.

Bright, Richard. *Original Papers of Richard Bright on Renal Disease.* Edited by A. Arnold Osman. London: Oxford University Press, 1937.

Cabot, Richard C. "Clinical Examination of the Urine. A Critical Study of the Commoner Methods." *Journal of the American Medical Association*, vol. 44 (1905), pp. 837–42, 943–50.

Friedenwald, Julius. "The Diazo Reaction of Ehrlich." *New York Medical Journal*, vol. 58 (1893), pp. 745–8.

Kiefer, Joseph H. "Uroscopy: The Clinical Laboratory of the Past." *Transactions of the American Association of Genito–Urinary Surgery*, vol. 50 (1958), pp. 161–72.

Neubauer, C., and Vogel, J. *A Guide to the Qualitative and Quantitative Analysis of the Urine.* Translated by W. O. Markham. London: New Sydenham Society, 1863.

Rees, George Owen. *On the Analysis of the Blood and Urine in Health and Disease; and on the Treatment of Urinary Diseases.* Philadelphia: Lea and Blanchard, 1848.

Roberts, William. "Lectures on Certain Points in the Clinical Examination of the Urine." *Lancet,* vol. 1 (1862), pp. 480–2, 507–10, 535–6.

Schaefer, Theodore W. "A Brief Historical Retrospect of the Examination of the Urine in Ancient and Modern Times." *Boston Medical and Surgical Journal,* vol. 136 (1897), pp. 623–6.

Sturgis, F. R. "On the Value of Albuminuria as a Means of Diagnosis." *International Medical Magazine,* vol. 1 (1892), pp. 152–8.

Wilks, Samuel. "Historical Notes on Bright's Disease, Addison's Disease, and Hodgkin's Disease." *Guy's Hospital Reports,* vol. 22 (1877), pp. 259–74.

Wood, Edward S. "Urinary Diagnosis." *Boston Medical and Surgical Journal,* vol. 130 (1894), pp. 484–7, 505–8.

Index

Index

Index